Clinical Trials in Surgical Oncology

Editors

SYED A. AHMAD
SHISHIR K. MAITHEL

SURGICAL ONCOLOGY CLINICS OF NORTH AMERICA

www.surgonc.theclinics.com

Consulting Editor
TIMOTHY M. PAWLIK

January 2023 • Volume 32 • Number 1

ELSEVIER

1600 John F. Kennedy Boulevard • Suite 1800 • Philadelphia, Pennsylvania, 19103-2899

http://www.theclinics.com

SURGICAL ONCOLOGY CLINICS OF NORTH AMERICA Volume 32, Number 1
January 2023 ISSN 1055-3207, ISBN-13: 978-0-323-96083-0

Editor: John Vassallo (j.vassallo@elsevier.com)
Developmental Editor: Diana Ang

Surgical Oncology Clinics of North America (ISSN 1055-3207) is published quarterly by Elsevier Inc., 360 Park Avenue South, New York, NY 10010-1710. Months of publication are January, April, July, and October. Business and Editorial Offices: 1600 John F. Kennedy Blvd., Ste. 1800, Philadelphia, PA 19103-2899. Customer Service Office: 3251 Riverport Lane, Maryland Heights, MO 63043. Periodicals postage paid at New York, NY and additional mailing offices. Subscription prices are $335.00 per year (US individuals), $651.00 (US institutions) $100.00 (US student/resident), $374.00 (Canadian individuals), $823.00 (Canadian institutions), $100.00 (Canadian student/resident), $484.00 (foreign individuals), $823.00 (foreign institutions), and $205.00 (foreign student/resident). Foreign air speed delivery is included in all *Clinics* subscription prices. All prices are subject to change without notice. **POSTMASTER**: Send address changes to *Surgical Oncology Clinics of North America*, Elsevier Health Science Division, Subscription Customer Service, 3251 Riverport Lane, Maryland Heights, MO 63043. **Customer Service: 1-800-654-2452 (US and Canada). 314-447-8871 (outside US and Canada). Fax: 314-447-8029. E-mail: journalscustomerservice-usa@elsevier.com (for print support); journalsonline support-usa@elsevier.com (for online support)**.

Reprints. For copies of 100 or more, of articles in this publication, please contact the Commercial Reprints Department, Elsevier Inc., 360 Park Avenue South, New York, New York 10010-1710. Tel. 212-633-3874; Fax: 212-633-3820; E-mail: reprints@elsevier.com.

Surgical Oncology Clinics of North America is covered in *MEDLINE/PubMed (Index Medicus)* and *EMBASE/ Excerpta Medica, Current Contents/Clinical Medicine, and ISI/BIOMED.*

Contributors

CONSULTING EDITOR

TIMOTHY M. PAWLIK, MD, PhD, MPH, MTS, MBA, FACS, FSSO, FRACS (Hon.)
Professor and Chair, Department of Surgery, The Urban Meyer III and Shelley Meyer Chair for Cancer Research, Professor of Surgery, Oncology, Health Services Management and Policy, The Ohio State University, Wexner Medical Center, Columbus, Ohio, USA

EDITORS

SYED A. AHMAD, MD, FACS
Professor of Surgery, The Hayden Family Endowed Chair for Cancer Research, Director, University of Cincinnati Cancer Center, Chief, Division Surgical Oncology, The University of Cincinnati College of Medicine, Cincinnati, Ohio, USA

SHISHIR K. MAITHEL, MD, FACS
Professor of Surgery, Scientific Director, Emory Liver and Pancreas Center, Director, Surgical Oncology Research Fellowship Program, Winship Cancer Institute, Division of Surgical Oncology, Department of Surgery, Emory University, Atlanta, Georgia, USA

AUTHORS

BERK AYKUT, MD
Department of Surgery, Division of Surgical Oncology, Duke University Medical Center, Durham, North Carolina, USA

GEORGIA M. BEASLEY, MD, MHS
Associate Professor, Department of Surgery, Duke University Medical Center, Durham, North Carolina, USA

ERIN E. BURKE, MD, MPH
Division of Surgical Oncology, University of Kentucky, Lexington, Kentucky, USA

EMILY B. CASSIM, BS
Division of Surgical Oncology, University of Kentucky, Lexington, Kentucky, USA

MICHAEL J. CAVNAR, MD
Division of Surgical Oncology, University of Kentucky, Lexington, Kentucky, USA

GLORIA Y. CHANG, MD
Department of Surgery, Division of Surgical Oncology, The University of Texas Southwestern Medical Center, Dallas, Texas, USA

AKHIL CHAWLA, MD
Division of Surgical Oncology, Department of Surgery, Northwestern Medicine Regional Medical Group, Northwestern University Feinberg School of Medicine, Robert H. Lurie Comprehensive Cancer Center, Chicago, Illinois, USA

ANGELENA CROWN, MD
Breast Surgery, True Family Women's Cancer Center, Swedish Cancer Institute, Seattle, Washington, USA

FAHIMA DOSSA, MD, PhD
Department of Surgery, University of Toronto, Toronto, Ontario, Canada

ALEXANDER DOWLI, MD
Clinical Fellow in Colorectal Surgery, Division of Colorectal Surgery, Department of Surgery, Baylor University Medical Center, Dallas, Texas, USA

CRISTINA R. FERRONE, MD
Department of Surgery, Massachusetts General Hospital, Boston, Massachusetts, USA

ALESSANDRO FICHERA, MD, FACS, FASCRS
FISS Surgery Safety and Quality Officer, Division Chief, Colon and Rectal Surgery, Baylor University Medical Center, Clinical Professor of Medical Education, Texas A&M University, Dallas, Texas, USA

SARAH B. FISHER, MD
Department of Surgical Oncology, The University of Texas MD Anderson Cancer Center, Houston, Texas, USA

JAMES FLESHMAN, MD, FACS, FASCRS
Sparkman Endowed Professor and Chair, Department of Surgery, Professor of Surgery, Texas A&M College of Medicine, Baylor University Medical Center, Dallas, Texas, USA

ALEXANDRA GANGI, MD
Department of Surgery, Cedars-Sinai Medical Center, Los Angeles, California, USA

REBECCA A. GLADDY, MD, PhD
Department of Surgery, University of Toronto, Division of Surgical Oncology, Department of Surgery, Mount Sinai Hospital and Princess Margaret Cancer Centre, Sinai Health System, Toronto, Ontario, Canada

MEGAN M. HARPER, MS, MD
Division of Surgical Oncology, University of Kentucky, Lexington, Kentucky, USA

BERNICE L. HUANG, MD
Department of Surgical Oncology, The University of Texas MD Anderson Cancer Center, Houston, Texas, USA

FABIAN M. JOHNSTON, MD, MHS, FACS, FSSO
Section of Gastrointestinal Surgical Oncology, Peritoneal Surface Malignancy Program, Division of Surgical Oncology, Johns Hopkins University, Baltimore, Maryland, USA

KATHIE-ANN JOSEPH, MD, MPH
Department of Surgery, New York University Grossman School of Medicine, NYC Health and Hospitals/Bellevue, NYU Langone Health's Institute for Excellence in Health Equity, New York, New York, USA

GIORGOS C. KARAKOUSIS, MD
Professor, Department of Surgery, Hospital of the University of Pennsylvania, Philadelphia, Pennsylvania, USA

MATTHEW H.G. KATZ, MD
Professor and Chair, Department of Surgical Oncology, The University of Texas MD Anderson Cancer Center, Houston, Texas, USA

GRACE KEEGAN, BS
University of Chicago, Pritzker School of Medicine, Chicago, Illinois, USA

JOSEPH KIM, MD
Division of Surgical Oncology, University of Kentucky, Lexington, Kentucky, USA

LAURA K. KRECKO, MD
Department of Surgery, University of Wisconsin Hospital and Clinics, Madison, Wisconsin, USA

MEEGHAN A. LAUTNER, MD, MSc
Department of Surgery, University of Wisconsin Hospital and Clinics, Madison, Wisconsin, USA

JANET LI, MD
Hepatopancreatobiliary Surgery Fellow, Division of Surgical Oncology, Department of Surgery, Oregon Health & Science University, Portland, Oregon, USA

MICHAEL E. LIDSKY, MD
Department of Surgery, Division of Surgical Oncology, Duke University Medical Center, Durham, North Carolina, USA

MICHAEL S. LUI, MD
Department of Surgical Oncology, The University of Texas MD Anderson Cancer Center, Houston, Texas, USA

EMILY F. MARCINKOWSKI, MD
Division of Surgical Oncology, University of Kentucky, Lexington, Kentucky, USA

SKYE C. MAYO, MD, MPH
Associate Professor of Surgery, Division of Surgical Oncology, Department of Surgery, Knight Cancer Institute, Oregon Health & Science University, Portland, Oregon, USA

HANNAH G. MCDONALD, MD
Division of Surgical Oncology, University of Kentucky, Lexington, Kentucky, USA

NICOLE M. NEVAREZ, MD
Department of Surgery, Division of Surgical Oncology, The University of Texas Southwestern Medical Center, Dallas, Texas, USA

PRAKASH K. PANDALAI, MD
Division of Surgical Oncology, University of Kentucky, Lexington, Kentucky, USA

NANCY D. PERRIER, MD
Department of Surgical Oncology, The University of Texas MD Anderson Cancer Center, Houston, Texas, USA

FLAVIO G. ROCHA, MD
Associate Professor of Surgery, Division Head of Surgical Oncology, Department of Surgery, Physician-in-Chief, Knight Cancer Institute, Oregon Health & Science University, Portland, Oregon, USA

ASHLEY RUSSO, MD
Department of Surgery, Cedars-Sinai Medical Center, Los Angeles, California, USA

CIMARRON E. SHARON, MD
Resident in General Surgery, Department of Surgery, Hospital of the University of Pennsylvania, Philadelphia, Pennsylvania, USA

ADITYA S. SHIRALI, MD
Department of Surgical Oncology, The University of Texas MD Anderson Cancer Center, Houston, Texas, USA

AMN SIDDIQI, MBBS
Department of Surgery, Johns Hopkins School of Medicine, Baltimore, Maryland, USA

REBECCA A. SNYDER, MD, MPH
Assistant Professor, Department of Surgery, Brody School of Medicine at East Carolina University, Greenville, North Carolina, USA

LEE G. WILKE, MD
Department of Surgery, University of Wisconsin Hospital and Clinics, Madison, Wisconsin, USA

ADAM C. YOPP, MD
Department of Surgery, Division of Surgical Oncology, The University of Texas Southwestern Medical Center, Dallas, Texas, USA

Contents

targeted and immune therapy, studies of adjuvant therapy for patients with resected stage III/IV melanoma have led to the approval of combined B-raf proto-oncogene (BRAF) and mitogen-activated protein kinase kinase inhibitors for patients with a BRAF mutation, and cytotoxic T-lymphocyte associated protein-4 or antiprogrammed cell death-1 therapy for patients without a BRAF mutation. This article discusses the details of the trials that have influenced these treatment decisions, in addition to discussing ongoing trials and possible future directions.

Optimal management of esophageal and gastric cancer during the perioperative period requires a coordinated multidisciplinary treatment effort. Accurate staging guides treatment strategy. Advances in minimally invasive surgery and endoscopy have reduced risks associated with resection while maintaining oncological standards. Although the standard perioperative chemo-and radiotherapy regimens have not yet been established, randomized control trials exploring this subject show promising results.

Most of the patients with gallbladder cancer (GBC), intrahepatic cholangiocarcinoma (iCCA), and peri-hilar cholangiocarcinoma (pCCA) present with advanced disease. Complete staging with multiphasic liver imaging is essential to determine the extent of disease. Operative goals should include a margin-negative resection, portal lymphadenectomy for staging, and sufficient remnant liver volume. Biliary tract malignancies have distinct mutational drivers (GBC and pCCA = ERBB2 in 20%; iCCA = fibroblast growth factor receptor 2 or isocitrate dehydrogenase 1 in 20%) amenable to therapy with inhibitors. Clinical trials assessing neoadjuvant, peri-operative, and adjuvant treatments continue to evolve and now include targeted inhibitors and the integration of hepatic arterial infusion.

Hepatocellular carcinoma (HCC) is one of the most common causes of cancer-related death worldwide. Partial hepatectomy, one of a few curative therapeutic modalities, is plagued by high recurrence rate of up to 70% at 5 years. Throughout the past 3 decades, many clinical trials have attempted to improve HCC recurrence rate following partial hepatectomy using adjuvant and neoadjuvant treatment modalities such as antiviral therapy, brachytherapy, systemic chemotherapy, immunotherapy, transarterial chemoembolization and radioembolization, and radiotherapy. The goal of this review is to discuss the clinical trials pertaining to resectable HCC including surgical technique considerations, adjuvant, and neoadjuvant treatment modalities.

Colorectal Cancer Liver Metastases: Multimodal Therapy   119

Berk Aykut and Michael E. Lidsky

Despite a steady decline in incidence and mortality rates, colorectal cancer (CRC) remains the second most common cancer diagnosis in women and the third most common in men worldwide. Notably, the liver is recognized as the most common site of CRC metastasis, and metastases to the liver remain the primary driver of disease-specific mortality for patients with CRC. Although hepatic resection is the backbone of curative-intent treatment, management of CRLM has become increasingly multimodal during the last decade and includes the use of downstaging chemotherapy, ablation techniques, and locoregional therapy, each of which are reviewed herein.

Surgeon-Led Clinical Trials in Pancreatic Cancer   143

Akhil Chawla and Cristina R. Ferrone

The review also highlights key landmark adjuvant, neoadjuvant and perioperative trials with an emphasis on surgeon-run clinical trials that have helped to define the pancreatic cancer treatment paradigms.

Primary Colorectal Cancer   153

Alexander Dowli, Alessandro Fichera, and James Fleshman

Over the last few decades, the colorectal surgery world has seen a paradigm shift in the care of patients. The introduction of minimally invasive techniques led to the development of procedures resulting in reduced patient morbidity and hospital stay. The vetting process of minimally invasive colorectal surgery involved rigorous studies to ensure that oncologic outcomes were not being compromised. In this chapter, we discuss the most relevant randomized controlled trials that support the practice of minimally invasive colorectal surgery. The multimodal treatment of rectal cancer has developed rapidly, resulting in improved survival and decreased morbidity and mortality. In this review, we also present the latest evidence behind the multidisciplinary approach to rectal cancer.

Evidence for the Current Management of Soft-tissue Sarcoma and Gastrointestinal Stromal Tumors and Emerging Directions   169

Fahima Dossa and Rebecca A. Gladdy

Soft-tissue sarcoma (STS) is not a single entity but, rather, a family of diseases with differing biologic behaviors and anatomic site- and histotype-specific responses to treatment. Whereas surgery remains the mainstay of treatment of primary, localized disease, evolving evidence is establishing the role of multimodality treatment of these tumors. This article summarizes prospective evidence to date informing our treatment of STS. Key future directions will include advancing our understanding of fundamental tumor biology and mechanisms of response and recurrence, as well as defining the optimal provision of regional, systemic, and targeted therapies, including the role of immunotherapy. Ongoing global collaborations will be integral to progress in treating these rare tumors.

Neuroendocrine tumors (NETs) represent a heterogeneous group of tumors, with variable presentation based on the location of origin and degree of metastatic spread. There are no randomized control trials to guide surgical management; however, surgery remains the mainstay of treatment for most gastroenteropancreatic NETs based on retrospective studies. Metastatic disease is common at the time of presentation, particularly in the liver. There is a role for cytoreduction for improvement of both symptoms and survival. Robust prospective randomized data exists to support the use of medical therapies to improve progression-free and overall survival in patients with advanced, metastatic, and unresectable NETs.

Recent changes in the landscape of endocrine surgery include a shift from total thyroidectomy for almost all patients with papillary thyroid cancer to the incorporation of thyroid lobectomy for well-selected patients with low-risk disease; minimally invasive parathyroidectomy with, and potentially without, intraoperative parathyroid hormone monitoring for patients with well-localized primary hyperparathyroidism; improvement in the management of parathyroid cancer with the incorporation of immune checkpoint blockade and/or targeted therapies; and the incorporation of minimally invasive techniques in the management of patients with benign tumors and selected secondary malignancies of the adrenal gland.

Minority groups are vastly underrepresented in clinical trial participants and leadership. Because these studies provide innovative and revolutionary treatment options to patients with cancer and have the potential to extend survival, it is imperative that public and private stakeholders, as well as hospital and clinical trial leadership, prioritize equity and inclusion of diverse populations in clinical trial development and recruitment strategies. Achieving equity in clinical trials could be an important step in reducing the overall cancer burden and mortality disparities in vulnerable populations.

SURGICAL ONCOLOGY CLINICS OF NORTH AMERICA

FORTHCOMING ISSUES

April 2023
Management of Endocrine Tumors
Nancy D. Perrier, *Editor*

July 2023
Advances in Radiotherapy
Terence M. Williams, *Editor*

October 2023
Personalizing Breast Cancer Care
Melissa Pilewskie, *Editor*

RECENT ISSUES

October 2022
Oncology Imaging: Updates and Advancements
Natalie S. Lui, *Editor*

July 2022
Sarcoma
Chandrajit Premanand Raut and Alessandro Gronchi, *Editors*

April 2022
Colorectal Cancer
Traci L. Hedrick, *Editor*

SERIES OF RELATED INTEREST

Advances in Surgery
https://www.advancessurgery.com
Surgical Clinics of North America
https://www.surgical.theclinics.com
Thoracic Surgery Clinics
https://www.thoracic.theclinics.com

Foreword

Clinical Trials in Surgical Oncology

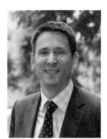

Timothy M. Pawlik, MD, PhD, MPH, MTS, MBA, FACS, FSSO, FRACS (Hon.)
Consulting Editor

This issue of the *Surgical Oncology Clinics of North America* focuses on clinical trials in oncology. Clinical trials are critical to develop and test new treatment modalities for a broad range of disease states. In fact, over the past two years we have witnessed and benefited from clinical trials related to COVID-19 that have made headlines, saved millions of lives, as well as given us the chance to return to some degree of normalcy. In the field of cancer, each of us has also witnessed the important "game-changing" and potentially lifesaving opportunities afforded to our patients through clinical trials. Clinical trials are the backbone of evidence-based treatment guidelines, translate research into clinical practice, and improve the quality of care. Data from clinical trials provide the "evidence" in "evidence-based medicine." In fact, it's estimated that almost one-half of phase 3 trials influence guideline care or new drug approvals. In turn, appropriately planned and well-executed clinical trials provide a unique opportunity to address gaps that still exist in patient care. Unfortunately, clinical trial participation among adults in the United States remains low at less than 5% and is even lower among racial/ethnic minority groups, as well as certain disenfranchised patient populations. The low rate of clinical trial participation has been attributed to limited knowledge about clinical trials, poor geographical access to trial locations, as well as skepticism and cynicism relative to trial participation among traditionally disadvantaged patient populations. The surgeon plays a central role in the conception, design, implementation, and accrual to clinical trials. In addition, surgeons need to be equipped to analyze and interpret clinical trial data in order to disseminate and apply new emerging therapeutic information to the care of their patients. Given the importance and central role of clinical trials to oncologic care, I am grateful to have Syed A. Ahmad, MD and Shishir K. Maithel, MD as the guest editors of this important issue of *Surgical Oncology Clinics of North America*. Dr Ahmad is the Hayden Family Endowed Chair for Research and Professor of Surgery at the University of Cincinnati College of Medicine. Dr Ahmad serves as the Division Chief of Surgical Oncology as well as the Director of

Surg Oncol Clin N Am 32 (2023) xiii–xiv
https://doi.org/10.1016/j.soc.2022.08.007
1055-3207/23/© 2022 Published by Elsevier Inc.

surgonc.theclinics.com

the University of Cincinnati Cancer Center. Dr Ahmad is the primary investigator of several national clinical trials as well as serves as the Surgical Chair for the Southwest Oncology Group. Dr Maithel is Professor of Surgery at Emory University where he is Scientific Director of the Liver and Pancreas Center. As chair of the Gastrointestinal Surgery Working Group of the Eastern Cooperative Oncology Group and the American College of Radiology Imaging Network Cancer Research Group, Dr Maithel evaluates the production of forward-looking clinical trials that focus on biomarker-driven cancer investigations. Both coeditors have extensive experience and leadership in the area of clinical trials and have published extensively in the field of oncology. As such, Dr Ahmad and Dr Maithel are imminently qualified to be the guest editors of this important issue of *Surgical Oncology Clinics of North America*.

The issue covers a range of important topics related to clinical trials. In particular, this issue highlights the fundamentals of conducting cooperative trials and how to leverage national trial networks as well as touches on investigator-initiated trials. In addition to these cross-cutting topics, the authors also provide a contemporary state-of-the-art update on clinical trials across a wide range of oncologic diseases. In particular, the team of expert coauthors provides data from clinical trials related to tumors, including breast cancer, melanoma, esophageal and gastric cancer, as well as hepatopancreaticobiliary malignancies, colorectal cancer, sarcoma, and neuroendocrine tumors. In addition, the important topic of diversity, equity, and inclusion in clinical trials is highlighted.

I wish to express my sincere gratitude to Dr Ahmad and Dr Maithel for their efforts to identify such a wonderful group of leaders in the field of clinical trials. These expert authors have done an incredible job emphasizing the various aspects of clinical trials as well as describing cancer-specific clinical trial data that will prove helpful to both trainees and faculty. I know that this issue of *Surgical Oncology Clinics of North America* will serve cancer providers well in acquainting them with the latest up-to-date data on clinical trials in oncology. I would like to thank Dr Ahmad and Dr Maithel and all the expert authors again for an outstanding issue of the *Surgical Oncology Clinics of North America*.

Timothy M. Pawlik, MD, PhD, MPH, MTS, MBA, FACS, FSSO, FRACS (Hon.)
Department of Surgery
The Ohio State University
Wexner Medical Center
395 West 12th Avenue, Suite 670
Columbus, OH 43210, USA

E-mail address:
tim.pawlik@osumc.edu

Preface

Clinical Trials in Surgical Oncology

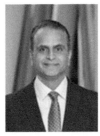 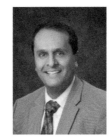

Syed A. Ahmad, MD, FACS   Shishir K. Maithel, MD, FACS
Editors

As physicians and research scientists, we can affect change and improve cancer outcomes in many ways. Historically, physicians work at the ground level managing individual patients. At this level, we diagnose their illness, help them make decisions, treat their cancers, and follow them long term. This interaction is noble and defines our profession. In addition to this, as researchers, we can also affect change at a population level. Research scientists can define new mechanisms and targets in the laboratory that can lead to drug development and new treatment options for patients. And, as clinical researchers, we can evaluate new drugs, biomarkers, and treatment sequencing in the context of clinical trials that can change existing paradigms and improve outcomes. The importance of clinical trials was recently highlighted by the Southwest Oncology Group (SWOG), which conducted a study evaluating all phase 3 trials from the adult National Clinical Trials Network (NCTN) groups (SWOG, Alliance, NRG, and ECOG-ACRIN) reported from 1980 onward, with statistically significant findings. In total, 163 trials that enrolled 108,102 patients were evaluated. These trials were estimated to have generated gains of 14 million life-years to patients with cancer. This analysis highlights the importance of clinical trials, the role of drug discovery, and the critical role of government-sponsored cancer research in extending and improving the lives of patients with cancer.

In this issue of *Surgical Oncology Clinics of North America*, we have asked some of the leading clinical researchers in the field of Surgical Oncology to discuss the importance and impact of conducting clinical trials. This issue can be used as a primer for trainees, as well as established surgeons, on how to develop clinical studies both at an institutional level and within the framework of the NCTN cooperative group structure. We have also summarized "The State of Science" with an update on the most surgically relevant clinical trials broken down by disease-based articles. Last, we also focus an article on the need to improve diversity and equity in conducting clinical trials.

Surg Oncol Clin N Am 32 (2023) xv–xvi
https://doi.org/10.1016/j.soc.2022.08.006
1055-3207/23/© 2022 Published by Elsevier Inc.

If results from these studies are to be applicable to broad populations, the trial partic-ipants need to reflect, as much as possible, the population of patients with the dis-ease. We know that differences in response to therapy can exist among different ethnic and racial populations based on nuclear polymorphisms, pharmacogenomics, and other factors. Thus, an emphasis on improving diversity and equity within clinical trial enrollment, as well as interpretation of results, will be necessary for future studies. In closing, we would like to dedicate this issue of *Surgical Oncology Clinics of North America* to all the patients with cancer and their families that have enrolled and partic-ipated in clinical trials with the goal of improving cancer care for future patients.

Syed A. Ahmad, MD, FACS
Division Surgical Oncology
The University of Cincinnati College of Medicine
231 Albert Sabin Way
ML 0558, Room 1466
Cincinnati, OH 45267, USA

Shishir K. Maithel, MD, FACS
Division of Surgical Oncology
Department of Surgery
Emory University
1365B Clifton Road, NE
Building B, Suite 4100, Office 4202
Atlanta, GA 30322, USA

E-mail addresses:
ahmadsy@ucmail.uc.edu (S.A. Ahmad)
smaithe@emory.edu (S.K. Maithel)

Fundamentals of Conducting Cooperative Group Trials Through the National Clinical Trials Network

Rebecca A. Snyder, MD, MPH[a], Matthew H.G. Katz, MD[b],*

KEYWORDS

- Clinical trials • Cooperative groups • National Clinical Trials Network
- Surgical oncology

KEY POINTS

- The cooperative group mechanism offers many benefits when performing multidisciplinary clinical oncology research, including a collaborative, multi-institutional infrastructure that can promote efficient accrual of a diverse population of patients to clinical trials.
- Designing and activating a National Clinical Trials Network clinical trial consists of a standard stepwise process outlined in this review.
- Cooperative group oncology trials have tremendous potential to generate practice-changing evidence to improve the care for patients with cancer. Surgeons are ideal leaders in this effort, as they bring unique experience and expertise to inform trial development and conduct.

INTRODUCTION

Multicenter randomized clinical trials generate the highest level of evidence to inform standard-of-care treatment guidelines for malignant solid tumors. Funding to support clinical trials is provided by a variety of sources, including industry sponsorship, institutional funds, foundations, and oncology cooperative groups. Clinical trials are often designed to test the safety and efficacy of novel therapeutic agents. However, studies can also generate evidence to address other clinical issues, such as optimal treatment sequencing, reduction in postoperative complications, improvement in patient quality of life, and optimal surveillance testing strategies.

[a] Department of Surgery, Brody School of Medicine at East Carolina University, 600 Moye Boulevard, Surgical Oncology Suite 4S-24, Greenville, NC 27834, USA; [b] Department of Surgical Oncology, Unit 1484, The University of Texas at MD Anderson Cancer Center, 1515 Holcombe Boulevard, Houston, TX 77030, USA
* Corresponding author.
E-mail address: mhgkatz@mdanderson.org

Surg Oncol Clin N Am 32 (2023) 1–12
https://doi.org/10.1016/j.soc.2022.07.002
1055-3207/23/Published by Elsevier Inc.
surgonc.theclinics.com

The cooperative group mechanism offers many advantages over single-institution or industry-sponsored trials when performing clinical trial research, including a collaborative, multi-institutional infrastructure that allows for accrual of diverse patients who are generalizable to the general population of patients with cancer. In addition, cooperative group trials can provide opportunities for adequate accrual of patients with rare tumor types or tumors with specific mutational profiles, which would be impractical within a single institution.

Surgeons are ideal leaders for multidisciplinary clinical trials, including in the cooperative group setting, as they bring unique experience and expertise to inform trial development and conduct, including trial feasibility, quality control, and outcome measurement. However, of 22,079 solid tumor clinical oncology trials registered at ClinicalTrials.gov from 2008 to 2020, only 7.6% involved a surgical intervention.[1] Importantly, among surgical trials, US government-funded trials had the lowest risk of early discontinuation when compared with industry-funded and academic-funded trials. These data clearly demonstrate an opportunity for growth in surgical oncology clinical trials, particularly through the National Clinical Trials Network (NCTN).

HISTORY OF THE NATIONAL CLINICAL TRIALS NETWORK

In the 1950s, the U.S. Congress designated funding within the National Cancer Institute (NCI) to develop the Cancer Chemotherapy National Service Center. Afterward, the NCI established the Clinical Trials Cooperative Group Program to create a mechanism for conducting multi-institutional oncology trials. The goal of the program was to create an infrastructure that could provide regulatory oversight for clinical trial conduct through the standardization of trial conduct, data collection, and statistical analysis. At that time, the Cooperative Group Program was composed of a member network of major academic institutions. Disease-site and specialty-specific cooperative groups formed over the next few decades, beginning with the Cancer and Leukemia Group B and including the National Surgical Adjuvant Breast and Bowel Project, Radiation Therapy Oncology Group, Eastern Cooperative Oncology Group (ECOG), Gynecologic Oncology Group, Southwest Oncology Group (SWOG), American College of Surgeons Clinical Oncology Group, Children's Oncology Group, American College of Radiology Imaging Network (ACRIN), and North Central Cancer Treatment Group.[2–14] In 1983, the NCI created the Community Clinical Oncology Program to enable community oncologists to participate in clinical trials and to support cancer control research across academic and community clinical settings.[15]

However, over time, the rapid pace of scientific discovery generated new challenges in conducting efficient clinical trials that could generate relevant and timely results. In 2009, an expert panel convened by the Institute of Medicine performed a comprehensive review of the Cooperative Group Program and recommended a redesign of its existing structure to reduce redundancy and improve effectiveness and efficiency in clinical trials.[16] Each cooperative group was asked to justify the group's contributions, as the role of the NCI in the Cooperative Group Program shifted from primarily providing oversight to facilitating clinical trial conduct, and the NCI replaced the Cooperative Group Program with the NCTN.

Ultimately, the NCI announced its intention to fund five US network operation group centers, which led to the formation of the five cooperative groups that exist today. Specifically, the American College of Surgeons Clinical Oncology Group, Cancer and Leukemia Group B, and the North Central Cancer Treatment Group merged to form the Alliance for Clinical Trials in Oncology; the ECOG and ACRIN merged to form ECOG-ACRIN; and the National Surgical Adjuvant Breast and Bowel Project,

Radiation Therapy Oncology Group, and Gynecologic Oncology Group merged to form NRG Oncology. The SWOG and Children's Oncology Group proceeded independently without a merger (**Table 1**). Finally, the NCI Community Oncology Research Program (NCORP) emerged from an alignment of the existing Community Clinical Oncology Program and Minority-Based Community Clinical Oncology Program and their research bases, and the NCI Community Cancer Centers Program (**Fig. 1**).[17]

During this reorganization, the NCI centralized data management, an institutional review board, imaging and radiation oncology quality, and other oversight. In addition, they established scientific oversight committees consisting of members of all of the cooperative groups to centralize trial review and to authorize the approval of new NCTN clinical trial concepts.[15] A tremendous benefit of the resulting NCTN infrastructure is that it provides a framework for collaboration across cooperative groups in the conduct of "intergroup trials," or NCTN trials led by one cooperative group and activated and championed by other groups as well. Today, the NCTN includes more than 14,000 oncology professionals across more than 2,200 unique sites and enrolls participants at both academic and community-based clinical centers across the United States.[18] Funding for the individual NCTN groups comes from the NCI in the form of a research cooperative agreement (U10 award).[19] The NCTN budget is an impressive $171 million and supports enrollment of 17,000 to 20,000 participants annually in both treatment and imaging protocols.[18]

NATIONAL CLINICAL TRIALS NETWORK ORGANIZATIONAL STRUCTURE

The NCTN consists of a well-defined and organized structure that is consistent across the five U.S. cooperative groups as well as the Canadian group, the National Cancer Institute of Canada Clinical Trials Group (see **Fig. 1**). Each cooperative group comprises specific committees, including disease-site (eg, gastrointestinal, breast, genitourinary) and cross-disciplinary (eg, health disparities, prevention, symptom control) committees, which can develop trial concepts, review proposals across cooperative groups, and make recommendations to the NCI Steering Committees. Within these committees are individual working groups focused on individual disease sites (eg, the Pancreas Cancer Working Group) or specific treatment modalities (eg, the Gastrointestinal Surgery Working Group). These groups provide investigators with a

Table 1
National Cancer Institute-funded network groups[26]

Current NCI Group	NCI Legacy Cooperative Group
Alliance for Clinical Trials in Oncology	American College of Surgeons Oncology Group Cancer and Leukemia Group B North Central Cancer Treatment Group
Children's Oncology Group	Children's Cancer Group Intergroup Rhabdomyosarcoma Study Group National Wilms Tumor Study Group Pediatric Oncology Group
ECOG-ACRIN	ACRIN ECOG
NRG Oncology	Gynecologic Oncology Group National Surgical Adjuvant Breast and Bowel Project Radiation Therapy Oncology Group
SWOG Cancer Research Network	SWOG

NCI National Clinical Trials Network Structure

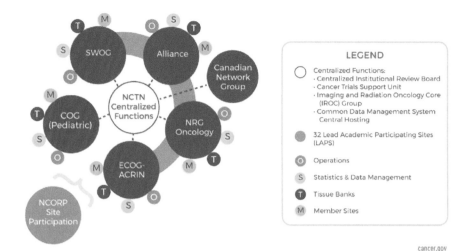

Fig. 1. NCI NCTN structure. Alliance, Alliance for Clinical Trials in Oncology; COG, Children's Oncology Group. (*Courtesy* of National Cancer Institute (NCI), https://www.cancer.gov/research/infrastructure/clinical-trials/nctn/nctn-clinical-trials-network.)

collaborative network within which to seek feedback and refine study concepts before presentation at larger committee meetings. Although most of these working groups do not formally sponsor trials, they serve as ideal entry points for young investigators interested in either serving as institutional principal investigators for cooperative group trials or lead principal investigators for new proposed studies. Senior working group members can often provide valuable mentorship and guidance to junior investigators navigating the process of trial design and approval.

The NCI Steering Committees consist of representatives from each cooperative group as well as other critical stakeholders, including NCORP representatives, community oncologists, patient advocates, biostatisticians, and other disease-site experts. These committees review trial proposals and make final decisions regarding the approval or disapproval of new trials in addition to establishing strategic priorities for the NCTN. Centralization of the trial approval process prevents the parallel development of similar trials and ensures that approved trials will not compete for the same patient population. Ultimately, the NCI Coordinating Center for Clinical Trials oversees and manages the Scientific Steering Committees and coordinates the Clinical Trials and Translational Research Advisory Committee, which is tasked with overseeing the organizational structure, funding, and strategic planning of precision medicine and translational trials.

Cooperative group membership is designated at the institutional level, and institutions can be members of more than one group. Institutional membership is defined based on the institution's size, administrative infrastructure, and accrual capabilities and includes Lead Academic Participating Sites (LAPS), main cooperative group members, and affiliate members. LAPS grants provide funding to major academic institutions, including NCI-Designated Cancer Centers, to fund the conduct of NCTN cooperative group trials, including the necessary institutional administrative infrastructure. Individual institutions can also be cooperative group main members or LAPS-affiliated members, and independent physician practices can maintain membership if they have shared access to the infrastructure of a main member institution or LAPS. In general, individual investigators at member institutions can initiate institutional participation in any trial led by any NCTN group.

The NCORP is an integrated NCI network designed to extend access to clinical trials beyond academic institutions into the community, especially to promote enrollment of patients underrepresented in trials historically conducted at centralized tertiary referral centers. The NCORP comprises 7 primary research bases and 46 community sites, 14 of which are minority or underserved community sites consisting of at least 30% racial or ethnic minorities or rural residents. The NCORP network participates in NCTN clinical trials and designs and conducts important clinical trials in the areas of cancer prevention and screening, supportive care, surveillance, and cancer care delivery.[17,20] Furthermore, a primary objective of the program is to integrate cancer disparities research across the continuum of NCORP research.[17]

Finally, the NCI does not fund every cooperative group study. Recently, cooperative groups have developed additional routes of funding to support trials through alternative mechanisms, including industry or pharmaceutical sponsorship, foundations, and other grant support. To do so, each cooperative group has established its own internal infrastructure to include an independent administrative core, statistics and data center, and biorepository in addition to the existing scientific review committees.

COOPERATIVE GROUP TRIALS: WHAT ARE THE BENEFITS?

The most obvious benefit of conducting a clinical trial through a cooperative group is the funding support provided by either the NCI or cooperative group foundation to allow for trial conduct across member institutions. NCTN-approved studies are conducted independently of industry support, which avoids associated conflicts of interest and industry oversight. Funding support may also cover costs of novel chemotherapeutic agents or drugs not currently approved by insurance companies as well as translational and correlative studies.

Another primary advantage of clinical trials conducted through the cooperative group mechanism is the opportunity to enroll patients across multiple centers participating in the NCTN. Investigators can accrue larger and more heterogeneous patient populations more quickly than single-institution studies, which allows for more timely completion and dissemination of study findings before the standard of care changes. Cooperative trials, especially those activated within the NCORP network, offer clinical trial access to patients in the community who may not otherwise have access to studies available only at major academic institutions.[21] In addition, enrollment of a more diverse study population when compared with that in single-institution or smaller consortium studies improves the external generalizability of the study results to real-world populations. The cooperative group network also enables the conduct of clinical trials specific to rare cancers, populations, or specific tumor subtypes, as accrual for these trials within a single-institution system would not be feasible.[22]

Quality control is a critical component of successful clinical trials, ensuring appropriate assessment of study eligibility as well as the primary outcome. The cooperative group infrastructure has evolved to include a robust central radiologic and pathologic review process, which allows for coordinated quality control across participating institutions. This can be critically important in surgical trials, both for quality control of surgical techniques and radiographic review to determine surgical eligibility. For example, the American College of Surgeons Clinical Oncology Group Z6051 randomized clinical trial of laparoscopic versus open resection for stage II or III rectal cancer required that surgeons submit an unedited laparoscopic video as well as operative and pathology reports for review by the credentialing committee to qualify for participation.[23] The trial investigators also provided technical instructions to ensure that surgeons followed a standardized sequence and approach to resection of rectal cancer and included a random audit of laparoscopic videos in the first 100 cases to confirm expertise in laparoscopic technique. The standardization of surgical quality control across institutions ensured that the trial could effectively answer the study question by minimizing variation in operative technique that could influence study outcomes, serving as an example of the benefits of performing a surgical trial within a cooperative group.

Similarly, the radiographic central review afforded within cooperative group trials can be critical for the successful conduct of a multi-institutional surgical trial. The recently completed Alliance for Clinical Trials in Oncology A021501 clinical trial was designed to investigate the therapeutic role of neoadjuvant radiation therapy in patients with borderline resectable pancreatic cancer.[24] Real-time central radiographic review was performed at study preregistration but before enrollment to ensure that all patients met radiographic anatomic criteria for borderline resectability status according to the National Comprehensive Cancer Network guidelines, thereby ensuring that the study question was tested in the appropriate patient population.

Participation in cooperative group studies also provides investigators with a unique opportunity to collaborate with multidisciplinary investigators and physician-researchers from diverse clinical and geographic settings, including clinicians providing care in community settings and in rural areas. The NCTN provides the ideal infrastructure to conduct multidisciplinary trials to test new therapeutic agents or procedural therapies by facilitating collaboration among medical oncologists, radiation oncologists, surgeons, and other key specialists in the trial design phase as well as during trial activation. Finally, the administrative infrastructure in place to perform data and safety monitoring and biostatistical analysis facilitates coordination and uniformity of trial activities across institutions.

To explore the clinical impact of cooperative group clinical trials, investigators performed a secondary analysis of 23 SWOG treatment trials that found a benefit of the experimental therapy from 1965 to 2012 and estimated that 3.34 million life-years were gained from these trials through 2015, at an estimated return on investment of only $125 per life-year gained.[25] Taken together, these results illustrated the tremendous value of the NCI cooperative group research program in advancing care that improves survival for the large population of patients with cancer in the United States.

TRIAL CONCEPT TO ACTIVATION

Clinical trial design and approval through NCTN cooperative groups consists of a standard process (**Fig. 2**). Any investigator can propose a concept within a cooperative group if the investigator's institution is a member institution of the group; the NCTN has no requirements about prior engagement, academic rank, or specialty. Following development of a study concept, an investigator must then categorize the study as either a cancer control or treatment trial to identify the appropriate committee responsible for trial review and approval. Cancer control trials focus on prevention and screening, health disparities, supportive care, symptom management, survivorship, and cancer care delivery research, whereas treatment trials focus on testing the safety or efficacy of new therapeutic agents and interventions.

In the early phase of study design, an investigator or the research team may choose to present the concept first to a smaller disease-site (eg, pancreas) or specialty-specific (eg, surgery) working group. Through an iterative process of feedback,

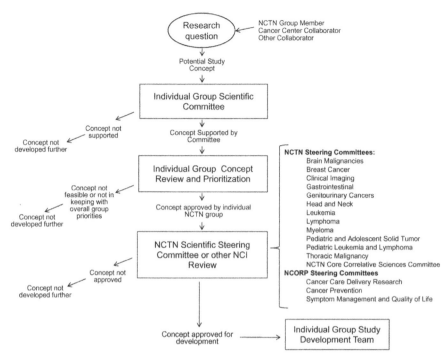

Fig. 2. Approval process for NCTN clinical trials.[19]

revision, and presentation within a working group, investigators may refine the proposal and garner support from colleagues before then presenting it to the appropriate scientific committee (eg, Gastrointestinal Committee) for feedback. Through discussion within the scientific committee, study leaders will typically revise and refine the trial further to address potential issues, such as clinical relevance, feasibility, analytical approach, consideration of potentially competing trials, and likelihood of changing clinical practice.

If the trial has adequate support from the scientific committee, the investigator then presents the study concept to the NCTN disease-specific task force (eg, NCTN Pancreas Task Force). This provides an opportunity to assess whether the trial would compete with other active NCTN trials, critically evaluate the potential clinical impact of the trial, and ensure that the concept is aligned with NCI priorities. The investigator may receive specific feedback to inform further revision of the trial and may be asked to represent the concept to the task force following additional changes. If supported by the disease-specific task force, the trial is then presented to the Scientific Steering Committee. At this point, the trial undergoes formal NCI review for approval, and the Cancer Therapy Evaluation Program committee centrally reviews the proposed study population size. If needed, the protocol is revised and finalized before activation and initiation of accrual.

The timeline from idea generation to study activation within the NCTN can vary tremendously depending on the simplicity of the trial design, feasibility of the study proposal, and extent of clinical equipoise. Although the process can be lengthy for complicated trials or trials investigating a treatment approach that is highly controversial, it can be streamlined and efficient for trials with a more straightforward study design.

Table 2
Resources for new investigators available through the National Clinical Trials Network groups

Group	Scientific Meetings	New Investigator-Specific Educational Offerings	Funding Opportunities	Information Sources
Alliance	Group meetings, twice yearly	Alliance new investigators committee Alliance new investigators workshop Committee-specific mentoring	Alliance career development awards Alliance executive officer training program Alliance travel awards	www.Allianceforclinicaltrialsinoncology.org
CCTG	Group meetings: spring-general fall-IND Scientific workshops	CCTG new investigators workshop CCTE new investigators clinical trial course (biennial) CCTG new investigators practicum Committee-specific mentoring Trial-specific mentoring	CCTG travel awards CCTG fellowships	www.Ctg.queensu.ca
COG	Group meetings, twice yearly	Twice-yearly COG young investigator committee COG young investigator career development lunch Committee-specific mentoring	The Aflac Archie Bleyer Young Investigator Award in Adolescent and Young Adult Oncology	www.childrensoncologygroup.org
ECOG-ACRIN	Group meetings, twice yearly	ECOG-ACRIN new investigator training PreCOG new investigator training Young investigator symposium ECOG-ACRIN fall meeting	The Paul Carbone Award ECOG Research and Education Foundation: Young Investigator Award ACRIN Young Investigator Award	www.ecog-acrin.org
NRG	Group meetings, twice yearly	NRG investigator training committee New investigator mentoring program New investigator educational workshop	—	www.NRGoncology.org

| SWOG | Group meetings, twice yearly | Young investigator training course Leadership academy | Charles A. Coltman, Jr Fellowship Rare Cancers Fellowship SWOG Development Awards SWOG/Hope Impact Award SWOG/Hope Early Exploration and Development (SEED) Fund SWOG Integrated Science Center Pilot Awards Grant Writing Award/Workshop | www.SWOG.org SWOG Oncology—Facebook |

Abbreviations: ACRIN, American College of Radiology Imaging Network; Alliance, Alliance for Clinical Trials in Oncology; CCTG, Canadian Clinical Trials Group; COG, Children's Oncology Group; NRG, NRG Oncology.

Adapted from Bertagnolli MM, Blaney SM, Blanke CD, et al. Current Activities of the Coalition of Cancer Cooperative Groups. J Natl Cancer Inst. 2019;111(1):11-18.

PROMOTING SURGEON INVOLVEMENT IN NATIONAL CLINICAL TRIALS NETWORK CLINICAL TRIALS

Surgeon involvement and leadership in cooperative group trials has numerous benefits, and in fact, some of the most impactful multidisciplinary trials over the past two decades have been led by surgeons. Surgeons are uniquely poised to design not only trials comparing surgical techniques or approaches but also multidisciplinary trials that include surgery or a procedural intervention combined with other therapy, as these trials require careful consideration of feasibility, particularly relating to a patient's candidacy for resection. Both in practice and in the clinical trial setting, patients must be evaluated for surgical candidacy, which may include determination of radiographic resectability as well as careful assessment of comorbidity, frailty, nutrition, and performance status. Surgeons accustomed to routinely conducting these assessments are uniquely equipped to estimate the feasibility of accrual. In addition, as a result of clinical experience, surgeons may be able to offer unique insight into patient preference, risk tolerability, and decision-making related to operative interventions and treatment sequencing, which is critical when determining trial feasibility. Surgeon expertise is also crucial to ensure that the study protocols are planned appropriately to include quality assessment to limit the effect of surgeon volume and experience or procedural variation on either immediate or long-term end points as discussed above.

Surgeons are also well suited for determining appropriate end points for multidisciplinary trials that include surgical intervention; these include postoperative complications, pathologic end points, and patient-reported measures in addition to traditional survival outcomes. For example, studies testing preoperative treatment strategies should also incorporate assessment of immediate postoperative outcomes. In addition, how to effectively define and assess adverse events in the postoperative setting may be best understood by experienced surgeons. Along with promoting accrual of surgical patients in clinical trials, surgeons can provide tissue samples for studies assessing translational end points. Finally, surgeons have historically proven to be successful leaders of landmark randomized NCTN clinical trials and are well positioned to champion future surgical and multidisciplinary oncology trials. Each cooperative group meets on a regular basis and has specific opportunities, such as funding awards and training courses, which are available to new or junior investigators, including surgeons (**Table 2**).

SUMMARY

As outlined in this review, performing multidisciplinary trials through the cooperative group mechanism has many benefits, including collaboration with national clinical and scientific experts, efficient accrual of a diverse and representative patient population given treatment in community and academic centers, and access to an established and streamlined administrative infrastructure. The process of study concept development to trial activation is effort-intensive and requires persistence on behalf of the investigators and study teams. However, the opportunity to generate practice-changing evidence to improve the care of patients with cancer is tremendous. Surgeons offer specific expertise in the development and design of innovative, multidisciplinary oncology trials and have a unique opportunity to be key leaders in the conduct of future practice-changing clinical trial research.

ACKNOWLEDGMENTS

The authors would like to acknowledge Don Norwood, Scientific Editor in The University of Texas MD Anderson Cancer Center Research Medical Library, for his assistance with article editing and formatting.

DISCLOSURE

The authors have nothing to disclose.

REFERENCES

1. Wong BO, Perera ND, Shen JZ, et al. Analysis of registered clinical trials in surgical oncology, 2008-2020. JAMA Netw Open 2022;5(1):e2145511.
2. Schilsky RL, McIntyre OR, Holland JF, et al. A concise history of the cancer and leukemia group B. Clin Cancer Res 2006;12(11 Pt 2):3553s–5s.
3. Children's Oncology Group. Our History. Available at: https://www.childrensoncologygroup.org/index.php/history. Accessed August 26, 2021.
4. SWOG Cancer Research Network: History & Impact. 2021. Available at: https://www.swog.org/about/history-impact. Accessed August 26, 2021.
5. Alliance for Clinical Trials in Oncology: History of the Alliance. Available at: https://www.allianceforclinicaltrialsinoncology.org/main/public/standard.xhtml?path=%2FPublic%2FHistory. Accessed August 26, 2021.
6. Wickerham DL, O'Connell MJ, Costantino JP, et al. The half century of clinical trials of the National Surgical Adjuvant Breast And Bowel Project. Semin Oncol 2008;35(5):522–9.
7. Cox JD. Evolution and accomplishments of the Radiation Therapy Oncology Group. Int J Radiat Oncol Biol Phys 1995;33(3):747–54.
8. ECOG-ACRIN Cancer Research Group: About Us. 2020. Available at: https://ecog-acrin.org/about-us. Accessed August 26, 2021.
9. NRG Oncology: Legacy Groups. Available at: https://www.nrgoncology.org/About-Us/Who-We-Are-What-We-Do/Legacy-Groups. Accessed August 26, 2021.
10. Grothey A, Adjei AA, Alberts SR, et al. North Central Cancer Treatment Group–achievements and perspectives. Semin Oncol 2008;35(5):530–44.
11. Coltman CA Jr. The Southwest Oncology Group: progress in cancer research. Semin Oncol 2008;35(5):545–52.
12. Giantonio BJ, Forastiere AA, Comis RL. The role of the Eastern Cooperative Oncology Group in establishing standards of cancer care: over 50 years of progress through clinical research. Semin Oncol 2008;35(5):494–506.
13. Green MR, George SL, Schilsky RL. Tomorrow's cancer treatments today: the first 50 years of the Cancer and Leukemia Group B. Semin Oncol 2008;35(5):470–83.
14. Boughey, Judy C, Kelly K Hunt. Chapter 44. The ACOSOG Experience. In: Kuerer HM, editor. Kuerer's Breast Surgical Oncology. New York, NY: McGraw Hill; 2010.
15. Bertagnolli MM, Blanke CD, Curran WJ, et al. What happened to the US cancer cooperative groups? A status update ten years after the Institute of Medicine report. Cancer 2020;126(23):5022–9.
16. Institute of Medicine (US) Committee on Cancer Clincial Trials and the National Cancer Institute (NCI) Cooperative Group Program. In: Nass S, Moses HL, Mendelsohn J, editors. A National Cancer Clinical Trials System for the 21st Century: Reinvigorating the NCI Cooperative Group Program. Washington, DC: National Academies Press; 2010.
17. McCaskill-Stevens W, Lyss AP, Good M, et al. The NCI Community Oncology Research Program: what every clinician needs to know. Am Soc Clin Oncol Educ Book 2013. https://doi.org/10.1200/EdBook_AM.2013.33.e84.
18. Schilsky RL. The national clinical trials network and the cooperative groups: the road not taken. Cancer 2020;126(23):5008–13.

19. Bertagnolli MM, Blaney SM, Blanke CD, et al. Current activities of the coalition of cancer cooperative groups. J Natl Cancer Inst 2019;111(1):11–8.
20. NIH National Cancer Institute Community Oncology Research Program (NCORP). Available at: https://ncorp.cancer.gov/about/. Accessed August 27, 2021.
21. Lloyd Wade J 3rd, Petrelli NJ, McCaskill-Stevens W. Cooperative group trials in the community setting. Semin Oncol 2015;42(5):686–92.
22. Schott AF, Welch JJ, Verschraegen CF, et al. The national clinical trials network: conducting successful clinical trials of new therapies for rare cancers. Semin Oncol 2015;42(5):731–9.
23. Fleshman J, Branda M, Sargent DJ, et al. Effect of laparoscopic-assisted resection vs open resection of stage II or III rectal Cancer on pathologic outcomes: the ACOSOG Z6051 randomized clinical trial. JAMA 2015;314(13):1346–55.
24. Katz MHG, Shi Q, Meyers JP, et al. Alliance A021501: preoperative mFOLFIRINOX or mFOLFIRINOX plus hypofractionated radiation therapy (RT) for borderline resectable (BR) adenocarcinoma of the pancreas. J Clin Oncol 2021; 39(3_suppl):377.
25. Unger JM, LeBlanc M, Blanke CD. The Effect of Positive SWOG Treatment trials on survival of patients with cancer in the US population. JAMA Oncol 2017;3(10): 1345–51.
26. St Germain D, Denicoff A, Torres A, et al. Reporting of health-related quality of life endpoints in National Cancer Institute-supported cancer treatment trials. Cancer 2020;126(11):2687–93.

The Development of Investigator-Initiated Clinical Trials in Surgical Oncology

Hannah G. McDonald, MD, Emily B. Cassim, BS,
Megan M. Harper, MS, MD, Erin E. Burke, MD, MPH,
Emily F. Marcinkowski, MD, Michael J. Cavnar, MD,
Prakash K. Pandalai, MD, Joseph Kim, MD*

KEYWORDS

- Investigator-initiated trials • Surgical oncology • Clinical trial protocol development

KEY POINTS

- Investigator-initiated trials (IITs) led by surgical oncologists advance cancer care by directly addressing knowledge gaps in treatment.
- Key stakeholders include the principal investigator, investigator team, research staff, industry partnerships, institutional and government regulatory bodies, and patients.
- There are challenges and barriers for surgical oncologists establishing and running IITs which can include lack of time, insufficient institutional support, difficulties securing funding, and meeting regulatory requirements.
- Understanding how to navigate the regulatory requirements of IITs can increase the number of surgical oncologists who can undertake leadership roles in IITs, thereby accelerating and expanding the impact of IITs for patients with cancer.

INTRODUCTION

Distinct from industry and cooperative group clinical trials, investigator-initiated trials (IITs) are unsolicited trials designed and led by physicians that positively impact current clinical practice.[1,2] Surgical oncologists traditionally have extensive training in hypothesis-driven investigations and are leaders of multidisciplinary clinical teams, making them poised to identify key clinical questions and design both surgical and

Division of Surgical Oncology, University of Kentucky, 800 Rose Street C224, Lexington, KY 40508, USA
* Corresponding author. Division of Surgical Oncology, Department of Surgery, University of Kentucky, 800 Rose Street, C223, Lexington, KY 40536.
E-mail address: joseph.kim@uky.edu
Twitter: @hpb.surgonc (J.K.)

Surg Oncol Clin N Am 32 (2023) 13–25
https://doi.org/10.1016/j.soc.2022.07.003
1055-3207/23/© 2022 Elsevier Inc. All rights reserved.

nonsurgical studies to answer them.[1,3] However, between 2001 to 2011 and 2008 to 2020 only 12.9% and 6.2%, respectively, of oncology trials involved surgical interventions.[4,5] The number of nonsurgical oncology trials led by surgeons is unknown, but they are also assumed to be underrepresented given the limited surgeon representation on National Institutes of Health (NIH) study sections and the disproportionately low NIH extramural grant funding rate of 2.3% versus 33.2% for other physicians in 2020.[6–8] Reasons for limited surgeon participation include time constraints due to increasing operative and clinical demands, inadequate institutional resources and support, and difficulty designing pragmatic oncologic trials.[3,6,9–11] In this article, we discuss the process of surgical oncologists developing and conducting IITs, provide examples of surgical oncology IITs at the University of Kentucky (UK), and address IIT challenges and pitfalls.

DEVELOPMENT OF INVESTIGATOR-INITIATED TRIALS

The steps in development, organization, and implementation of IITs can be exhaustive. We discuss the requisite components of IITs through the framework of a successfully completed IIT (NCT04088786) at UK. This IIT was a phase 1 clinical trial evaluating the safety of nanoliposomal irinotecan (Nal-IRI) as a hyperthermic intraperitoneal chemotherapy (HIPEC) agent.

Overview

The process of designing and conducting an IIT involves multiple steps involving the principal investigator (PI) and management of regulatory matters (**Fig. 1**). IIT design begins when the PI generates an innovative hypothesis based on clinical observations (**Fig. 2**). The PI then develops a trial protocol to test the hypothesis. The protocol includes study design, inclusion/exclusion criteria, defined endpoints, target enrollment, anticipated timeline, feasibility, and budget. Often, preliminary data or published studies are needed to support the rationale to conduct the study. Typically, a biostatistician performs a power calculation based on the estimated effect of the intervention, with interim analyses built into the protocol that allow for early closure if the intervention is deemed futile. Financial support can be secured through institutional, government, nonprofit, or industry sources (**Fig. 3**). Institutions may provide infrastructural support to facilitate detailed protocol design, feasibility analyses, funding approvals, data safety monitoring board (DSMB) review, external contractual agreements, and fulfillment of regulatory requirements (**Fig. 4**). Then, the institutional review board (IRB) reviews the complete clinical trial proposal. After IRB approval, resources and staffing must be organized before patient enrollment. This may include receipt of study drug(s) or equipment and recruitment of all research team members, such as phlebotomists, clinical trial nurse(s), trial coordinator(s), and statisticians. During the study, predetermined safety and efficacy analyses are performed by the research team and DSMB to assess efficacy/futility and to ensure that study continuation is ethical. Depending on the study design and endpoint(s) chosen, final data analysis may occur months or years after the trial has closed. After final data collection and analysis, the

STEP 1: TRIAL DESIGN	STEP 2: TRIAL OPENS	STEP 3: TRIAL CLOSES	STEP 4: TRIAL COMPLETE
• Protocol development • Funding acquisition • Regulatory approval • Establish agreements	• Enrollment, accrual, clinical monitoring • Data collection • Ongoing safety analysis • Intermittent data analysis	• Preliminary clinical conclusions • Long-term follow-up data collection • Data verification • Final data analysis and statistics	• Clinical conclusions • Publish/present results • Evaluate next steps to implement new clinical knowledge (efficacy, multicenter trials)

Fig. 1. IIT process overview.

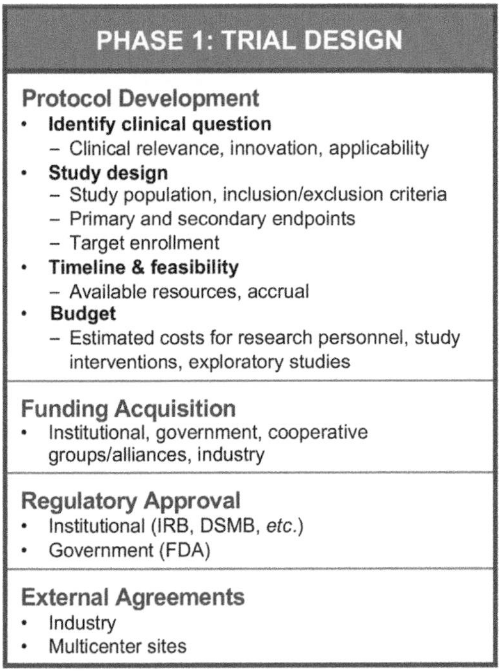

PHASE 1: TRIAL DESIGN
Protocol Development
Identify clinical question
– Clinical relevance, innovation, applicability
Study design
– Study population, inclusion/exclusion criteria
– Primary and secondary endpoints
– Target enrollment
Timeline & feasibility
– Available resources, accrual
Budget
– Estimated costs for research personnel, study interventions, exploratory studies
Funding Acquisition
Institutional, government, cooperative groups/alliances, industry
Regulatory Approval
Institutional (IRB, DSMB, etc.)
Government (FDA)
External Agreements
Industry
Multicenter sites

Fig. 2. Successfully establishing an IIT. DSMB, data and safety monitoring board; FDA, Food and Drug Administration; IRB, institutional review board.

completed trial results and clinical conclusions can be disseminated. The publication and presentation of trial results allow for changes to clinical practice and inform future areas for investigation such as larger, later phase confirmatory trials.

Investigator-Initiated Trial Stakeholders

Principle investigator

IIT PIs include practicing physicians who oversee all aspects of the IIT including trial design, protocol development, funding acquisition, accrual, recruitment, patient monitoring, data analysis, and publication of trial results (see **Fig. 1**).[1,2,12] Because our model IIT involved two treatment sites, there was a co-PI for each participating site

Funding Acquisition
Institutional
Operative techniques
Small, early phase, or regional-specific studies
External Non-profit
Large, multicenter and community trials
Smaller awards (can support exploratory studies)
Industry
New drugs or devices
New indications for approved drugs/devices

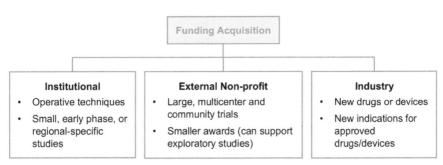

Fig. 3. IIT funding options based on study design.

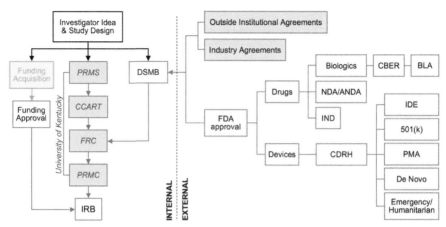

Fig. 4. Institutional and external regulatory requirements for IIT approval. BLA, biologics license application; CBER, Center for Biologics Evaluation and Research; CCART, Clinical Care and Research Team; CDRH, Center for Devices and Radiological Health; DSMB, data and safety monitoring board; FDA, Food and Drug Administration; FRC, Feasibility Review Committee; IDE, investigational device exemption; IND, investigational new drug; IRB, institutional review board; NDA/ANDA, new drug application/abbreviated NDA; PMA, premarket approval; PRMC, Protocol Review and Monitoring Committee; PRMS, Protocol Review and Monitoring System.

and a trial PI. Surgical oncologists are uniquely experienced to serve as PIs of IITs because they are well-positioned define gaps in current standards-of-care as they closely follow patients through all aspects of treatment.

Coinvestigators
Coinvestigators (co-Is) can include other clinicians who help recruit, monitor, or evaluate patients within clinical trials, or staff who provide contributions to protocol design or data collection (eg, statisticians). In the case of our model HIPEC IIT, co-Is included medical and surgical oncologists as well as a central radiologist.

Clinical research staff
Study coordinators help to screen patients for trial eligibility, coordinate study and clinical visits, and communicate with institutional regulatory bodies to ensure protocol compliance and data maintenance. Data collection is managed by clinical research nurses and associates who perform individual chart reviews and compile data (eg, central laboratory). Clinical staff including nursing, laboratory, pathology, and radiology personnel also assist with collection of trial-specific data. In our model HIPEC IIT, anesthesia staff obtained timed venous blood samples throughout surgery and clinical nurses obtained postoperative blood samples.

Basic and translational research science staff
Research scientists and laboratories may perform exploratory studies to generate data for future clinical trials. In our model HIPEC IIT, we used a central laboratory to obtain pharmacokinetic data correlating plasma drug levels with adverse events (AEs). One of the added benefits of PI surgical oncologists leading the basic and translational research efforts of the study is their ability to obtain (IRB-approved) research samples directly in the operating room.

Regulatory bodies

To ensure safety in clinical trials, institutional and government authorities evaluate trial design and progress (see **Fig. 4**). Although IRBs and DSMBs are common for most institutions, other clinical research offices can vary in structure, function, and name. For example, additional oversight by a Protocol Review and Monitoring System (PRMS) is required at the National Cancer Institute (NCI)-designated cancer centers. Government regulation comes from the Food and Drug Administration (FDA) to ensure that the drugs and devices in clinical trials are safe. For our IIT, we obtained an investigational new drug (IND) exemption from the FDA to use nal-IRI in our clinical trial.

Sponsors

IITs cannot be implemented without financial support. Trial sponsors include the host institution, external nonprofit groups, or industry sponsors (see **Fig. 3**). Our model HIPEC IIT was supported by industry (IPSEN).

Patients and families

Patient participation in oncology clinical trials has recently improved but remains a considerable challenge for successful execution of IITs.[3,13] Local catchment areas, selective exclusion criteria, and limited patient recruitment efforts present the largest barriers to oncology trial participation.13,38,39 In fact, when offered to participate in clinical trials, greater than 50% of patients agree to enroll in oncology clinical trials, regardless of race/ethnicity.[14] In surgical oncology, IITs provide patients with access to interventions that are otherwise unavailable and can provide hope for diseases with few standard-of-care regimens and poor outcomes, such as with peritoneal carcinomatosis (PC) in our model HIPEC IIT.

Protocol Design

Importance of the clinical question

The inception of every IIT occurs when an investigator identifies an important, clinically meaningful question that can be answered with available resources. In the case of our HIPEC IIT, the drugs used during HIPEC have changed little over the past decades and vary widely.[15] Because standard-of-care systemic regimens for many gastrointestinal (GI) cancers include an irinotecan backbone (eg, FOLFIRINOX, FOLFIRI),[16] this was identified as a candidate HIPEC agent for patients with PC from GI tumors. In 2015, the FDA approved a novel nal-IRI formulation that demonstrated higher efficacy at lower doses and with improved toxicity profile.[17-25] Subsequently, Dr Joseph Kim (PI) designed a clinical trial to evaluate the safety of nal-IRI as a HIPEC agent.

Choosing the study design

Clinical trials can be categorized as treatment, prevention, supportive, palliation, screening, or diagnostic.[26] To study a drug/device in humans, preclinical animal data must demonstrate reasonable anticipated safety in humans.[27] The FDA then designates clinical trials by phase, which can only progress to higher levels if prior studies demonstrate safety and promising clinical outcomes.[27] In general, phase 0 trials are uncommon except in cancer studies, involve very few participants (<15), and evaluate a limited number of low doses to determine if investigational drugs have mechanisms congruent with preclinical data. Phase 1 trials evaluate safety in humans. Phase 2 and 3 studies evaluate efficacy, with phase 2 typically evaluating for initial signs of efficacy, and phase 3 studies determining if the intervention is more efficacious than current standard of care or placebo. Phase 4 studies are large, long-term, population after-marketing studies.

Determining primary and secondary endpoints

Studies are designed to meet primary endpoints, which focus on the most important outcomes of each study (eg, survival).[28,29] Secondary endpoints include other important clinical measures, but may not be able to determine statistical significance because studies are not powered to meet these goals. Exploratory studies can be included to generate data for future clinical trials (eg, evaluation of molecular and genomic characteristics of disease). It is important to consult with biostatisticians to determine clinically meaningful, significant endpoints prior to enrollment.

Inclusion and exclusion criteria

Inclusion/exclusion criteria determine the study population, which impacts future applicability of trial results. A major problem of modern clinical trials is creating inclusion/exclusion criteria that are so narrow that accrual becomes unattainable, resulting in trial closure and wasted resources.[14,30]

Determining target enrollment

Target enrollment is determined based on the proposed treatment effect size. Regional and institutional disease incidence/prevalence will provide a realistic estimate of patients eligible to participate in trials. If the disease or disease characteristic prevalence is low, the investigator should consider a multicenter design to expedite accrual and ensure that target enrollment is achieved in the specified time period.

Study timeline

The study timeline should be estimated so that target accrual, complete data collection and analysis, publication, and dissemination can be achieved. Time from enrollment to intervention is impacted by availability of resources and staffing. Length of follow-up required to complete data collection should be clearly defined. During the follow-up period, long-term AEs and overall, progression-free, and disease-free survival may be assessed.

Trial Types

Trial sponsors (investigator, cooperative group and industry)

Although IITs are developed and led by physician PIs, cooperative group clinical trials are overseen by a central committee of clinical experts in a particular field with site-specific PIs to oversee and manage the trial at each institution.[1,2,31] IITs can be multicenter studies, but often involve fewer patients and sites than large multicenter cooperative group trials.[1,2,31] The endpoints of cooperative group trials are applicable to a broader patient population due to higher accrual and wider geographic distribution of patients.[2,31]

Industry-initiated trials have financial interests which can introduce bias. Historically, industry-based studies have shown higher rates of favorable results compared with nonindustry-sponsored studies. This may reflect the need for companies to see returns on large financial investments.[32] The goal of most industry-initiated trials is to show the success of a drug or device that can be marketed, rather than to answer current clinical questions.[33] However, industry-sponsored trials (ISTs), which include IITs, can defray the costs of investigational drugs/devices.[34] To limit industry biases, industry involvement can be limited to funding and overview of final results to ensure scientific accuracy, without input into study design, data analysis, or clinical conclusions.

Single-center versus multicenter investigator-initiated trials

Single-center trials involve a PI and patients from one institution. Because only one clinical site is involved, many aspects of the study design and oversight are simplified and easier to navigate, such as the protocol approval process. Unless the disease or condition being studied is very common, these studies are optimal for smaller, non-randomized trials because of the limited ability to accrue patients.[1,2] This may narrow the study scope and limit applicability to broader patient populations.[1,2] However, single-institution studies are the building blocks to larger multicenter clinical trials.

Multicenter IITs involve multiple institutions with site-specific PIs to manage the trial at the institutional level. These sub-PIs report to the main PI who performs all the tasks required in establishing any IIT. The primary PI of a multicenter trial ensures institutional approval and compliance at all sites and successful accrual to meet each site's goals and performs final data analysis and interpretation. With larger accrual targets/sample size, these studies can generate clinically meaningful data representing larger patient populations. Disadvantages include increased protocol approval times and need for ongoing contractual agreements between institutions (eg, data sharing).[1,2,35] Many of these issues have been addressed by the creation of clinical research organizations (CROs), which develop master contracts between main study sites and all member institutions and oversee study progress and coordination.[1] CROs also assist with regulatory processes such as filing IND applications with the FDA and data management across all centers.[1]

Regulatory Requirements and Protocol Approval

Overview of the National Clinical Trials Network
In 2014, the NCI developed the National Clinical Trials Network (NCTN) for clinical trials management at the NCI-designated cancer centers. The NCTN has a centralized IRB and the cancer trials support unit as part of the Cancer Therapy Evaluation Program, Imaging and Radiation Oncology Core, and a common data management system. The NCTN is a network of five cooperative groups: the Southwest Oncology Group, Alliance for Clinical Trials in Oncology, Eastern Cooperative Oncology Group American College of Radiology and Imaging network, NRG Oncology, and Children's Oncology Group. NCI provides oversight with scientific steering committees that facilitate information exchange across cooperative groups and improve trial design and conduct efficiency.

Institutional requirements
At the UK Markey Cancer Center (MCC), the PRMS is composed of four entities: the PRMS administrative office, disease working groups or Clinical Care and Research Teams, the Feasibility Review Committee, and the Protocol Review and Monitoring Committee. Collectively, these entities provide oversight and rigorous review for scientific merit, feasibility, inclusivity, and impact before IRB review (see **Fig. 4**).

Institutional review board
IRBs are designated to monitor research involving humans and determine whether trial protocols have met the scientific, ethical, and regulatory requirements of the institution, scientific community, and government.

Data safety monitoring board
DSMBs assure patient safety and protocol compliance for clinical trials. At MCC, the internal DSMB is a committee, which meets monthly to review study-specific reports including status updates, safety, and progress. They analyze protocol deviations, subject accruals, and analyze serious AEs. External DSMBs are required by the NCI for all phase III randomized trials.

Additional institutional resources

The MCC Clinical Resarch Office can assist investigators with protocol design, approval, budget development and management of pre-grant and post-grant ascertainment before submission to the PMRS.

The MCC Investigational Drug Service (IDS) is managed by the Department of Pharmacy. The IDS supports all clinical drug-related research and reviews protocols for study drug concerns. This entity also receives, maintains, prepares, verifies, and dispenses study drugs.

Government regulatory requirements

As outlined in **Fig. 4**, the FDA requires different approvals for new drug use depending on the rigor of prior research and intended use.[27] First, IND applications are needed before initiating phase I clinical trials and require promising preclinical data or applicable/corresponding human studies. When investigators want to evaluate a drug for a new indication, IND exemptions may be granted, as was the case with our HIPEC IIT. INDs must be submitted at least 30 days before the planned start of a clinical trial and are required before shipping any new drug across state lines. After completion of phase 2/3 studies and before US commercialization, a new drug application (NDA) is required. NDAs aim to evaluate new drug safety, efficacy of the proposed use, and benefits/risks. Abbreviated NDAs enable approval of generic formulations of medications. Biologics require additional approval including the therapeutic biologics application by the FDA and approval by the Center for Biologics Evaluation and Research.

Medical devices are regulated by the FDAs Center for Devices and Radiological Health. Medical devices require investigational device exemption (IDE) approval based on preclinical safety data before initiation of phase I studies. When adequate preclinical data are not feasible, early feasibility studies (EFS) are required at the same time as IDEs. After safety in humans has been confirmed, the pathway for medical devices diverges into three classes based on the level of risk. Class I and II devices generally require premarket notification (501(k)) before commercialization. Class II devices require additional oversight termed "special controls," which vary depending on the specific device. Class III, the highest risk devices generally require more thorough premarket approvals instead of 501(k)s. Other application processes may be required for novel devices or those for emergency/humanitarian use.

Funding acquisition

As experimental therapies are not covered by insurance, financial support is necessary to limit patient burden. Funding may be obtained from the primary institution, government, nonprofit groups, or industry. Institutional funding may include start-up funds, cancer center or institutional foundations, and investigator awards. Government or nonprofit group funding (such as NIH, NCI, Veterans Affairs, and Department of Defense) is best for larger or multicenter trials, which are the most expensive to manage but are expected to have broader impact and applicability. Funding may also be obtained from private research foundations (eg, the Lustgarten Foundation). Industry funding is helpful when using drugs or devices for new indications or efficacy studies as these can only be obtained from these entities, which is the mechanism of funding our model HIPEC IIT. This has the potential to directly benefit industry as new indications for drugs/devices can extend patents and market share (see **Fig. 3**).

Current Investigator-Initiated Trials at the University of Kentucky

In addition to the previously referenced ITT led by Dr Joseph Kim which was completed in April 2020 (NCT04088786), many of our surgical oncology faculty are successful IIT PIs (**Table 1**).

				Target
PI	ID	Phase	Study Type	Accrual
Joseph Kim	NCT05052723	2	Interventional	21
Prakash Pandalai	NCT04779554	2	Interventional	100
Emily Marcinkowski	NCT05150652	2	Interventional	65
Michael Cavnar	NCT04276090	1	Interventional	34

Table 1
Current surgical oncology investigator-initiated trials at University of Kentucky

Cabozantinib and pembrolizumab in metastatic pancreatic cancer

The Kim laboratory has shown the synergistic effect of the anti-PD-1 antibody, pembrolizumab (PEMBRO) and multi-kinase inhibitor, cabozantinib (CABO) using pancreatic adenocarcinoma (PDAC) cells, patient-derived organoids, and patient-derived xenografts. NCT05052723, a phase 2 trial evaluating CABO/PEMBRO as second-line therapy for advanced PDAC, began recruitment in January 2022. This trial has a targeted accrual of 21 patients with primary endpoint of progression-free survival in patients with advanced PDAC treated with pembrolizumab and cabozantinib.

Flat dose versus weight-based intraperitoneal chemotherapy for CRS/hyperthermic intraperitoneal chemotherapy

Mitomycin C (MMC) is the most commonly used HIPEC agent worldwide, although significant variability exists between regimens.36,37 There is no direct comparison between flat dosing and weight-based dosing to inform clinical practice. NCT04779554 is a phase 2 IIT led by Dr Prakash Pandalai which opened in February 2021, comparing flat versus weight-based dosing of intraperitoneal MMC during CRS/HIPEC for patients with peritoneal carcinomatosis from GI malignancies. The primary endpoints include characterizing the pharmacokinetic profile associated with each dosing strategy and measuring the incidence of neutropenia. The goal enrollment is 100 patients.

Neoadjuvant endocrine therapy in ER-positive, HER2-negative early-stage breast cancer

Up to 50% of patients treated with breast conservation surgery (BCS) will undergo re-excision of an involved margin resulting in greater psychosocial burden, adjuvant therapy delays, and increased health care costs.[40,41] Data suggest lower margin positivity and decreased re-excision rates when BCS follows neoadjuvant chemotherapy. However, data regarding BCS margin status with neoadjuvant endocrine therapy (NaET) are lacking.[42,43] Therefore, Dr Emily Marcinkowski designed a phase 2 IIT (NCT05150652) to evaluate the effect of NaET on margin positivity status following BCS for women with early-stage (I–II), low-risk ER/PR + HER2-breast cancer. Enrollment target is 65 patients for this trial, which opened in February 2022.

Hepatic Artery Infusion Chemotherapy using the Synchromed II Pump/Codman Catheter device combination for Unresectable Colorectal Metastases/Intrahepatic Cholangiocarcinoma

Hepatic artery infusion (HAI) delivers regional chemotherapy directly into the liver via the hepatic artery, typically for colorectal cancer liver metastases or unresectable intrahepatic cholangiocarcinoma.[44] After discontinuation of the widely used Codman C3000 pump, the only FDA-approved device for HAI, an alternate device was necessary to continue serving patients in need of HAI chemotherapy. This study initially aimed to test the safety and efficacy of HAI pump placement and intra-arterial standard-of-care floxuridine initiation using a novel combination, the Medtronic Syn-chromed II pump combined with the Codman vascular catheter (which remained available). Patients with unresectable liver metastases from colorectal cancer and unresectable intrahepatic cholangiocarcinoma were included. The primary endpoint was the percentage of patients who completed the first cycle of hepatic artery chemotherapy. Goal accrual for this study was 34, however, since Dr Michael Cavnar opened this IIT (NCT04276090) in May 2020, the Codman C3000 pump has become available as the Intera 3000 pump, which is now FDA approved.

DISCUSSION

IITs developed by surgical oncologists generate essential data to test innovative treatments that improve clinical practice. Surgical oncologists are uniquely poised to be effective PIs of IITs due to the ability to identify key gaps in the treatment of patients with cancer and their experience as leaders of multidisciplinary teams. IITs can be difficult to design, establish, and complete due to the rigor of simultaneous clinical practice, extensive regulatory processes, and funding acquisition. These processes may be streamlined for future investigators by including formal clinical trials training in surgical oncology fellowship curricula to help navigate this complex field, strengthening networking and mentorship in trial design, harmonizing and simplifying regulatory processes, generating appropriate recruitment targets, and increasing public funding of IITs. It is essential for surgical oncologists to continue to advance our field through hypothesis-driven investigations.

FUNDING

This research was supported by NIH training grant T32CA160003 (M.M. Harper). P.K. Pandalai received research funding from the University of Kentucky (UK) Markey Cancer Center (MCC) to conduct clinical trial NCT04779554. M.J. Cavnar received research funding from the UK MCC and the American Cancer Society to conduct clinical trial NCT04276090. E.F. Marcinkowski received research funding from the UK MCC to conduct clinical trial NCT05150652. J. Kim received research funding from Merck and Exelixis to conduct clinical trial NCT05052723 and Ipsen to conduct clinical trial NCT04088786.

CONTRIBUTIONS

Conceptualization, supervision: J.K.; methodology, H.G. McDonald., E.B. Cassim, and M.M. Harper; data acquisition: H.G. McDonald., E.B. Cassim, and M.M. Harper; clinical efforts: E.E. Burke, E.F. Marcinkowsi, M.J. Cavnar., P.K. Pandalai, and J. Kim; writing-original draft: H.G. McDonald, E.B. Cassim, and M.M. Harper; writing-review and editing: all authors; visualization: H.G. McDonald and M.M. Harper. All authors have read and agreed to the published article version.

ACKNOWLEDGMENTS

The authors would like to thank Donna Gilbreath for her assistance with editing the figures used in this publication.

DISCLOSURE

No financial support was received from any commercial interest in the production of this research. The remaining authors declare no potential conflicts of interest.

REFERENCES

1. Park KU, Mamounas EP, Katz MHG, et al. Clinical Trials for the Surgical Oncologist: Opportunities and Hurdles. Ann Surg Oncol 2020;27(7):2269–75. https://doi.org/10.1245/s10434-020-08472-z.

2. Tsai S, Evans DB. Lessons learned from investigator-initiated clinical trials for localized pancreatic cancer. J Surg Oncol 2022;125(1):69–74. https://doi.org/10.1002/jso.26756.

3. Roland CL, Grubbs EG, Katz MHG, et al. Clinical trials-Designing, implementing, and collaborating. J Surg Oncol 2020;122(1):25–8. https://doi.org/10.1002/jso.25889.

4. Menezes AS, Barnes A, Scheer AS, et al. Clinical research in surgical oncology: an analysis of ClinicalTrials.gov. Ann Surg Oncol 2013;20(12):3725–31. https://doi.org/10.1245/s10434-013-3054-y.

5. Wong BO, Perera ND, Shen JZ, et al. Analysis of Registered Clinical Trials in Surgical Oncology, 2008-2020. JAMA Netw Open 2022;5(1):e2145511. https://doi.org/10.1001/jamanetworkopen.2021.45511.

6. Fisher G, O'Dwyer P. Importance of surgeons in cooperative groups: Perspectives from the medical oncologists. J Surg Oncol 2022;125(1):93–4. https://doi.org/10.1002/jso.26754.

7. Demblowski LA, Busse B, Santangelo G, et al. NIH Funding for Surgeon-Scientists in the US: What Is the Current Status? J Am Coll Surg 2021;232(3):265–74.e2. https://doi.org/10.1016/j.jamcollsurg.2020.12.015.

8. Lewit RA, Black CM, Camp L, et al. Association of Surgeon Representation on NIH Study Sections With Receipt of Funding by Surgeon-scientists. Ann Surg 2021;273(6):1042–8. https://doi.org/10.1097/sla.0000000000004836.

9. Fanfan D, Ehrlich H, Elkbuli A. The Future of the surgeon-scientist: A Journey Funneled through inspiration, Roadblocks and Resilience. Ann Med Surg (Lond) 2021;62:65–7. https://doi.org/10.1016/j.amsu.2020.12.047.

10. Keswani SG, Moles CM, Morowitz M, et al. The Future of Basic Science in Academic Surgery: Identifying Barriers to Success for Surgeon-scientists. Ann Surg 2017;265(6):1053–9. https://doi.org/10.1097/sla.0000000000002009.

11. McLennan S, Nussbaumer-Streit B, Hemkens LG, et al. Barriers and Facilitating Factors for Conducting Systematic Evidence Assessments in Academic Clinical Trials. JAMA Netw Open 2021;4(11):e2136577. https://doi.org/10.1001/jamanetworkopen.2021.36577.

12. Feehan AK, Garcia-Diaz J. Investigator Responsibilities in Clinical Research. The Ochsner journal. Spring 2020;20(1):44–9. https://doi.org/10.31486/toj.19.0085.

13. Unger JM, Vaidya R, Hershman DL, et al. Systematic Review and Meta-Analysis of the Magnitude of Structural, Clinical, and Physician and Patient Barriers to Cancer Clinical Trial Participation. J Natl Cancer Inst 2019;111(3):245–55. https://doi.org/10.1093/jnci/djy221.

14. Unger JM, Hershman DL, Till C, et al. When Offered to Participate": A Systematic Review and Meta-Analysis of Patient Agreement to Participate in Cancer Clinical Trials. J Natl Cancer Inst 2021;113(3):244–57. https://doi.org/10.1093/jnci/djaa155.

15. Harper MM, Kim J, Pandalai PK. Current Trends in Cytoreductive Surgery (CRS) and Hyperthermic Intraperitoneal Chemotherapy (HIPEC) for Peritoneal Disease from Appendiceal and Colorectal Malignancies. J Clin Med 2022;(10):11. https://doi.org/10.3390/jcm11102840.

16. Benson AB, Venook AP, Al-Hawary MM, et al. Colon Cancer, Version 2.2021, NCCN Clinical Practice Guidelines in Oncology. J Natl Compr Canc Netw 2021;19(3):329–59. https://doi.org/10.6004/jnccn.2021.0012.

17. Highlights FDA. of Prescribing Information, ONYVIDE (liposomal irinotecan) for injection. Drugs@FDA 2015;1–18.

18. Santos A, Zanetta S, Cresteil T, et al. Metabolism of irinotecan (CPT-11) by CYP3A4 and CYP3A5 in humans. Clin Cancer Res 2000;6(5):2012–20.

19. Kalra AV, Kim J, Klinz SG, et al. Preclinical activity of nanoliposomal irinotecan is governed by tumor deposition and intratumor prodrug conversion. Cancer Res 2014;74(23):7003–13. https://doi.org/10.1158/0008-5472.Can-14-0572.

20. Wang-Gillam A, Li CP, Bodoky G, et al. Nanoliposomal irinotecan with fluorouracil and folinic acid in metastatic pancreatic cancer after previous gemcitabine-based therapy (NAPOLI-1): a global, randomised, open-label, phase 3 trial. Lancet 2016;387(10018):545–57. https://doi.org/10.1016/s0140-6736(15)00986-1.

21. Wöll E, Thaler J, Keil F, et al. Oxaliplatin/Irinotecan/Bevacizumab Followed by Docetaxel/Bevacizumab in Inoperable Locally Advanced or Metastatic Gastric Cancer Patients - AGMT_GASTRIC-3. Anticancer Res 2017;37(10):5553–8. https://doi.org/10.21873/anticanres.11987.

22. Adiwijaya BS, Kim J, Lang I, et al. Population Pharmacokinetics of Liposomal Irinotecan in Patients With Cancer. Clin Pharmacol Ther 2017;102(6):997–1005. https://doi.org/10.1002/cpt.720.

23. Frøysnes IS, Andersson Y, Larsen SG, et al. Novel Treatment with Intraperitoneal MOC31PE Immunotoxin in Colorectal Peritoneal Metastasis: Results From the ImmunoPeCa Phase 1 Trial. Ann Surg Oncol 2017;24(7):1916–22. https://doi.org/10.1245/s10434-017-5814-6.

24. Leonard SC, Lee H, Gaddy DF, et al. Extended topoisomerase 1 inhibition through liposomal irinotecan results in improved efficacy over topotecan and irinotecan in models of small-cell lung cancer. Anticancer Drugs 2017;28(10):1086–96. https://doi.org/10.1097/cad.0000000000000545.

25. Tossey JC, Reardon J, VanDeusen JB, et al. Comparison of conventional versus liposomal irinotecan in combination with fluorouracil for advanced pancreatic cancer: a single-institution experience. Med Oncol 2019;36(10):87. https://doi.org/10.1007/s12032-019-1309-6.

26. Hulley SBCSR, Browner WS, Grady DG, et al. Designing clinical research. 4 edition. Lippincott Williams and Wilkins; 2013.

27. FDA. The FDA's Drug Review Process: Ensuring Drugs Are Safe and Effective. 2022. https://www.fda.gov/drugs/information-consumers-and-patients-drugs/fdas-drug-review-process-ensuring-drugs-are-safe-and-effective.

28. Cumpston MS, Webb SA, Middleton P, et al. Understanding implementability in clinical trials: a pragmatic review and concept map. Trials 2021;22(1):232. https://doi.org/10.1186/s13063-021-05185-w.

29. McCoy CE. Understanding the Use of Composite Endpoints in Clinical Trials. West J Emerg Med 2018;19(4):631–4. https://doi.org/10.5811/westjem.2018.4.38383.

30. Kelly D, Spreafico A, Siu LL. Increasing operational and scientific efficiency in clinical trials. Br J Cancer 2020;123(8):1207–8. https://doi.org/10.1038/s41416-020-0990-8.

31. Snyder RA, Ahmad S, Katz MHG. Pancreas cancer trials for early stage disease: Surgeons leading therapeutic cooperative group trials. J Surg Oncol 2022;125(1):75–83. https://doi.org/10.1002/jso.26701.

32. Lundh A, Lexchin J, Mintzes B, et al. Industry sponsorship and research outcome. Cochrane Database Syst Rev 2017;2(2):Mr000033. https://doi.org/10.1002/14651858.MR000033.pub3.

33. Blümle A, Wollmann K, Bischoff K, et al. Investigator initiated trials versus industry sponsored trials - translation of randomized controlled trials into clinical practice (IMPACT). BMC Med Res Methodol 2021;21(1):182. https://doi.org/10.1186/s12874-021-01359-x.

34. Santamaria-Barria JA, Stern S, Khader A, et al. Changing Trends in Industry Funding for Surgical Oncologists. Ann Surg Oncol 2019;26(8):2327–35. https://doi.org/10.1245/s10434-019-07380-1.

35. Herfarth HH, Jackson S, Schliebe BG, et al. Investigator-Initiated IBD Trials in the United States: Facts, Obstacles, and Answers. Inflamm Bowel Dis 2017;23(1):14–22. https://doi.org/10.1097/mib.0000000000000907.

36. Yurttas C, Hoffmann G, Tolios A, et al. Systematic Review of Variations in Hyperthermic Intraperitoneal Chemotherapy (HIPEC) for Peritoneal Metastasis from Colorectal Cancer. J Clin Med 2018;7(12):567. https://doi.org/10.3390/jcm7120567.

37. Turaga K, Levine E, Barone R, et al. Consensus guidelines from The American Society of Peritoneal Surface Malignancies on standardizing the delivery of hyperthermic intraperitoneal chemotherapy (HIPEC) in colorectal cancer patients in the United States. Ann Surg Oncol 2014;21(5):1501–5. https://doi.org/10.1245/s10434-013-3061-z.

38. Somkin CP, Ackerson L, Husson G, et al. Effect of medical oncologists' attitudes on accrual to clinical trials in a community setting. J Oncol Pract 2013;9(6):e275–83. https://doi.org/10.1200/jop.2013.001120.

39. Mahmud A, Zalay O, Springer A, et al. Barriers to participation in clinical trials: a physician survey. Curr Oncol 2018;25(2):119–25. https://doi.org/10.3747/co.25.3857.

40. Landercasper J, Attai D, Atisha D, et al. Toolbox to Reduce Lumpectomy Reoperations and Improve Cosmetic Outcome in Breast Cancer Patients: The American Society of Breast Surgeons Consensus Conference. Ann Surg Oncol 2015;22(10):3174–83.

41. Grant Y, Al-Khudairi R, St John E, et al. Patient-level costs in margin re-excision for breast-conserving surgery. Br J Surg 2019;106(4):384–94.

42. Torabi R, Hsu C-H, Patel P, et al. Predictors of margin status after breast-conserving operations in an underscreened population. Langenbecks Arch Surg 2013;398(3):455–62.

43. Landercasper J, Bennie B, Ahmad H, et al. Opportunities to reduce reoperations and to improve inter-facility profiling after initial breast-conserving surgery for cancer. A report from the NCDB. Eur Surg Oncol 2019;45(11):2026–36.

44. Thiels C, D'Angelica M. Hepatic artery infusion pumps. Journal of Surgical Oncology 2020;1:70–7.

Clinical Trials That Have Informed the Modern Management of Breast Cancer

Laura K. Krecko, MD[a], Meeghan A. Lautner, MD, MSc[b],
Lee G. Wilke, MD[b],*

KEYWORDS

- Breast cancer • Clinical trials • Adjuvant • Neoadjuvant • Endocrine
- Chemotherapy • Axilla

KEY POINTS

- With surgical, medical, technological, and genomic advancements, the treatment of breast cancer has become less morbid yet more complex.
- Randomized controlled trials form the backbone of current practices in: Breast surgery; axillary management; selection of neoadjuvant and adjuvant therapies; and selection of chemotherapy and endocrine therapies via application of genomic assays.
- This article explores trials conducted by key national and international groups, including but not limited to: National Surgical Adjuvant Breast and Bowel Project B-01, B-04, B-06, B-51, B-19, B-31, B-18, B-27, B-14, B-20, B-33; Alliance for Clinical Trials in Oncology Z0010, Z0011, Z1071, Z1031; and European Organization for Research and Treatment of Cancer 10801, 10041.

INTRODUCTION

Breast cancer (BC) management has undergone a dramatic transformation in the past century. Early BC care involved extensive surgical debulking and chemotherapy regimens to gain control over what was historically a debilitating disease. Although early innovations led to improved survival, efforts to sustain life came at the price of morbidity. Distilling operative and nonoperative treatments to the minimum necessary to achieve disease control and improve survival—while maximizing quality of life and minimizing complications—has led to the nuanced and individualized treatment paradigms that define BC management today. This modern approach has evolved largely

Funding sources: Dr L.K. Krecko is supported by the National Cancer Institute of the NIH, grant T32CA090217. The content is solely the responsibility of the authors and does not necessarily represent the official views of the National Institutes of Health.
[a] Department of Surgery, University of Wisconsin Hospital and Clinics, 600 Highland Avenue K4/642, Madison, WI 53792, USA; [b] Department of Surgery, University of Wisconsin Hospital and Clinics, 600 Highland Avenue K4/624, Madison, WI 53792, USA
* Corresponding author.
E-mail address: wilke@surgery.wisc.edu
Twitter: @LauraKrecko (L.K.K.); @mlautnermd (M.A.L.); @LeeWilke (L.G.W.)

due to the rigorous conduct of randomized controlled trials (RCTs). The authors summarize key trials investigating the following: (a) extent of breast surgery; (b) axillary management; (c) the transition from adjuvant to neoadjuvant therapies; and (d) selection for chemotherapy and endocrine therapies.

Extent of Breast Surgery

Radical mastectomy and total mastectomy confer comparable survival

In the 1890s, Dr William Halsted developed the radical mastectomy (RM), which included en bloc removal of all breast tissue, chest wall muscles, and axillary lymph nodes, for the surgical treatment of breast malignancy.[1] This approach became the standard until the mid-1900s when the utility of this operation was questioned.[2,3] Proposals for less extensive operations (with or without the addition of adjuvant therapies such as radium[4]) centered on the hypothesis that a smaller amount of tissue could be removed and still provide oncologic benefit while decreasing morbidity. These alternatives included total mastectomy (TM), quadrantectomy (excision of an entire quadrant of the breast), and lumpectomy/partial mastectomy (excision of only the tumor with a smaller surrounding margin). The Milan study (1973), conducted at the National Cancer Institute (NCI) in Milan, randomized 701 women (mean age 50, tumor <2 cm, no palpable axillary nodes) to (1) RM or (2) quadrantectomy with axillary lymph node dissection (ALND) and radiotherapy to the ipsilateral breast. Twenty year follow-up found no difference in long-term survival between the groups.[5,6] In the United States, National Surgical Adjuvant Breast and Bowel Project (NSABP) B-04 (1971), conducted by one of the first NCI Cancer Cooperative groups, randomized women (1079) with clinically negative axillary nodes to (1) RM, (2) TM without ALND but with postoperative radiation, or (3) TM plus ALND if their nodes became clinically positive in follow-up.[1] Women with positive axillary nodes (n = 586) underwent (1) RM or (2) TM without ALND but with postoperative radiation.[1] After 25 years of follow-up, no survival advantage from RM or from radiation therapy after TM in women with clinically negative nodes was found.[1] Patients with clinically positive nodes with axillary radiation alone had higher rates of axillary recurrence compared with ALND with RM (11% vs 8%).[1,7] Leaving positive nodes in situ, however, did not increase the rate of distant recurrence or BC-related mortality,[1] inspiring less invasive axillary management strategies.

Total mastectomy and breast conservation therapy confer comparable survival

As the results of the Milan and NSABP B-04 studies were maturing in the 1980s, 10-year results of an RCT at the Institut Gustave-Roussy (1972) of 179 patients comparing modified RM (MRM) (retained pectoralis muscles) and breast conservation therapy (BCT, defined as breast-conserving surgery [BCS] plus radiation) also showed no difference in overall survival (OS) or locoregional recurrence (LRR).[8] Of note, in trials of this era, BCT included ALND. A comparison between TM, BCT, and lumpectomy alone, with all arms receiving ALND, occurred in the NSABP B-06 trial (1973). NSABP B-06 found that women with breast tumors less than 4 cm had identical survival and disease-free recurrence after 20 years, regardless of nodal status. Highlighting the role of radiation, BCT patients had the lowest local recurrence risk at less than 3%.[9,10] The European Organization for Research and Treatment of Cancer (EORTC) 10801 trial (1980), a phase III RCT comparing MRM with BCT (including axillary clearance and breast/tumor bed radiotherapy) for patients with tumors ≤5 cm and axillary node negative or positive disease,[11] also found similar OS. These trials, among others,[12–14] highlighted the equivalence of BCT and mastectomy for local/regional BC and provided a less invasive operative option by the latter half of the twentieth century.[15]

Utilization of radiation after breast-conserving surgery for invasive breast cancer and ductal carcinoma in situ
The outcomes of adding radiation to BCS to improve local control was further explored by several studies in the 1990s to early 2000s (**Table 1**).[16–25] Most trials found that radiotherapy improves LRR but does not improve OS for invasive BC; several trials also concluded that the addition of endocrine therapy for estrogen receptor (ER)-positive disease reduces LRR and distant recurrence. The progression of these trials led to an important finding further refining the extent of surgery and radiation that postmenopausal clinically node-negative women with low-grade, ER-positive disease may be able to avoid radiation despite breast preservation for those who adhere to 5 years of endocrine therapy.

Tumor margins and breast conservation
There remains a paucity of RCTs evaluating the difference in outcomes by margin width. Of the RCTs comparing mastectomy with BCT, only NSABP B-06 required microscopically clear margins (no ink on tumor),[9] whereas others specified only gross removal.[26] The National Comprehensive Cancer Network (NCCN) guidelines[27] for resection margins for invasive BC cite the Society of Surgical Oncology-American Society for Radiation Oncology (SSO-ASTRO) consensus guidelines (based on a meta-analysis of 33 studies), stating that for stage I and II invasive BC treated with BCT, no tumor on ink provides equivalent LRR to wider margins.[28]

A similar meta-analysis for patients with ductal carcinoma in situ (DCIS) identified a 2-mm margin as the most likely to lower LRR risk.[29] Of four RCTs of patients receiving radiotherapy following DCIS, three defined margins as no ink on tumor[30–32] but one Swedish Ductal Carcinoma In Situ (SweDCIS) did not mandate microscopically clear margins.[33] The time to evaluate margin width for BCT in RCTs has likely passed, but review of longer term outcomes from these margin guidelines will provide an insight into their ability to reduce re-excision and evaluate the impact on LRR in the era of modern systemic therapy.

Axillary Management

As surgical management of the breast saw a shift from RM to BCT, attention was similarly turned to de-escalation of axillary surgery. The concept of the sentinel lymph node biopsy (SLNB), or removing only the first draining lymph node(s) of the breast, revolutionized the axillary management of BC. The efficacy and safety of SLNB in women with clinically node-negative BC to allow avoidance of ALND was established by several key trials (**Table 2**).[34–41]

The utility of SLNB in patients with 1 to 2 positive sentinel lymph nodes (SLNs) was then evaluated. ACOSOG (American College of Surgeons Oncology Group; now Alliance for Clinical Trials) Z0011 (1999) randomized 891 patients with 1 to 2 positive SLNs to completion ALND or no further surgery and though it did not reach prespecified accrual, short- and long-term follow-up found no differences in regional recurrence, OS or disease-free survival (DFS).[42,43] Several other trials (AMAROS, OTOASOR, and MA-20) evaluated the role of axillary with breast radiotherapy in those with positive SLNs and found equivalence to ALND with less morbidity (see **Table 2**).[44–46] Unlike Z0011, which included BCT-only patients, AMAROS included a subset (248 of 1425), who had a mastectomy. Reviewers of this study note that most of the patients had only one positive SLN (75%–78%); however, this study supports limiting the use of ALND in those with mastectomy for which radiation therapy is recommended. It should be noted that for the majority of patients eligible for Z0011, regional nodal radiation, as described in AMAROS, OTOASOR, and MA-20, may not

Table 1
Radiation after breast-conserving surgery for invasive breast cancer and ductal carcinoma in situ

Study (Trial Start Year)	Number of Patients	Tumor Characteristics	Randomization Arms	Local Recurrence [95% CI]	Survival	Key Findings
Liljegren et al, "10 y results after Sector Resection with or Without Postoperative Radiotherapy for Stage I Breast Cancer: A Randomized Trial (1981)[16]	381	Unifocal BC <2 cm; no histopathologic signs of axillary metastasis	Sector resection + ALND followed by: 1. XRT (n = 184) 2. No XRT (n = 197)	1. XRT: 8.5% [3.9%–13.1%] 2. No XRT: 24.0% [17.6%–30.4%]	OS: 1. XRT 77.5% [70.9%–84.1%] 2. No XRT 78% [71.7%–84.3%]	Women > 55 y of age without comedo or lobular carcinomas had a low risk of local recurrence.
Clark et al, "Randomized Clinical Trial of Breast Irradiation Following Lumpectomy and Axillary Dissection for Node-Negative Breast Cancer: an Update" (Ontario Clinical Oncology Group, 1984)[17,18]	837	Node-negative BC ≤ 4 cm; local excision microscopically complete; histologically negative ALNs	Lumpectomy + ALND followed by: 1. XRT (n = 416) 2. No XRT (n = 421)	Local recurrence only: 1. XRT: 6.3% 2. No XRT: 18.8%	Death: 1. XRT 20.9% 2. No XRT 23.5%	Tumor size (>2 cm), age (<40), and poor nuclear grade predicted for breast relapse.
Veronesi et al, "Radiotherapy after breast-conserving surgery in small breast carcinoma: Long-term results of a randomized trial" (Milan National Cancer Institute, 1987)[19]	579	Invasive carcinoma <2.5 cm	1. Quadrantectomy, ALND, + XRT (n = 299) 2. Quadrantectomy, ALND, no XRT (n = 280)	Intra-breast Tumor Reappearance 1. XRT: 16/294 (5.4%) 2. No XRT: 59/273 (21.6%)	All-cause mortality: 1. XRT: 2.0% (n = 52) 2. No XRT: 2.4% (n = 57)	XRT indicated in all patients up to 55 y; XRT may be avoided in patients >65 and optional in women 56–65 y with negative nodes.

Study	No.	Inclusion criteria	Intervention	Outcome	Outcome	Conclusion
Fisher et al, "Tamoxifen, radiation therapy, or both for prevention of ipsilateral breast tumor recurrence after lumpectomy in women with invasive breast cancers of 1 cm or less" (NSABP B-21, 1989)[25]	1009	Primary invasive tumor <1 cm; ALNs negative on histologic examination	Lumpectomy + ALND followed by: 1. XRT + placebo (n = 332) 2. XRT + TAM (n = 334) 3. TAM alone (n = 334)	Ipsilateral BC recurrence as first event: 1. XRT + placebo: 6.9% (n = 23) 2. XRT + TAM: 2.7% (n = 9) 3. TAM alone: 13.5% (n = 45)	Alive, event-free: 1. XRT + placebo: 81.6% (n = 271) 2. XRT + TAM: 84.4% (n = 282) 3. TAM alone: 77.8% (n = 260)	XRT after breast conservation (with or without TAM) should be considered for women with tumors <1 cm given rates of ipsilateral breast tumor recurrence.
Kunkler et al, "Breast-conserving surgery with or without irradiation in women aged 65 y or older with early breast cancer (PRIME II): a randomized controlled trial." (PRIME II, 2003)[22]	1326	Early BC, HR+, axillary node negative, T1–T2 (≤ 3 cm); either grade 3 or lymphovascular invasion	BCS + adjuvant endocrine treatment plus: 1. XRT (n = 658) 2. No XRT (n = 668)	Local recurrence: 1. XRT: 1% (n = 5) 2. No XRT: 4% (n = 26) Ipsilateral breast tumor recurrence 1. XRT: 1.3% [0.2%–2.3%] 2. No XRT: 4.1 [2.4%–5.7%]	5-y OS: 93.9% [91.8%–96.0%] in both groups	Lower BC recurrence at 5 y in ER-rich tumors compared with total study population.
Hughes et al, "Lumpectomy plus Tamoxifen with or without Irradiation in Women 70 y of Age or Older with Early Breast Cancer" (Cancer and Leukemia Group B 9343 [1994]; Eastern Cooperative Oncology Group and Radiation Therapy Oncology Group [1996])[20,21]	636 (≥ 70 y)	Clinical stage I (T1N0M0), ER+	Lumpectomy followed by: 1. TAM + XRT (n = 317) 2. TAM alone (n = 319)	Local or regional recurrence at 5 y 1. TAM + XRT: 1% (n = 2) 2. TAM alone: 4% (n = 16)	5-y OS: 1. TAM + XRT: 87% 2. TAM alone: 86%	TAM alone reasonable adjuvant treatment for women ≥70 y with early ER + BC.

(continued on next page)

Table 1 (continued)						
Study (Trial Start Year)	**Number of Patients**	**Tumor Characteristics**	**Randomization Arms**	**Local Recurrence [95% CI]**	**Survival**	**Key Findings**
Fisher et al, "Lumpectomy compared with lumpectomy and radiation therapy for the treatment of intraductal breast cancer" (NSABP B-17, 1985)[23]	818	DCIS	1. Lumpectomy + XRT (n = 413) 2. Lumpectomy alone (n = 405)	Ipsilateral BC 1. XRT: 2.1% (n = 28) 2. No XRT: 5.1% (n = 64)	EFS: 1. XRT: 84.4% 2. No XRT: 73.8%	XRT reduced incidence of noninvasive and invasive second tumors (to 7.5% and 2.9%, respectively).
Fisher et al., "Tamoxifen in treatment of intraductal breast cancer: National Surgical Adjuvant Breast and Bowel Project B-24 randomized controlled trial (NSABP B-24, 1991)[24]	1804 Stratified by age ($\leq$ 49 or > 49 y)	DCIS; if ALND performed, all LNs histologically negative	Lumpectomy followed by: 1. XRT + TAM (n = 902) 2. XRT + placebo (n = 902)	Ipsilateral BC 1. XRT + TAM: 13.75% 2. XRT + placebo: 19.62%	5-y OS: 97% [96%–98%] for both groups	Positive sample margins and comedonecrosis associated with increased risk of ipsilateral BC.

Abbreviations: ALND, axillary lymph node dissection; BC, breast cancer; BCS, breast-conserving surgery; CI, confidence interval; DCIS, ductal carcinoma in situ; EFS, event-free survival; HR, hormone receptor; OS, overall survival; TAM, tamoxifen; XRT, radiation therapy.

Table 2
Safety and efficacy of sentinel lymph node biopsy as an alternative to axillary lymph node dissection

Trial (Start Year)	Patient Characteristics	Treatment	Key Findings	Conclusions
NSABP B-32 (1999)[34,35]	Invasive BC, clinically node negative 5611 patients randomized	1. SLNB (plus ALND if positive node found) 2. SLNB alone (if node negative)	OS, DFS, and regional control equivalent between groups.	In patients with clinically negative axillary nodes and negative SLNB, no further ALND is necessary.
Sentinella/GIVOM (1999)[36]	BC ≤ 3 cm 749 patients randomized	1. SLNB + ALND (ALND arm) 2. SLNB + ALND only if SLN metastatic (SLN arm)	Significantly less postoperative side effects in SLN arm. DFS and OS slightly worse in SLN group; insufficient sample to draw definitive conclusions.	SLNB is effective and well tolerated.
European Institute of Oncology Milan (1998)[37,38]	BC < 2 cm undergoing BCS 516 patients randomized	1. SLNB + ALND 2. SLNB + ALND only if SLN involved	Similar BC-related EFS in both groups.	ALND can be avoided in patients with negative SLNs.
National Cancer Research Institute of Genoa trial (1998)[39]	BC ≤ 3 cm with clinically negative axillary LNs 248 patients randomized	1. SLNB and ALND 2. SLNB plus ALND if SLNs contained metastases	No significant difference in OS and EFS between two arms.	SLNB is non-inferior to ALND.
American College of Surgeons Oncology Group Z0010 (1999)[40]	T1-2N0M0 BC 5327 patients assessed	BCT, bilateral anterior iliac crest bone marrow aspiration, SLNB	SLNB complication rate <10%.	SLNB is safe with low overall rate of complications.
American College of Surgeons Oncology Group Z0011 (1999)[42,43]	T1-2 BC with 1–2 positive SLNs and no palpable axillary LNs 891 patients randomized	BCT and adjuvant systemic therapy plus: 1. Completion ALND 2. No further axillary-specific treatment	No differences between groups in regional recurrence, OS, or DFS.	ALND should not be routinely performed in this population.

(continued on next page)

Table 2
(continued)

Trial (Start Year)	Patient Characteristics	Treatment	Key Findings	Conclusions
International Breast Cancer Study Group (IBCSG) trial 23–01 (2001)[41]	Patients with non-palpable ALNs and primary tumor <5 cm; after SLNB had 1 or more micrometastatic (<2 mm) LNs 934 patients randomized	1. ALND 2. No ALND Note: 9% underwent mastectomy	No difference in DFS or OS between groups.	ALND should be avoided for those with early BC and minimal SLN involvement.
AMAROS (EORTC 10981–22023) (2001)[44]	T1-2 BC with no palpable LNs Included subset (248 of 1425 with positive SLN) who had a mastectomy 4806 randomized; 1425 with positive SLN	1. ALND* 2. Axillary radiotherapy[a] [a]If positive SLN	Equivalent DFS and OS between groups, with less morbidity from radiotherapy	ALND and axillary radiotherapy after positive SLN provide confer similar axillary control; ALND may be limited in patients undergoing mastectomy for whom radiation therapy is recommended.
OTOASOR (2002)[45]	Invasive BC (cN0, cT ≤ 3 cm) and SLN metastasis 2106 patients randomized	1. ALND 2. Regional nodal irradiation	Radiotherapy noninferior to ALND in preventing axillary recurrence.	Axillary radiotherapy is a reasonable alternative treatment of select patients with early-stage invasive BC and SLN metastasis.
MA-20 (2000)[46]	Node-positive or high-risk node-negative BC 1832 patients randomized	BCS + adjuvant systemic therapy and: 1. Whole-breast irradiation + regional nodal irradiation 2. Whole-breast irradiation alone	Regional irradiation reduced rate of BC recurrence but did not improve OS.	For patients with node-positive or high-risk node-negative BC, addition of regional nodal irradiation to whole-breast irradiation reduces BC recurrence.

SN FNAC (2009)[51]	Stage II to IIIA biopsy-proven, node-positive BC 153 patients included	SLNB + ALND with required immunohistochemistry (IHC) after NAT	Low FNR (8.4%) for SLNB with mandatory IHC	Low FNR of SLNB after NAT can be achieved with mandatory use of IHC.
GANEA 2 (2010)[52]	Early BC patients treated with NAT 957 patients scheduled for NAT included	After NAT: 1. pN1 (cytologically proven node involvement): SLN + ALND 2. CN0: SLND + ALND only if mapping failure or SLN involvement	Patients with negative SLN after NAT (and no lymphovascular invasion; remaining tumor size 5 mm): 3.7% risk of positive ALND	Safe to avoid ALND in node negative patients with negative SLNB after NAT.

Abbreviations: ALND, axillary lymph node dissection; BC, breast cancer; BCS, breast-conserving surgery; BCT, breast conservation therapy; DFS, disease-free survival; EFS, event-free survival; FNR, false negative rate; NAT, neoadjuvant therapy; OS, overall survival; RCT, randomized controlled trial; SLNB, sentinel lymph node biopsy.

be needed, though it was used in up to 15% of patients in the ACOSOG study. This remains an area of evaluation and recent use of nomograms may provide support for radiation oncologists until further stratification is available.[47]

Prospective studies next turned to evaluate the role of SLNB in patients undergoing neoadjuvant therapy (NAT). ACOSOG Z1071 (2009) evaluated patients with clinical node (cN1) disease who had completed NAT and underwent SLNB and ALND and found that SLNB alone had a high false negative rate (FNR) (12.6%), exceeding the prespecified threshold of 10%.[48] The FNR, however, could be reduced below 10% with the use of dual tracer, removal of at least three nodes, and when a node with a biopsy clip placed before therapy is removed.[48] The importance of evaluating clipped nodes following NAT was reiterated in a prospective trial by Caudle and colleagues (2011) showing improved accuracy of axillary staging (FNR 4.2%) in clinically node-positive patients who received targeted ALND (ie, SLN dissection with removal of a clip placed pretreatment to mark biopsy-proven metastatic disease).[49] SENTINA (2009) similarly found that after NAT, SLNB had higher FNR compared with SLNB before NAT, but that FNR decreased with removal of three or more nodes and with the use of dual tracer.[50] Based on the results of these and other studies (see **Table 2**),[51,52] SLNB with the use of dual tracer and finding at least three SLNs and a clipped node after NAT has become more widespread due to the high likelihood of a pathologic complete response (pCR), especially in patients with triple-negative or HER2-positive disease.[53,54] The NSABP B-51, SENOMAC,[55] and Alliance A011202 trials[56] seek to build on the substantial progress being made identifying sub-groups of patients, including those having completed NAT, who may safely avoid ALND.

From Adjuvant to Neoadjuvant Chemotherapy and Impact on Breast Surgery

NSABP B-01 (1958) was the first RCT to evaluate adjuvant chemotherapy (Thiotepa) in BC after RM and revealed a significant decrease in recurrence in premenopausal women with greater than three positive axillary nodes.[57] Other early adjuvant trials established the importance of systemic therapy for survival but required prolonged follow-up and incorporated patient populations who frequently did not need cytotoxic therapy. The following sections summarize the adjuvant treatment of BC and how these trials built the foundation for subsequent neoadjuvant and combination neoad-juvant/adjuvant approaches.

Adjuvant chemotherapy improves survival

The next trial after NSABP B-01 demonstrating an OS improvement from the addition of chemotherapy (cyclophosphamide, methotrexate, and fluorouracil) was conducted by Bonadonna and colleagues (1973).[58] Although chemotherapy regimens are now tailored to BC subtype (ie, ER, progesterone receptor [PR], and HER2 status), the premise of administering adjuvant chemotherapy to improve survival was grounded by these early seminal studies. The NSABP, now a pillar in the NCIs NSABP/RTOG/GOG National Surgical Adjuvant Breast and Bowel Project [NSABP], the Radiation Therapy Oncology Group [RTOG], and the Gynecologic Oncology Group [GOG] (NRG), remained a key group in evaluating novel agents with, for example, NSABP B-19 (1988) documenting a survival advantage for cyclophosphamide.[59] The Early Breast Cancer Trialists Group has performed meta-analyses to highlight the current recommendations for adjuvant and, more recently, NAT. A review of 26 trials evalu-ating the current "third generation" of combination adjuvant chemotherapy has shown that anthracyclines with taxanes delivered in a dose-dense manner reduce the 10 year risk of recurrence and BC mortality and are now the backbone of NAT.[60,61]

Adjuvant anti-HER2 therapy improves survival for HER2-positive breast cancer

The role for immunotherapy in cancer treatment moved to the forefront with the discovery the anti-HER2 therapy (eg, trastuzumab). A joint analysis of NSABP B-31 (2000) and the North Central Cancer Treatment Group Trial N9831 (2000) found that adding trastuzumab to paclitaxel after postoperative receipt of doxorubicin and cyclophosphamide leads to significant improvements in survival and decreased recurrence.[62,63] The HERA (Breast International Group [BIG] 1–01) trial (2001) was a phase III RCT of 5102 women with HER2-positive, early-stage BC randomized to receive trastuzumab for 1 or 2 years or observation.[64] Women receiving 1 year of adjuvant trastuzumab had improved long-term DFS, with a second treatment year found to not add benefit.[64] A second anti-HER2 therapeutic, pertuzumab, was evaluated in APHINITIY (2011). Patients with node-positive or high-risk node-negative HER2-positive disease who received adjuvant chemotherapy plus 1 year of trastuzumab were randomly assigned to pertuzumab or placebo; those treated with pertuzumab had significantly improved DFS.[65] These studies demonstrated the improved survival of HER2-positive patients receiving adjuvant anti-HER2 therapies.

Comparison of adjuvant and neoadjuvant therapies

Until the late 1980s, the standard for evaluation of new oncologic agents was performance in the adjuvant setting. However, after several neoadjuvant trials, it became apparent that the "medical treatment before surgery" design could offer several advantages for the patient and surgeon namely, axillary downstaging and increased eligibility for BCT. It also became apparent that the pCR rate could be a reliable surrogate marker of long-term outcomes and offer a rapid readout of primary endpoints.[66] NSABP B-18 (1988) evaluated how the same chemotherapy regimen would affect outcomes when given in adjuvant versus neoadjuvant settings. Women (1523) with operable BC (T1-3, N0-1 tumors) received either neoadjuvant or adjuvant doxorubicin and cyclophosphamide (AC); the neoadjuvant group showed high clinical responses, a 9% pCR, nodal downstaging, and higher rates of BCT with no difference in OS.[3,67,68] NSABP B-27 (1995) examined adding docetaxel preoperatively or postoperatively to patients undergoing neoadjuvant AC. Compared with preoperative AC alone, the addition of preoperative docetaxel increased rates of pCR and decreased pathologic node positivity but did not improve DFS or OS.[68] Analyses of B-18 and B-27 have contributed to the understanding of how breast and axillary pathologic response to NAT can predict LRR risk.[69]

The next generation of trials focused on treating specific BC phenotypes. For HER2-positive patients, several phase II trials validated the benefit of dual HER2 targeting. NeoSphere (2007) was a 4 × 4 design with one arm using both trastuzumab and pertuzumab with docetaxel followed postoperatively by fluorouracil, epirubicin, and cyclophosphamide.[70] The pCR rates were significantly higher in the trastuzumab, pertuzumab with docetaxel arm and, importantly, the combination was shown to be safe, with pCR providing an early indication of long-term outcomes. The TRYPHAENA study (2009) was primarily designed to assess the cardiac safety of dual HER2 blockade, but similarly showed a high pCR (55%–64%) with trastuzumab/pertuzumab containing regimens and equivalent long-term outcomes.[71] Such trials inspired further study of de-escalation of NAT for HER2-positive patients.[72]

For patients with triple-negative BC (ie, ER-, PR-, and HER2-negative), recent trials evaluated the use of immune checkpoint inhibitors. KEYNOTE-52221 (2017) was a phase III RCT for patients with clinical stage II–III disease who received pembrolizumab or placebo with carboplatin plus paclitaxel followed by standard anthracycline-based regimen.[73] Both pCR and event-free survival (EFS) were improved with pembrolizumab (pCR: 64.8% vs 51.2%; 18-month EFS: 91.3% vs 85.4%). ISPY2 (Investigation of Serial Studies to Predict Your Therapeutic Response with Imaging and Molecular Analysis 2) and IMpassion031 similarly evaluated NAT for triple-negative disease and identified immunotherapy regimens as potential benefits for this unique patient population.[72] ISPY2 (2010) added veliparib poly (ADP-ribose) polymerase (PARP inhibitor)-carboplatin to standard therapy for those with HER2-negative tumors and found that although this regimen had higher toxicity, it led to higher pCR than standard therapy alone, particularly for those with triple-negative BC.[74,75]

Knowing that not all patients will have a complete response to NAT, attention has turned to improving the adjuvant approaches for those that have residual disease at surgery. The CREATE-X trial (2007) randomized 910 patients treated with standard NAT with residual disease to adjuvant capecitabine for six to eight cycles or no additional therapy.[76] The trial was terminated early due to improvement in the treatment arm, and the use of capecitabine for patients with triple-negative BC who have residual disease after NAT has become a frequent recommendation. As the targeted therapy approaches for NAT for BC improve, there will continue to be efforts to downstage the surgical approaches both in the breast and axilla, potentially to the point of no surgical interventions.[77]

Adjuvant endocrine therapy for estrogen receptor-positive cancer

Endocrine responsive BC is the most common disease subtype, representing over 70% of BC. There are two primary endocrine therapy modalities: aromatase inhibitors (AIs) and selective ER modulators or degraders, such as tamoxifen or fulvestrant, which can be used in premenopausal or postmenopausal patients. The use of adjuvant and/or neoadjuvant endocrine therapy has revolutionized the approach to the care of BC patients, offering decreased recurrence and long-term survival.[78] NSABP B-14 (1982) found that adding 5 years of tamoxifen conferred a significant benefit in DFS and OS and reduced likelihood for contralateral BC.[79] In 1988, NSABP B-20 randomized women (with node-negative, ER-positive BC) to tamoxifen alone or tamoxifen plus six cycles of chemotherapy (cyclophosphamide, methotrexate, and 5-fluorouracil) and found that the combination of chemotherapy plus tamoxifen was superior to tamoxifen alone in improving DFS and OS.[80] Of note, samples from this study were used to develop the 21-gene Genomic Assay (Oncotype DX), enabling identification of those patients who could avoid chemotherapy and be treated with endocrine therapy alone; this is described in more detail in Section "Selection for Chemotherapy Versus Endocrine Therapy."

Once the efficacy of adjuvant endocrine therapy was established, the phase III study of the International Letrozole Breast Cancer group (1996) found that the AI letrozole was superior to tamoxifen.[81,82] The extent of endocrine therapy needed for decreased recurrence was evaluated by the National Cancer Information Center (NCIC) NCIC MA.17 (1998), which demonstrated that administering letrozole to postmenopausal women with hormone receptor (HR)-positive BC following 5 years of tamoxifen offered protection against recurrent BC.[83]

Multiple studies have validated the importance of endocrine therapy for decreasing BC recurrence and reducing contralateral disease, highlighting that the duration and type of endocrine therapy may differ depending on the patient's menopausal and nodal status, as well as tumor features. The American Society of Clinical Oncology provides clinical practice guideline updates based on the results of published trials which are too numerous to delineate in detail; examples include: ATAC, BIG 1-98, NSABP B-33, SOFT, and TEXT.[84,85] Neoadjuvant endocrine therapy has also been evaluated in a series of trials in postmenopausal patients and shown to facilitate

BCT with less impact on axillary downstaging. For example, the ACOSOG Z1031 trial (2006), an RCT comparing letrozole, anastrozole, and exemestane for women with ER-positive stage II–III BC, found that of women who had been considered for mastectomy at presentation, 51% were able to undergo BCT following neoadjuvant endocrine therapy.[3,86]

Selection for Chemotherapy Versus Endocrine Therapy

With increasing understanding of tumor biology and genomics came to the realization that tumors with the same receptor status may react differently to the same therapy. The development of genomic-based prognostic assays for an individual's risk revolutionized BC treatment. The utility of two of the most commonly used assays, the Oncotype DX (21-gene) and Mamma Print (70-gene), has been established in several trials. TAILORx (Trial Assigning Individualized Options for Treatment) (2006) evaluated the benefit of chemotherapy for patients with mid-range (11–25) Oncotype DX scores by enrolling patients with HR-positive, HER2-negative, node-negative BC who met NCCN guidelines for adjuvant chemotherapy to receive either chemotherapy and endocrine therapy or endocrine therapy alone. This trial found equivalent DFS, OS, and local and distance BC recurrence.[87] A similar study but with women with node-positive disease was conducted in the Southwest Oncology Group SWOG S1007 RxPonder trial (2011), with results showing that postmenopausal women with 1 to 3 positive axillary nodes and a recurrence score 0 to 25 do not benefit from chemotherapy and thus can forego adjuvant chemotherapy.[88,89]

The EORTC 10041/BIG 3-04 MINDACT study (2007) evaluated the utility of the Mamma Print (70-gene) assay. This multicenter RCT enrolled patients with invasive BC (T1-2 or operable T3) with up to three positive nodes to receive chemotherapy or not based on their clinical or genomic risk. The study concluded that approximately 46% of women with high clinical risk BC may not benefit from chemotherapy[90] and that the 70-gene signature can identify those with low genomic risk who may undergo endocrine therapy alone.[91] The ability to assess both genomic and clinical risk promises to further personalize BC care to avoid overtreatment and associated morbidity.

SUMMARY

This article offers a summary of pivotal clinical trials that defined current standards for BC management. The evolution of BC care—from RM to individualized, genomic-based care designed for unique tumor and patient characteristics—is a triumph resulting from the rigorous conduct of clinical trials. The generosity of those who have participated in clinical trials, combined with the dedication of those collaborating to implement them, continues to result in remarkable improvements in the way patients with BC receive care.

CLINICS CARE POINTS

- Total mastectomy and breast conservation therapy confer comparable survival. Postmenopausal women who are clinically node negative and have low-grade, ER-positive disease may be able to avoid radiation despite breast preservation with the use of endocrine therapy.

- Sentinel lymph node biopsy (SLNB) is a safe and effective alternative to axillary lymph node dissection (ALND) for patients with clinically node-negative breast cancer (BC) or 1 to 2 positive SLNs. Patients with high-risk positive sentinel nodes may undergo axillary radiotherapy with less morbidity and similar outcomes to ALND.

- For patients who undergo SLNB following neoadjuvant therapy, acceptable false negative rates are achieved by using dual tracer, finding at least three SLNs, and identifying a clipped node.
- HER2 blockade can be used in both neoadjuvant and adjuvant settings to improve long-term outcomes for HER2-positive patients.
- Newer agents such as PARP inhibitors and immunotherapies may be particularly beneficial in patients with triple-negative BC.
- Endocrine therapies improve survival for patients with hormone receptor-positive BC in the adjuvant setting and improve eligibility for breast conservation in the neoadjuvant setting.
- Genomic assays identify patients receiving endocrine therapy who will not derive benefit from chemotherapy and thus can be spared its associated morbidities.

DISCLOSURE

L.G. Wilke: Founder and Minority Stock Owner Elucent Medical (not discussed in this publication). The remaining authors have nothing to disclose.

REFERENCES

1. Fisher B, Jeong JH, Anderson S, et al. Twenty-Five-Year Follow-up of a Randomized Trial Comparing Radical Mastectomy, Total Mastectomy, and Total Mastectomy Followed by Irradiation. N Engl J Med 2002;347(8):567–75.
2. Fentiman IS. Long-term follow-up of the first breast conservation trial: Guy' wide excision study. Breast Edinb Scotl 2000;9(1):5–8.
3. Mathis KL, Nelson H. Randomized Controlled Trials in Surgical Oncology. Surg Oncol Clin N Am 2012;21(3):449–66.
4. Keynes G. The Radium Treatment of Primary Carcinoma of the Breast *Read 25th November 1930. Edinb Med J 1931;38(2):T19–36.
5. Veronesi U, Saccozzi R, Del Vecchio M, et al. Comparing Radical Mastectomy with Quadrantectomy, Axillary Dissection, and Radiotherapy in Patients with Small Cancers of the Breast. N Engl J Med 1981;305(1):6–11.
6. Veronesi U, Cascinelli N, Mariani L, et al. Twenty-Year Follow-up of a Randomized Study Comparing Breast-Conserving Surgery with Radical Mastectomy for Early Breast Cancer. N Engl J Med 2002;347(16):1227–32.
7. Review of Breast Cancer Clinical Trials Conducted by the National Surgical Adjuvant Breast Project - ClinicalKey. Available at: https://www-clinicalkey-com.ezproxy.library.wisc.edu/#!/content/playContent/1-s2.0-S0039610907000199?returnurl=null&referrer=null. Accessed November 30, 2021.
8. Sarrazin D, Lê MG, Arriagada R, et al. Ten-year results of a randomized trial comparing a conservative treatment to mastectomy in early breast cancer. Radiother Oncol J Eur Soc Ther Radiol Oncol 1989;14(3):177–84.
9. Fisher B, Anderson S, Bryant J, et al. Twenty-Year Follow-up of a Randomized Trial Comparing Total Mastectomy, Lumpectomy, and Lumpectomy plus Irradiation for the Treatment of Invasive Breast Cancer. N Engl J Med 2002;347(16):1233–41.
10. Fisher B, Anderson S, Redmond CK, et al. Reanalysis and Results after 12 Years of Follow-up in a Randomized Clinical Trial Comparing Total Mastectomy with Lumpectomy with or without Irradiation in the Treatment of Breast Cancer. N Engl J Med 1995;333(22):1456–61.

11. Litière S, Werutsky G, Fentiman IS, et al. Breast conserving therapy versus mastectomy for stage I-II breast cancer: 20 year follow-up of the EORTC 10801 phase 3 randomised trial. Lancet Oncol 2012;13(4):412–9.

12. Jacobson JA, Danforth DN, Cowan KH, et al. Ten-year results of a comparison of conservation with mastectomy in the treatment of stage I and II breast cancer. N Engl J Med 1995;332(14):907–11.

13. Poggi MM, Danforth DN, Sciuto LC, et al. Eighteen-year results in the treatment of early breast carcinoma with mastectomy versus breast conservation therapy: the National Cancer Institute Randomized Trial. Cancer 2003;98(4):697–702.

14. Blichert-Toft M, Rose C, Andersen JA, et al. Danish randomized trial comparing breast conservation therapy with mastectomy: six years of life-table analysis. Danish Breast Cancer Cooperative Group. J Natl Cancer Inst Monogr 1992;11:19–25.

15. Effects of Radiotherapy and Surgery in Early Breast Cancer — An Overview of the Randomized Trials | NEJM. Available at: https://www.nejm.org/doi/full/10.1056/nejm199511303332202. Accessed December 3, 2021.

16. Liljegren G, Holmberg L, Bergh J, et al. 10-Year results after sector resection with or without postoperative radiotherapy for stage I breast cancer: a randomized trial. J Clin Oncol 1999;17(8):2326–33.

17. Clark RM, McCulloch PB, Levine MN, et al. Randomized clinical trial to assess the effectiveness of breast irradiation following lumpectomy and axillary dissection for node-negative breast cancer. J Natl Cancer Inst 1992;84(9):683–9.

18. Clark RM, Whelan T, Levine M, et al. Randomized Clinical Trial of Breast Irradiation Following Lumpectomy and Axillary Dissection for Node-Negative Breast Cancer: an Update. JNCI J Natl Cancer Inst 1996;88(22):1659–64.

19. Veronesi U, Marubini E, Mariani L, et al. Radiotherapy after breast-conserving surgery in small breast carcinoma: long-term results of a randomized trial. Ann Oncol 2001;12(7):997–1003.

20. Hughes KS, Schnaper LA, Berry D, et al. Lumpectomy plus Tamoxifen with or without Irradiation in Women 70 Years of Age or Older with Early Breast Cancer. N Engl J Med 2004;351(10):971–7.

21. Hughes KS, Schnaper LA, Bellon JR, et al. Lumpectomy Plus Tamoxifen With or Without Irradiation in Women Age 70 Years or Older With Early Breast Cancer: Long-Term Follow-Up of CALGB 9343. J Clin Oncol 2013;31(19):2382–7.

22. Kunkler IH, Williams LJ, Jack WJL, et al. PRIME II investigators. Breast-conserving surgery with or without irradiation in women aged 65 years or older with early breast cancer (PRIME II): a randomised controlled trial. Lancet Oncol 2015;16(3):266–73.

23. Fisher B, Costantino J, Redmond C, et al. Lumpectomy Compared with Lumpectomy and Radiation Therapy for the Treatment of Intraductal Breast Cancer. N Engl J Med 1993;328(22):1581–6.

24. Fisher B, Dignam J, Wolmark N, et al. Tamoxifen in treatment of intraductal breast cancer: National Surgical Adjuvant Breast and Bowel Project B-24 randomised controlled trial. Lancet Lond Engl 1999;353(9169):1993–2000.

25. Fisher B, Bryant J, Dignam JJ, et al. Tamoxifen, radiation therapy, or both for prevention of ipsilateral breast tumor recurrence after lumpectomy in women with invasive breast cancers of one centimeter or less. J Clin Oncol 2002;20(20):4141–9.

26. Moran MS, Schnitt SJ, Giuliano AE, et al. SSO-ASTRO Consensus Guideline on Margins for Breast-Conserving Surgery with Whole Breast Irradiation in Stage I and II Invasive Breast Cancer. Int J Radiat Oncol Biol Phys 2014;88(3):553–64.

27. Guidelines Detail. NCCN. Available at: https://www.nccn.org/guidelines/guidelines-detail. Accessed January 19, 2022.

28. Houssami N, Macaskill P, Luke Marinovich M, et al. The Association of Surgical Margins and Local Recurrence in Women with Early-Stage Invasive Breast Cancer Treated with Breast-Conserving Therapy: A Meta-Analysis. Ann Surg Oncol 2014;21(3):717–30.

29. Morrow M, Van Zee KJ, Solin LJ, et al. Society of Surgical Oncology-American Society for Radiation Oncology-American Society of Clinical Oncology Consensus Guideline on Margins for Breast-Conserving Surgery With Whole-Breast Irradiation in Ductal Carcinoma In Situ. J Clin Oncol 2016;34(33):4040–6.

30. Wapnir IL, Dignam JJ, Fisher B, et al. Long-term outcomes of invasive ipsilateral breast tumor recurrences after lumpectomy in NSABP B-17 and B-24 randomized clinical trials for DCIS. J Natl Cancer Inst 2011;103(6):478–88.

31. Houghton J, George WD, Cuzick J, et al. Radiotherapy and tamoxifen in women with completely excised ductal carcinoma in situ of the breast in the UK, Australia, and New Zealand: randomised controlled trial. Lancet Lond Engl 2003;362(9378):95–102.

32. Julien JP, Bijker N, Fentiman IS, et al. Radiotherapy in breast-conserving treatment for ductal carcinoma in situ: first results of the EORTC randomised phase III trial 10853. EORTC Breast Cancer Cooperative Group and EORTC Radiotherapy Group. Lancet Lond Engl 2000;355(9203):528–33.

33. Emdin SO, Granstrand B, Ringberg A, et al. SweDCIS: Radiotherapy after sector resection for ductal carcinoma in situ of the breast. Results of a randomised trial in a population offered mammography screening. Acta Oncol Stockh Swed 2006;45(5):536–43.

34. Krag DN, Anderson SJ, Julian TB, et al. Technical outcomes of sentinel-lymph-node resection and conventional axillary-lymph-node dissection in patients with clinically node-negative breast cancer: results from the NSABP B-32 randomised phase III trial. Lancet Oncol 2007;8(10):881–8.

35. Krag DN, Anderson SJ, Julian TB, et al. Sentinel-lymph-node resection compared with conventional axillary-lymph-node dissection in clinically node-negative patients with breast cancer: overall survival findings from the NSABP B-32 randomised phase 3 trial. Lancet Oncol 2010;11(10):927–33.

36. Zavagno G, De Salvo GL, Scalco G, et al. A Randomized clinical trial on sentinel lymph node biopsy versus axillary lymph node dissection in breast cancer: results of the Sentinella/GIVOM trial. Ann Surg 2008;247(2):207–13.

37. Veronesi U, Paganelli G, Viale G, et al. Sentinel-lymph-node biopsy as a staging procedure in breast cancer: update of a randomised controlled study. Lancet Oncol 2006;7(12):983–90.

38. Veronesi U, Viale G, Paganelli G, et al. Sentinel lymph node biopsy in breast cancer: ten-year results of a randomized controlled study. Ann Surg 2010;251(4):595–600.

39. Canavese G, Catturich A, Vecchio C, et al. Sentinel node biopsy compared with complete axillary dissection for staging early breast cancer with clinically negative lymph nodes: results of randomized trial. Ann Oncol 2009;20(6):1001–7.

40. Wilke LG, McCall LM, Posther KE, et al. Surgical complications associated with sentinel lymph node biopsy: results from a prospective international cooperative group trial. Ann Surg Oncol 2006;13(4):491–500.

41. Galimberti V, Cole BF, Zurrida S, et al. Axillary dissection versus no axillary dissection in patients with sentinel-node micrometastases (IBCSG 23-01): A phase 3 randomised controlled trial. Lancet Oncol 2013;14(4):297–305.

42. Giuliano AE, Hunt KK, Ballman KV, et al. Axillary Dissection vs No Axillary Dissection in Women With Invasive Breast Cancer and Sentinel Node Metastasis: A Randomized Clinical Trial. JAMA 2011;305(6):569–75.

43. Giuliano AE, Ballman KV, McCall L, et al. Effect of Axillary Dissection vs No Axillary Dissection on 10-Year Overall Survival Among Women With Invasive Breast Cancer and Sentinel Node Metastasis: The ACOSOG Z0011 (Alliance) Randomized Clinical Trial. JAMA 2017;318(10):918–26.

44. Donker M, van Tienhoven G, Straver ME, et al. Radiotherapy or surgery of the axilla after a positive sentinel node in breast cancer (EORTC 10981-22023 AMAROS): a randomised, multicentre, open-label, phase 3 non-inferiority trial. Lancet Oncol 2014;15(12):1303–10.

45. Sávolt Á, Péley G, Polgár C, et al. Eight-year follow up result of the OTOASOR trial: The Optimal Treatment Of the Axilla - Surgery Or Radiotherapy after positive sentinel lymph node biopsy in early-stage breast cancer: A randomized, single centre, phase III, non-inferiority trial. Eur J Surg Oncol 2017;43(4):672–9.

46. Whelan TJ, Olivotto IA, Parulekar WR, et al. Regional Nodal Irradiation in Early-Stage Breast Cancer. N Engl J Med 2015;373(4):307–16.

47. Katz MS, McCall L, Ballman K, et al. Nomogram-based estimate of axillary nodal involvement in ACOSOG Z0011 (Alliance): validation and association with radiation protocol variations. Breast Cancer Res Treat 2020;180(2):429–36.

48. Boughey JC, Suman VJ, Mittendorf EA, et al. Sentinel lymph node surgery after neoadjuvant chemotherapy in patients with node-positive breast cancer: the ACOSOG Z1071 (Alliance) clinical trial. JAMA 2013;310(14):1455–61.

49. Caudle AS, Yang WT, Krishnamurthy S, et al. Improved Axillary Evaluation Following Neoadjuvant Therapy for Patients With Node-Positive Breast Cancer Using Selective Evaluation of Clipped Nodes: Implementation of Targeted Axillary Dissection. J Clin Oncol 2016;34(10):1072–8.

50. Kuehn T, Bauerfeind I, Fehm T, et al. Sentinel-lymph-node biopsy in patients with breast cancer before and after neoadjuvant chemotherapy (SENTINA): a prospective, multicentre cohort study. Lancet Oncol 2013;14(7):609–18.

51. Boileau JF, Poirier B, Basik M, et al. Sentinel Node Biopsy After Neoadjuvant Chemotherapy in Biopsy-Proven Node-Positive Breast Cancer: The SN FNAC Study. J Clin Oncol 2015;33(3):258–64.

52. Classe JM, Loaec C, Gimbergues P, et al. Sentinel lymph node biopsy without axillary lymphadenectomy after neoadjuvant chemotherapy is accurate and safe for selected patients: the GANEA 2 study. Breast Cancer Res Treat 2019; 173(2):343–52.

53. Boughey JC, Ballman KV, McCall LM, et al. Tumor Biology and Response to Chemotherapy Impact Breast Cancer-Specific Survival in Node-Positive Breast Cancer Patients Treated with Neoadjuvant Chemotherapy: Long-term Follow-up from ACOSOG Z1071 (Alliance). Ann Surg 2017;266(4):667–76.

54. Samiei S, Simons JM, Engelen SME, et al. Axillary Pathologic Complete Response After Neoadjuvant Systemic Therapy by Breast Cancer Subtype in Patients With Initially Clinically Node-Positive Disease: A Systematic Review and Meta-analysis. JAMA Surg 2021;156(6):e210891.

55. de Boniface J, Frisell J, Andersson Y, et al. Survival and axillary recurrence following sentinel node-positive breast cancer without completion axillary lymph node dissection: the randomized controlled SENOMAC trial. BMC Cancer 2017;17:379.

56. Alliance for Clinical Trials in Oncology. A Randomized Phase III Trial Comparing Axillary Lymph Node Dissection to Axillary Radiation in Breast Cancer Patients

(CT1-3 N1) Who Have Positive Sentinel Lymph Node Disease After Neoadjuvant Chemotherapy. clinicaltrials.gov; 2022. Available at: https://clinicaltrials.gov/ct2/show/NCT01901094. Accessed March 1, 2022.

57. Fisher B, Ravdin RG, Ausman RK, et al. Surgical adjuvant chemotherapy in cancer of the breast: results of a decade of cooperative investigation. Ann Surg 1968; 168(3):337–56.

58. Bonadonna G, Valagussa P, Moliterni A, et al. Adjuvant cyclophosphamide, methotrexate, and fluorouracil in node-positive breast cancer: the results of 20 years of follow-up. N Engl J Med 1995;332(14):901–6.

59. Fisher B, Dignam J, Mamounas EP, et al. Sequential methotrexate and fluorouracil for the treatment of node-negative breast cancer patients with estrogen receptor-negative tumors: eight-year results from National Surgical Adjuvant Breast and Bowel Project (NSABP) B-13 and first report of findings from NSABP B-19 comparing methotrexate and fluorouracil with conventional cyclophosphamide, methotrexate, and fluorouracil. J Clin Oncol 1996;14(7):1982–92.

60. Early Breast Cancer Trialists' Collaborative Group (EBCTCG). Increasing the dose intensity of chemotherapy by more frequent administration or sequential scheduling: a patient-level meta-analysis of 37 298 women with early breast cancer in 26 randomised trials. Lancet Lond Engl 2019;393(10179):1440–52.

61. Anampa J, Makower D, Sparano JA. Progress in adjuvant chemotherapy for breast cancer: an overview. BMC Med 2015;13:195.

62. Perez EA, Romond EH, Suman VJ, et al. Trastuzumab plus adjuvant chemotherapy for human epidermal growth factor receptor 2-positive breast cancer: planned joint analysis of overall survival from NSABP B-31 and NCCTG N9831. J Clin Oncol 2014;32(33):3744–52.

63. Romond EH, Perez EA, Bryant J, et al. Trastuzumab plus Adjuvant Chemotherapy for Operable HER2-Positive Breast Cancer. N Engl J Med 2005;353(16):1673–84.

64. Cameron D, Piccart-Gebhart MJ, Gelber RD, et al. 11 years' follow-up of trastuzumab after adjuvant chemotherapy in HER2-positive early breast cancer: final analysis of the HERceptin Adjuvant (HERA) trial. Lancet Lond Engl 2017; 389(10075):1195–205.

65. von Minckwitz G, Procter M, de Azambuja E, et al. Adjuvant Pertuzumab and Trastuzumab in Early HER2-Positive Breast Cancer. N Engl J Med 2017;377(2): 122–31.

66. Hurvitz SA, Gelmon KA, Tolaney SM. Optimal Management of Early and Advanced HER2 Breast Cancer. Am Soc Clin Oncol Educ Book Am Soc Clin Oncol Annu Meet 2017;37:76–92.

67. Fisher B, Bryant J, Wolmark N, et al. Effect of preoperative chemotherapy on the outcome of women with operable breast cancer. J Clin Oncol 1998;16(8): 2672–85.

68. Rastogi P, Anderson SJ, Bear HD, et al. Preoperative chemotherapy: updates of National Surgical Adjuvant Breast and Bowel Project Protocols B-18 and B-27. J Clin Oncol 2008;26(5):778–85.

69. Mamounas EP, Anderson SJ, Dignam JJ, et al. Predictors of Locoregional Recurrence After Neoadjuvant Chemotherapy: Results From Combined Analysis of National Surgical Adjuvant Breast and Bowel Project B-18 and B-27. J Clin Oncol 2012;30(32):3960–6.

70. Gianni L, Pienkowski T, Im YH, et al. 5-year analysis of neoadjuvant pertuzumab and trastuzumab in patients with locally advanced, inflammatory, or early-stage HER2-positive breast cancer (NeoSphere): a multicentre, open-label, phase 2 randomised trial. Lancet Oncol 2016;17(6):791–800.

71. Schneeweiss A, Chia S, Hickish T, et al. Long-term efficacy analysis of the randomised, phase II TRYPHAENA cardiac safety study: Evaluating pertuzumab and trastuzumab plus standard neoadjuvant anthracycline-containing and anthracycline-free chemotherapy regimens in patients with HER2-positive early breast cancer. Eur J Cancer Oxf Engl 1990 2018;89:27–35.
72. Leon-Ferre RA, Hieken TJ, Boughey JC. The Landmark Series: Neoadjuvant Chemotherapy for Triple-Negative and HER2-Positive Breast Cancer. Ann Surg Oncol 2021;28(4):2111–9.
73. Schmid P, Cortes J, Pusztai L, et al. Pembrolizumab for Early Triple-Negative Breast Cancer. N Engl J Med 2020;382(9):810–21.
74. Barnard K, Klimberg VS. An Update on Randomized Clinical Trials in Breast Cancer. Surg Oncol Clin N Am 2017;26(4):587–620.
75. Rugo HS, Olopade OI, DeMichele A, et al. Adaptive Randomization of Veliparib–Carboplatin Treatment in Breast Cancer. N Engl J Med 2016. https://doi.org/10.1056/NEJMoa1513749.
76. Masuda N, Lee SJ, Ohtani S, et al. Adjuvant Capecitabine for Breast Cancer after Preoperative Chemotherapy. N Engl J Med 2017;376(22):2147–59.
77. M.D. Anderson Cancer Center. Multicenter Trial for Eliminating Breast Cancer Surgery or Radiotherapy in Exceptional Responders to Neoadjuvant Systemic Therapy. clinicaltrials.gov; 2021. Available at: https://clinicaltrials.gov/ct2/show/NCT02945579. Accessed March 2, 2022.
78. Early Breast Cancer Trialists' Collaborative Group (EBCTCG). Effects of chemotherapy and hormonal therapy for early breast cancer on recurrence and 15-year survival: an overview of the randomised trials. Lancet Lond Engl 2005;365(9472):1687–717.
79. Fisher B, Dignam J, Bryant J, et al. Five versus more than five years of tamoxifen therapy for breast cancer patients with negative lymph nodes and estrogen receptor-positive tumors. J Natl Cancer Inst 1996;88(21):1529–42.
80. Fisher B, Dignam J, Emir B, et al. Tamoxifen and Chemotherapy for Lymph Node-Negative, Estrogen Receptor-Positive Breast Cancer. JNCI J Natl Cancer Inst 1997;89(22):1673–82.
81. Mouridsen H, Gershanovich M, Sun Y, et al. Phase III study of letrozole versus tamoxifen as first-line therapy of advanced breast cancer in postmenopausal women: analysis of survival and update of efficacy from the International Letrozole Breast Cancer Group. J Clin Oncol 2003;21(11):2101–9.
82. Mouridsen H, Gershanovich M, Sun Y, et al. Superior efficacy of letrozole versus tamoxifen as first-line therapy for postmenopausal women with advanced breast cancer: results of a phase III study of the International Letrozole Breast Cancer Group. J Clin Oncol 2001;19(10):2596–606.
83. Goss PE, Ingle JN, Martino S, et al. Randomized trial of letrozole following tamoxifen as extended adjuvant therapy in receptor-positive breast cancer: updated findings from NCIC CTG MA.17. J Natl Cancer Inst 2005;97(17):1262–71.
84. Burstein HJ, Lacchetti C, Anderson H, et al. Adjuvant Endocrine Therapy for Women With Hormone Receptor-Positive Breast Cancer: ASCO Clinical Practice Guideline Focused Update. J Clin Oncol 2019;37(5):423–38.
85. Burstein HJ, Lacchetti C, Anderson H, et al. Adjuvant Endocrine Therapy for Women With Hormone Receptor-Positive Breast Cancer: American Society of Clinical Oncology Clinical Practice Guideline Update on Ovarian Suppression. J Clin Oncol 2016;34(14):1689–701.
86. Ellis MJ, Suman VJ, Hoog J, et al. Randomized phase II neoadjuvant comparison between letrozole, anastrozole, and exemestane for postmenopausal women with

estrogen receptor-rich stage 2 to 3 breast cancer: clinical and biomarker outcomes and predictive value of the baseline PAM50-based intrinsic subtype–ACOSOG Z1031. J Clin Oncol 2011;29(17):2342–9.

87. Sparano JA, Gray RJ, Makower DF, et al. Adjuvant Chemotherapy Guided by a 21-Gene Expression Assay in Breast Cancer. N Engl J Med 2018;379(2):111–21.

88. Postmenopausal Women with HR+/HER2– Early Breast Cancer, 1–3 Positive Nodes, and a Low Risk of Recurrence Can Safely Forego Chemotherapy. Oncologist 2021;26(Suppl 2):S11–2.

89. Kalinsky K, Barlow WE, Gralow JR, et al. 21-Gene Assay to Inform Chemotherapy Benefit in Node-Positive Breast Cancer. N Engl J Med 2021;385(25):2336–47.

90. Cardoso F, van't Veer LJ, Bogaerts J, et al. 70-Gene Signature as an Aid to Treatment Decisions in Early-Stage Breast Cancer. N Engl J Med 2016;375(8):717–29.

91. Piccart M, van 't Veer LJ, Poncet C, et al. 70-gene signature as an aid for treatment decisions in early breast cancer: updated results of the phase 3 randomised MINDACT trial with an exploratory analysis by age. Lancet Oncol 2021; 22(4):476–88.

Clinical Trials in Melanoma

Margins, Lymph Nodes, Targeted and Immunotherapy

Cimarron E. Sharon, MD[a],*, Georgia M. Beasley, MD, MHS[b],
Giorgos C. Karakousis, MD[c]

KEYWORDS

- Melanoma • Surgical margins • Sentinel lymph node • Targeted therapy
- Immunotherapy

KEY POINTS

- The current guidelines for wide local excision of cutaneous melanoma, recommending no larger than a 2 cm margin, are based on 6 randomized control trials (RCTs).
- The first Multicenter Selective Lymphadenectomy Trial led to widespread adaptation of sentinel lymph node biopsy, reaffirming the important prognostic utility of this procedure.
- Two RCTs of patients with positive sentinel lymph node biopsies demonstrated safety in observing the nodal basin with serial ultrasounds rather than proceeding to an immediate completion lymph node dissection.
- Studies of adjuvant-targeted therapy have led to the approval of using combined BRAF and MEK inhibitors for patients with resected stage III/IV melanoma with a BRAF mutation.
- Four major clinical trials of immune therapy support the use of adjuvant CTLA-4 or anti-PD-1 therapy for patients with resected stage III/IV melanoma without a BRAF mutation.

INTRODUCTION

The surgical treatment of cutaneous melanoma has changed dramatically during the past 100 years, with a current focus on delivering optimal care while minimizing surgical morbidity. In this article, we discuss the most significant clinical trials that have affected the surgical care of melanoma, including surgical excision margins, management of the regional nodal basin, and adjuvant treatment of patients with resected high-risk melanoma.

---

[a] Department of Surgery, Hospital of the University of Pennsylvania, 3400 Spruce Street – Maloney 4, Philadelphia, PA 19104, USA; [b] Department of Surgery, Duke University Medical Center, 20 Duke Medicine Circle, Durham, NC 27710, USA; [c] Department of Surgery, Hospital of the University of Pennsylvania, 3400 Spruce Street – Silverstein 4, Philadelphia, PA 19104, USA
* Corresponding author.
E-mail address: Cimarron.sharon@pennmedicine.upenn.edu

Surg Oncol Clin N Am 32 (2023) 47–63
https://doi.org/10.1016/j.soc.2022.07.005

MARGINS

The current National Comprehensive Cancer Center (NCCN) guidelines for cutaneous melanoma,[1] recommending no larger than a 2 cm margin, are based on 6 randomized control trials (RCTs) performed between 1980 and 2004. For the larger part of the twentieth century, the standard treatment of cutaneous melanoma was wide local excision (WLE) with a 5-cm margin.[2] As our understanding of melanoma progressed, it became clear that aggressive local management of melanoma (whose prognosis was significantly associated with tumor thickness) did not necessarily prevent the development of distant metastases and their associated morbidity and mortality.[3–5] However, local recurrence (LR) remained a concern for high-risk melanomas, prompting extensive research into optimal excision margins to both reduce surgical morbidity and optimize oncologic outcomes. Six completed RCTs, which examined excision margins and their relationship with LR and survival, have largely influenced the current recommendations for WLE of cutaneous melanoma (**Table 1**). Importantly, no study found a difference in overall survival (OS) or LR rates between narrower and wider excision margins, although one study performed in patients not undergoing sentinel lymph node biopsy (SLNB) found a higher rate of locoregional recurrence with narrower margin excision.

World Health Organization Melanoma Trial

The World Health Organization Melanoma Program was the first to perform an RCT analyzing a narrow excision margin for cutaneous melanoma.[6,7] This RCT, performed between July 1, 1980, and April 15, 1985, was an international, multicenter study of 612 patients with clinical stage I melanoma and a thickness of 2 mm or less, who were randomized into either a 1 cm (N = 305) or 3 cm (N = 307) margin. Following WLE, patients were seen every 2 months for the first 2 years, every 3 months for years 3 to 5, and every 6 months for the remaining study period. The study outcomes were OS, disease-free survival (DFS), and LR rate.

This study found no difference in OS, or DFS between the 2 groups. Although there was no statistically significant difference in LR rates for the cohorts, the LR rate was 2.6% for the narrow excision group, compared with 1% for patients who had a wider excision margin. Seven locoregional recurrences (5 [4.2%] patients in the 1 cm cohort vs 2 [1.5%] in the 3 cm cohort) were noted in patients with a melanoma thickness of 1.01 to 2 mm, compared with 4 recurrences (3 [1.6%] patients in the 1 cm cohort vs 1 [0.6%] in the 3 cm cohort) for patients with a melanoma 1.0 mm or lesser. The authors concluded that a 1-cm excision margin is safe for patients with a melanoma thickness of 2 mm or lesser.

Intergroup Melanoma Trial

The Intergroup Melanoma Trial (1983–1992),[8–10] an international multi-institutional study of 740 patients from 77 institutions, analyzed optimal wide excision margins for patients with intermediate thickness melanomas ranging from 1 to 4 mm in Breslow depth. Patients were divided into 2 groups based on the location of their primary melanoma. Group A consisted of patients with truncal and proximal extremity melanoma, and group B of patients with head/neck and distal extremity tumors. Patients in group A were randomized to either 2 or 4 cm margins, whereas all patients in group B received 2 cm margins. Patients were followed every 3 months for the first 2 years, every 6 months for years 3 to 5, and then yearly thereafter for the primary end points of OS, DFS, and LR. The most recent publication from this trial included 94% of patients with a median follow-up time of 10 years.[8]

Table 1
Description of clinical trials investigating wide local excision margins for cutaneous melanoma

Study	Year/Study Type	No. of Patients/Clinical Characteristics	Arms	Endpoints/Results
WHO Melanoma Trial	1980–1985 / RCT	612 / Melanomas ≤ 2 mm	1-cm margin 3-cm margin	OS—no difference DFS—no difference LRR—no difference
Intergroup Melanoma Trial	1983–1992 / RCT	740 / Intermediate thickness melanomas 1–4 mm	2-cm margin 4-cm margin	OS—no difference DFS—no difference LRR—no difference Worse 5-y OS for patients who recurred (35%) compared to those who did not (85%)
Swedish Melanoma Group Trial I	1982–1991 / RCT	989 / Intermediate thickness melanomas 0.8–2 mm	2-cmmargin 5-cm margin	OS—no difference RFS—no difference LRR—no difference
Swedish Melanoma Group Trial II	1992–2004 / RCT	936 / Thick Melanomas >2mm	2-cm margin 4-cm margin	OS – no difference DFS – no difference LRR – no difference
European Group Trial	1981–2000 / RCT	325 / Melanomas <2mm	2-cm margin 5-cm margin	OS – no difference DFS – no difference LRR – no difference
UK Trial	1992–2001 / RCT	900 / Thick Melanomas >2mm	1-cm margin 3-cm margin	OS – no difference DFS – improved for patients with 3cm margin LRR – improved for patients with 3cm margin

Abbreviations: DFS, disease-free survival; LRR, local recurrence rate; OS, overall survival; RCT, randomized controlled trial; WHO, World Health Organization.

In group A, there was no difference in LR rates for patients with a 2 versus 4 cm margin (0.8% vs 1.7%, P>.05), although patients in group B had a higher recurrence rate of 6.2% overall. Additionally, for both groups combined there was no difference in 10-year DFS between patients with 2 or 4 cm margins (70% vs 77% P = .12). Importantly, the patients that locally recurred had a significantly worse 5-year OS than patients who never had a LR (35% vs 85%, P<.001), and all patients who locally recurred died of metastatic melanoma within 10 years. Factors associated with increased LR in this study included ulceration and head/neck primary site. Overall, the results of this study confirmed the safety of a 2-cm margin and provided insight into the biology of tumors with a high risk of LR.

Swedish Melanoma Group Trial I

The Swedish Melanoma Group Trial I,[11,12] performed on 989 patients between 1982 and 1991, investigated the safety of 2 cm versus the traditional 5 cm margins for melanomas between 0.8 and 2 mm. Patients were randomized to either 2 (N = 476) or 5 cm (N = 513) margins, and the study outcomes were OS, DFS, and LR. Patients were followed every 3 months for the first 3 years, and every 6 months for years 3 to 5.

This RCT produced 2 publications, with the most recent showing a median follow-up time of 11 years. There was no difference between the 2 and 5 cm margin groups for LR (0.6% vs 1.0%), DFS, or OS. This study reinforced the safety of a 2 cm margin, compared with the traditional 5 cm margin for melanomas between 0.8 and 2 mm in Breslow depth.

Swedish Melanoma Group Trial II

In this trial, the Swedish Melanoma Group studied the safety of 2 versus 4 cm margins for 936 patients with thick melanomas greater than 2 mm.[13,14] Patients were randomized to either 2 cm (N = 465) or 4 cm (N = 471) margins and were followed every 3 months for the first 2 years, and every 6 months for years 2 to 5. The study outcomes were OS, DFS, and LR.

Patients with a 2 cm margin had a LR of 4.3%, compared with 1.9% of patients with 4 cm margins, although this difference was not statistically significant (P = .06). There was no difference in 5-year OS (65% in both groups), 5-year DFS (56% in both groups), and 10-year OS (50% in both groups). Extended data with a median follow-up time of 19.6 years demonstrated no difference in DFS or OS. This study represents the largest RCT of excision margins for melanomas greater than 2 mm, reaffirming that a 2 cm margin is adequate for these thicker lesions.

European Group Trial

Similar to the Swedish Melanoma Group Trial I, the European Group Trial[15] (1981–2000) evaluated the adequacy of 2 cm versus 5 cm margins for 326 patients with melanomas 2 mm or lesser. There was no significant difference in LR rates between the 2 excision margin groups (0.6% 2 cm vs 2.4% 5 cm, P = .22). Additionally, 10-year DFS (85% 2 cm vs 83% 5 cm) and 10-year OS (87% 2 cm vs 86% 5 cm) were no different in the 2 cm versus 5 cm groups (P = .83 and P = .56, respectively). Again, this study confirmed the safety of a 2 cm margin over the traditional 5 cm margin.

UK Trial

Between 1992 and 2001 the United Kingdom Melanoma Study Group, The British Association of Plastic, Reconstructive, and Aesthetic surgeons, and the Scottish Cancer Therapy Network performed a study of 900 patients evaluating optimal margins for thick melanomas greater than 2 mm.[16,17] Patients with melanoma of the trunk or extremity were randomized to either 1 or 3 cm margins. Study endpoints were locoregional recurrence and DFS. Patients were followed every 3 months for the first 2 years, every 6 months for years 3 to 5, and then yearly.

With a median follow-up of 5 years, patients in the 1 cm group had a higher locoregional (local, in-transit, and/or nodal) recurrence rate compared with the 3 cm group [hazard ratio (HR) 1.34, P = .02], although there was no difference in disease-specific survival (DSS) or OS. At a longer follow-up, with a median of 8.8 years, patients with a 3 cm margin had an improved DSS, although no difference in OS.

This was the first study to show that a wider surgical margin (3 cm) improved DSS for melanoma greater than 2 mm, and that a 1 cm margin increased the risk of recurrence. However, it is important to note that their recurrence variable included nodal recurrence, and most recurrences in this study (67%) were in the regional nodal basin. This study was performed before the routine performance of SLNB, which is currently indicated for tumors greater than 2 mm, which likely affected the magnitude of nodal recurrences. The authors performed additional analyses comparing local/in transit to nodal recurrences and found no differences between the 2 groups. Overall, this study shows no difference in OS rates between narrow and wide excision margins but an increase in locoregional recurrence rates in the narrow margin group. The significance of these results in the era of SLNB is unclear.

LYMPH NODES

The management of regional lymph nodes in melanoma has been the subject of considerable controversy and has evolved dramatically during recent years. Until the advent of SLNB techniques in the late 1990s, patients with melanoma were routinely offered an elective lymph node dissection. However, multiple trials found no survival benefit to elective lymphadenectomy,[18–20] prompting more frequent utilization of SLNB. Three landmark surgical trials have informed the current practice of SLNB for patients without clinical evidence of nodal disease[21] **(Table 2)**.

Multicenter Selective Lymphadenectomy Trial

The first Multicenter Selective Lymphadenectomy Trial (MSLT I) was designed to investigate the utility of SLNB for patients with localized melanoma.[22,23] The primary study group included patients with melanoma between 1.2 and 3.5 mm in Breslow thickness, who were randomized to either WLE alone with completion lymph node dissection (CLND) only in the event of clinical nodal recurrence (observation group), or WLE with SLNB, with immediate lymph node dissection (LND) in the case of a positive sentinel node (biopsy group). The endpoints included melanoma-specific survival (MSS), DFS, OS, and rates of nodal metastases. The study included 1347 patients with melanomas between 1.2 and 3.5 mm (intermediate thickness), and 314 patients with melanoma greater than 3.5 mm (thick).

For the overall study population, there was no difference in 10-year MSS between the observation and biopsy groups. However, patients who received a SLNB had a significantly improved DFS: 71% versus 65% for intermediate-thickness melanomas, and 51% versus 41% for thick melanomas. The study reaffirmed the incredibly important prognostic utility of the SLNB procedure: Patients with a positive sentinel node had a worse 10-year MSS than patients without nodal disease: 62% versus 85% (P<.001) for intermediate-thickness melanomas and 48% versus 65% (P = .03) for thick melanomas. Although there was no difference in MSS between the 2 study groups overall, in subgroup analysis, for patients with intermediate-thickness

Table 2
Description of clinical trials investigating management of the nodal basin in cutaneous melanoma

Study	Year/Study Type	No. of Patients/Clinical Characteristics	Arms	Endpoints/Results
MSLT I	1993–2012 / RCT	1347—intermediate thickness melanomas (1.2–3.5 mm) 314—thick melanomas >3.5 mm	WLE alone—CLND in the event of nodal recurrence (observation) WLE w/SLNB—CLND if positive SLN (biopsy)	MSS—no difference overall. Patients with a positive SLNB had worse MSS (62% vs 85% for intermediate-thickness melanomas; 48% vs 65% for thick melanomas) DFS—improved for patients who received an SLNB (HR 0.62, $P = .02$)
DeCOG-SLT	2005–2018 / RCT	483/positive SLNB	Immediate CLND Nodal observation with ultrasound (q 4 mo)	OS—no difference DMFS—no difference RFS—no difference
MSLT II	2004–2019 / RCT	1939/positive SLNB	Immediate CLND Nodal observation with ultrasound (q 4 mo for years 1–2, q6 months for years 3–5, yearly thereafter)	MSS—no difference DFS—higher for patients who underwent CLND (68% vs 65%, $P = .05$) Nonsentinel lymph node metastases predicted recurrence (HR 1.78, $P = .005$)

Abbreviations: CLND, completion lymph node dissection; DFS, disease-free survival; HR, hazard ratio; ; MSS, melanoma specific survival; OS, overall survival; RCT, randomized controlled trial; RFS, recurrence-free survival; SLN, sentinel lymph node; SLNB, sentinel lymph node biopsy melanomas and nodal metastases, those who received SLNB demonstrated an improved rate of 10-year distant DFS (HR 0.62, P = .02), and 10-year MSS (HR 0.56, P = .006) compared with patients in the nodal observation group. Interestingly, this difference in MSS was not observed among patients with nodal metastases and thick melanomas.

This trial demonstrated that the practice of SLNB improved DFS for all patients, primarily by virtue of reducing the incidence of nodal recurrences. Moreover, among patients with intermediate-thickness melanomas and nodal metastases, it demonstrated a potential advantage of early nodal intervention by SLNB and immediate completion nodal dissection on distant DFS and MSS. Again, these analyses were subgroup analyses and not the primary endpoints of the trial. Importantly, this study highlighted the role of SLNB with regard to prognostication because patients with nodal positivity had a significantly worse MSS compared with sentinel lymph node (SLN)-negative patients.

German Dermatologic Cooperative Oncology Group Selective Lymphadenectomy Trial

The aim of the German Dermatologic Cooperative Oncology Group Selective Lymphadenectomy Trial (DeCOG-SLT) was to evaluate whether CLND was beneficial and affected the survival for patients with positive sentinel lymph nodes.[24] The context of this study question is that in most cases, no additional positive lymph nodes were identified on CLND after a positive SLN, and even when discovered, non-SLN positivity was associated with a negative prognosis with high risk of distant relapse.[25] This trial included 483 patients with positive sentinel lymph nodes, who were randomized to either immediate CLND (n = 242) or nodal observation with ultrasound (n = 241) every 3 months. The primary endpoint was distant metastasis-free survival (DMFS).

This study showed no significant difference in 3-year DMFS, OS, or recurrence-free survival (RFS). Additionally, there was no difference in regional recurrence rates between the 2 groups. Notably, one of the strongest predictors of OS was tumor burden in the SLN of 1 mm or less. Unfortunately, because of difficulty enrolling patients and the overall low event rate, the trial was concluded early and was thus underpowered. Moreover, the study did not enroll patients with head and neck primaries. Regardless, the authors concluded that nodal surveillance with ultrasound rather than CLND is a safe option for patients, particularly with sentinel nodal tumor deposits less than 1 mm.

Multicenter Selective Lymphadenectomy Trial II

Given the small patient numbers in the DeCOG trial, results from the second MSLT (MSLT-II) were eagerly awaited. Similar to the DeCOG trial, MSLT-II was designed to assess whether CLND was beneficial in patients with positive sentinel lymph nodes, and whether it improved MSS compared with ultrasound surveillance of the nodal basin (every 4 months for years 1–2, every 6 months for years 3–5, and yearly thereafter).[26] Secondary study endpoints included DFS and the rate of nonsentinel lymph node metastases. Patients with a positive sentinel lymph node were randomized to either immediate CLND or nodal observation with ultrasound.

With a median follow-up time of 43 months, there was no difference found in MSS between the CLND and the observation groups. However, at 3 years, patients who underwent a CLND had a higher DFS (68% vs 65%, P = .05), due to lower rates of disease recurrence in the nodal basin. Additionally, nonsentinel lymph node metastases were an independent predictor of recurrence (HR 1.78, P = .005). Notably, a relatively small proportion of patients were included in the trial with a high SLN microscopic tumor burden or with multiple positive SLNs.

The MSLT-II trial demonstrated that ultrasound surveillance of the nodal basin is a safe option for patients with a positive sentinel lymph node, based on the lack of difference in MSS. However, CLND can improve DFS by improving control of regional nodal disease. Moreover, CLND can offer additional prognostic information because patients with positive nonsentinel lymph nodes demonstrated higher rates of recurrence. Even so, given the lack of benefit in MSS and the morbidity associated with CLND, practice paradigm has almost universally shifted toward ultrasound nodal surveillance in patients with SLN metastasis.

ADJUVANT TARGETED AND IMMUNOTHERAPY

In parallel to our understanding of surgical margins and management of the nodal basin, breakthroughs in immunology and cellular biology have led to the development of targeted cancer therapy. This type of treatment is designed to identify and interact with molecular targets to inhibit the growth and progression of cancer cells, resulting in a low rate of systemic toxicity.[27] A common mutation in cutaneous melanoma, with a prevalence of approximately 50%[28], is in the B-raf proto-oncogene (BRAF) protein (V600 E/K), which regulates the mitogen-activated protein kinase pathway, responsible for cell division.[29] Targeted therapy is designed to inhibit this BRAF pathway and downstream mitogen-activated protein kinase (MEK) protein. Alternatively, patients may be treated with immune therapy in the form of checkpoint inhibitors, which assist the patient's own immune system in targeting the melanoma by blocking negative regulators of the immune system.[30] Immune therapy for melanoma typically includes monoclonal antibodies to cytotoxic T-lymphocyte associated protein-4 (CTLA-4; ipilimumab) or programmed cell death-1 (PD-1; nivolumab, pembrolizumab).[30] Development of these therapies has led to dramatic improvements in the treatment of patients with advanced disease.

Targeted Therapy

Multiple clinical trials have investigated the BRAF inhibitors vemurafenib and dabrafenib in patients with metastatic melanoma, noting a response rate of up to 75%.[31–34] Unfortunately, progression-free survival is limited due to the rapid development of acquired resistance, with median time to resistance of approximately 6 months.[31,34,35] Subsequent clinical trials have focused on combination targeted therapy with BRAF and MEK inhibitors, in order to delay the development of resistance (**Table 3**).

BRIM-8
BRIM-8 was a phase 3, double-blind, placebo-control trial of vemurafenib monotherapy for patients with resected stage IIC/IIIA/IIIB (cohort 1) or stage IIIC (cohort 2) melanoma.[36] The study enrolled 314 patients in cohort 1, and 184 patients in cohort 2, with a median follow-up of 33.5 and 30.8 months, respectively. As the primary endpoint of DFS was not met for cohort 2, the DFS advantage of vemurafenib seen in cohort 1 [HR 0.80, 95% confidence intervals (CI) 0.37 to 0.78, $P = .001$] was considered only exploratory. Notably, grade 3 to 4 adverse events occurred in 57% of patients who received vemurafenib compared with 15% in placebo group.

COMBI-AD
Similar to BRIM-8, COMBI-AD was a phase 3, double-blind, placebo control trial of patients with resected stage III melanoma with a BRAF mutation.[37] This trial compared adjuvant combination dabrafenib (BRAF inhibitor) and trametinib (MEK inhibitor)

Table 3
Description of clinical trials investigating adjuvant targeted/immunotherapy of resected stage III/IV cutaneous melanoma

Study	Year/Study Type	No. of Patients/Stage	Arms	RFS	OS	DMFS
BRIM-8	2018 / Phase III	489 / IIC, IIIA-C	Cohort 1: IIC/IIIA/IIIB Cohort 2: IIIC Vemurafenib vs placebo	Cohort 1: endpoint not met Cohort 2: Vemurafenib HR 0.80 P = .26	-	-
COMBI D	2017 / Phase III	879 / IIIA-C w/BRAF mutations	Dabrafenib plus trametinib vs placebo	Dabrafenib/trametinib HR 0.47 P<.001	Dabrafenib/trametinib HR 0.57 P = .0006	Dabrafenib/trametinib HR 0.51 P<.001
EORTC 18071	2015 / Phase III	951 / IIIA-C	Ipilimumab vs placebo	Ipilimumab HR 0.75 (P = .001)	-	-
EORTC 1325/KEYNOTE-054	2021 / Phase III	1019 / IIIA-C	Pembro vs placebo	Pembro. HR 0.59 P<.05	-	Pembro. HR 0.60 P<.001
Checkmate 238	2017 / Phase III	906 / IIIB-C, IV	Ipilimumab vs nivolumab	Nivolumab HR 0.65 P<.001	-	-
E 1609	2019 / Phase III	1670 / IIIB-C, M1a-b	Ipilimumab (3 or 10 mg/kg vs HDI	Ipi3 HR 0.85 P = .065 Ipi10 HR 0.84 P>.05	Ipi 3 HR 0.78 P = .044 Ipi10 HR 0.88 P>.05	-
S1404	ASCO 2021 / Phase III	1301 / IIIA-IIIC, IV	Pembro vs Investigator's Choice (HDI/Ipi 10)	Pembro HR 0.77 P = .002	Pembro HR 0.82 P = .15	-

Abbreviations: ASCO, American Society of Clinical Oncology; HDI, high dose interferon; HR, hazard ratio; Pembro, pembrolizumab.

versus placebo. A total of 870 patients were enrolled, with a primary endpoint of relapse-free survival, and secondary endpoints of OS, DMFS, freedom from relapse, and safety.

The 3-year rate of relapse-free survival was 58% in the combination-therapy group and 39% for patients who received placebo (P<.001). Rates of 3-year OS, DMFS, and freedom from relapse were all higher in the combination-therapy group. The rates of grade 3 to 4 adverse events were 36% in the combination-therapy group, and 10% in the placebo group. This led to the combination BRAF/MEK inhibitor approval by the Food and Drug Administration (FDA) in the adjuvant stage III setting (**Fig. 1**).

Immunotherapy

With the efficacy of immune checkpoint inhibitors (in the form of either anti-CTLA-4 or anti-PD-1 antibody therapy) demonstrated in the metastatic melanoma setting, these therapies have now been brought into the adjuvant setting based on the results of several randomized trials (see **Table 3**). Notably, in order to be included in these trials, patients with nodal disease generally required a CLND. With the apparent improved efficacy and more favorable toxicity profile, anti-PD-1 therapy is generally used in practice as adjuvant immunotherapy for resected metastatic stage III/IV melanoma. Recently, pembrolizumab (anti-PD-1) has received FDA approval for usage in patients with pathologic stage IIB/C melanoma (see **Fig. 1**).

European Organization for Research and Treatment of Cancer 18071

This study, performed by the European Organization for Research and Treatment of Cancer (EORTC) was an intention-to treat (ITT), double-blind, placebo-controlled, phase III trial of adjuvant ipilimumab 10 mg/kg (antibody to CTLA-4) in 951 patients with resected stage III melanoma, with a primary endpoint of RFS.[38] With a median follow-up of 2.74 years, median RFS was 26.1 months for patients who received ipilimumab, versus 17.1 months in the placebo group. Additionally, the 3-year RFS was 46.5% in the ipilimumab group, compared with 34.8% in the placebo group. Adverse events led to discontinuation of treatment in 52% of patients who started ipilimumab, and there was a 1% treatment-related mortality. The authors concluded that adjuvant ipilimumab significantly improved RFS for patients with resected stage III melanoma but the risk–benefit ratio required further evaluation to its utilization in this setting due to its high toxicity profile.

European Organization for Research and Treatment of Cancer 1325/KEYNOTE-054

This trial, also performed by the EORTC, was a double-blind, placebo-controlled, stage III trial of adjuvant pembrolizumab (anti-PD-1 therapy) in patients with resected stage III melanoma.[39] The primary study endpoint was RFS in an ITT population and in

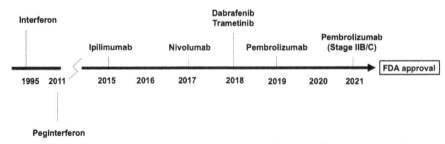

Fig. 1. Timeline to FDA approval of adjuvant therapies for resectable metastatic melanoma.

patients with PD-L1-positive melanomas. The secondary endpoint was DMFS in both cohorts. With a median-follow up of 42.3 months, patients in the pembrolizumab group had a higher 3.5-year DMFS than patients in the placebo group for both cohorts (ITT 65.3% pembrolizumab vs 49.4% placebo, HR 0.60, $P<.0001$; PD-L1 66.7% pembrolizumab vs 51.6% placebo, HR 0.61, $P<.0001$). Additionally, RFS was longer for patients who received pembrolizumab compared with placebo (ITT 59.8% pembrolizumab vs 41.4% placebo, HR 0.59, $P<.0001$; PD-L1 61.4% pembrolizumab vs 44.1% placebo, HR 0.59, $P<.0001$). The results of this trial supported the use of adjuvant pembrolizumab for patients with resected stage III melanoma.

CheckMate 238
The goal of this randomized, double-blind, phase III trial was to analyze the effectiveness of adjuvant ipilimumab versus nivolumab (anti-PD-1 therapy) for resected stage III/IV melanoma.[40] The primary study endpoint was RFS in the ITT population. The 12-month RFS rate was 70.5% in the nivolumab group compared with 60.8% in the ipilimumab group, $P<.001$. Additionally, the rate of grade 3 to 4 adverse events was 14.4% in the nivolumab group and 45.9% in the ipilimumab group. Treatment was discontinued due to adverse events in 9.7% of nivolumab patients, compared with 42.6% of ipilimumab patients. The authors concluded that adjuvant nivolumab increased RFS with a lower rate of grade 3 to 4 adverse events than ipilimumab. Following this study, nivolumab received FDA approval for adjuvant treatment of cutaneous melanoma in patients with stage III or higher resected disease (see **Fig. 1**).

E 1609
This randomized phase III trial by the North American Intergroup compared adjuvant ipilimumab (3 or 10 mg/kg) to high-dose interferon (HDI) for 1670 patients with resected stage III–IV cutaneous melanoma. In an ITT analysis, ipilimumab at 3 mg/kg (ipi3) had an improved OS (HR 0.78, $P = .044$), whereas ipilimumab at 10 mg/kg (ipi10) had no advantage over HDI. Additionally, grade 3 or greater events occurred in 37% of patients receiving ipi3 and 58% receiving ipi10. This study showed that the approved ipilimumab at 10 mg/kg was more toxic than ipi3, and was not more efficacious than HDI, whereas ipi3 demonstrated an improved OS compared with HDI.

Keynote-716
The previously discussed Keynote-054 trial[39] demonstrated a significantly improved RFS for patients with resected stage III melanoma who were treated with adjuvant pembrolizumab. The recently published Keynote-716 trial[41] investigated the role of adjuvant pembrolizumab in surgically resected, high-risk stage II melanoma.

Keynote-716 was a randomized, double-blind placebo-controlled, multicenter phase III study of adjuvant pembrolizumab in patients with resected pathologic stage IIB or IIC melanoma. Patients were randomized to receive adjuvant therapy with either pembrolizumab or saline placebo every 3 weeks for up to 17 cycles, with allowance for crossover in patients in the nontreatment arm on recurrence. The primary outcome measure was RFS, and secondary outcomes were DMFS and OS. At the first interim analysis with a median follow-up of 14.4 months, patients in the adjuvant pembrolizumab intention to treat arm demonstrated an improved risk of recurrence or death of approximately 6% compared with placebo (11% vs 17%, HR 0.65, $P = .0066$). At the second interim analysis, relative risk of recurrence or death was reduced by approximately 9% in the pembrolizumab arm versus placebo (85% vs 76%, HR 0.61). Results of this trial led to the recent approval of adjuvant pembrolizumab in patients with resected pathologic stage IIB/C melanoma (see **Fig. 1**).

S1404

The phase III, randomized, Intergroup S1404 trial[42,43] compared either adjuvant HDI or ipilimumab to pembrolizumab for patients with resected stage III/IV melanoma. The results of the patients who received HDI or ipilimumab were pooled as the "control" group. The primary outcomes were RFS and OS among all patients and OS among patients with baseline PD-L1 positive biopsies. Results were reported 3.5 years following randomization. Patients who received pembrolizumab had a significantly improved RFS (HR 0.77, 99.6% CI 0.59 to 0.99, P = .002), with no improvement in OS among all patients (HR 0.82, 96.3% CI 0.61–1.09, P = .15), or patients with PD-L1 positive biopsies (HR 0.84, 97.8% CI 0.59–1.22, P = .29). Additionally, pembrolizumab had a lower rate of grade 3 to 5 adverse events (32%) compared with HDI (72%) and ipilimumab (57%). Overall, pembrolizumab improved RFS and was a better-tolerated adjuvant regiment than HDI or ipilimumab.

FUTURE DIRECTIONS

Several randomized clinical trials in melanoma are currently enrolling. Although the final data may not be available, preliminary studies show promising results, which could continue to change the landscape of melanoma treatment in the coming years.

MelMarT

The previously discussed RCTs analyzing optimal resection margins in melanoma were performed before the routine practice of SLNB, which may have unknown impact on patterns of recurrence and survival. The Australian and New Zealand Medical Trials Group designed an RCT evaluating 1-cm versus 2-cm margins for patients with melanoma greater than 1 mm, who would also undergo SLNB.[44] To accurately power the study for the endpoints of recurrence and DSS, a sample size of 10,000 patients is needed.

A pilot study recruited patients from 17 centers between January 2015 and June 2016. Of the 718 patients who met study criteria, 400 were randomized to a 1 or 2 cm margin. Although there has not been a sufficient amount of follow-up time to evaluate oncologic outcomes, short-term data showed that patients in the 2-cm group had a more than 2-fold higher rate of skin graft or flap (35% vs 14%) to address the primary excision wound, compared with patients in the 1-cm group. Additionally, patients with a 2-cm margin had a significantly higher rate of wound necrosis (3.6% vs 0.5%). These results highlight the importance of identifying the optimal surgical margin to balance oncologic outcomes with morbidity. If 1-cm and 2-cm margins are found to be equivalent with regards to local recurrence and survival, a subsequent practice change could have profound effects on patient morbidity and quality of life.[45] Finally, although there are increasing reports of using the Mohs micrographic surgery technique, there has never been a randomized controlled clinical trial examining outcomes between WLE and the Mohs surgery technique for invasive melanoma.

CheckMate-915

CheckMate-915 is a randomized, placebo-controlled, double-blind phase 3 trial of adjuvant nivolumab plus low-dose ipilimumab versus nivolumab alone in 1943 patients with resected stage IIIB/C/D or stage IV melanoma. The results of this trial have not yet been published. However, a recent press release noted that the addition of ipilimumab did not improve RFS for patients with tumors expressing PD-L1.[46] The study is ongoing, with the goal of assessing RFS in the overall study population.

NADINA

Increasingly, there has been an interest in the benefit of neoadjuvant immuno-therapy approaches in the treatment of resectable melanoma. The goal of the ran-domized, phase III NADINA trial[47] is to compare neoadjuvant combination ipilimumab and nivolumab to adjuvant nivolumab alone for patients with macro-scopic stage III melanoma. Patients will be randomized to receive either 2 cycles of neoadjuvant ipilimumab (80 mg) and nivolumab (240 mg) every 3 weeks followed by LND, or up front LND followed by 12 cycles of adjuvant nivolumab (480 mg) every 4 weeks. The primary outcome measure is event-free survival (EFS), defined as progression of melanoma to irresectable stage III/IV disease, disease recur-rence, and death. The secondary outcome measures include RFS, DMFS, OS, and pathologic response rate in the neoadjuvant arm. This study will provide much needed insight into optimal timing of immunotherapy for patients with resect-able stage III melanoma. The study is currently recruiting, with an estimated completion date of January 2027.

SWOG/S1801

Similar to the NADINA study, the active SWOG trial[48] aims to compare neoadjuvant to adjuvant pembrolizumab for patients with stage III/IV melanoma. The neoadjuvant cohort will receive IV pembrolizumab every 3 weeks for 3 cycles followed by surgical resection within 3 weeks, followed by adjuvant pembrolizumab every 3 weeks for 15 cycles. The patients in the adjuvant arm will receive IV pembrolizumab every 3 weeks for 18 cycles within 17 days following surgical resection. The primary objective is EFS, and the secondary objectives include OS and toxicities. The trial is currently active, with an estimated completion date of September 1, 2022.

CheckMate 76k

Trials are ongoing to determine the role of adjuvant targeted/immunotherapy for high-risk stage IIB-C disease. Presented at the American Society of Clinical Oncology (ASCO) meeting in 2021, Wilson and colleagues[49] discussed preliminary results of their phase 2 trial of adjuvant nivolumab for patients with IIB/C melanoma. At the time of presentation, the 26 patients enrolled demonstrated a 2-year RFS of 87.8%, compared with a historic 2-year RFS of 70%. The patients are continuing to be moni-tored; however, the preliminary results show a trend toward improved RFS in patients treated with adjuvant nivolumab.

SUMMARY

The current guidelines for the surgical care of cutaneous melanoma have been shaped by multiple randomized controlled clinical trials. Six prospective randomized trials per-formed between 1980 and 2004 have informed the current NCCN guidelines for margin excision in melanoma, and the currently enrolling MelMarT trial will provide important information on the safety of narrower surgical margins for thicker lesions in the era of SLNB. MSLT-I led to the common practice of SLNB for patients with in-termediate thickness and thick melanomas primarily for prognostication and staging, and MSLT-II and DECOG-SLT demonstrated safety in observing the nodal basin with serial ultrasound compared with immediate CLND in patients with a positive sentinel node. Additionally, for patients with nodal disease (stage III), recent developments in targeted and immune therapy have led to effective adjuvant therapy options with demonstrated improvements in RFS. As the melanoma landscape continues to evolve with an increasing interest in neoadjuvant therapy approaches, it is anticipated that future clinical trials will continue to change practice, improving the care for patients with cutaneous melanoma.

CLINICS CARE POINTS

- Wide local excision margins for melanoma should be no larger than 2 cm, based on the results of 6 randomized trials.
- Although CLND can offer helpful insight regarding prognostication for patients with positive sentinel lymph node biopsies, 2 randomized trials have demonstrated that nodal surveillance with serial ultrasounds is a safe option, as CLND offers no improvement in MSS. As such, given the lack of benefit and the morbidity of lymph node dissection, practice paradigm has almost universally shifted to nodal surveillance in patients with positive sentinel lymph nodes.
- For stage III/IV patients with a BRAF mutation, adjuvant treatment with a combination BRAF/MEK inhibitor can decrease recurrence rates, and improve overall and distant-metastasis free survival.
- For stage III/IV patients without a BRAF mutation, adjuvant treatment with anti-PD-1 therapy can improve RFS and distant-metastasis free survival, with a tolerable toxicity profile.

DISCLOSURE

Dr Beasley: received clinical trial funding from Istari Oncology, Delcath, Oncosec Medical, Replimune, and Checkmate Pharmaceuticals paid to Duke University. Served one time on the advisory boards for Cardinal Health and Regeneron. Giorgos Karakousis: PI of Investigator Initiated Trial with institutional support by Merck. Advisory board: Merck.

REFERENCES

1. Coit DG, Thompson JA, Albertini MR, et al. Cutaneous Melanoma, Version 2.2019, NCCN Clinical Practice Guidelines in Oncology. J Natl Compr Canc Netw 2019;17(4):367–402.
2. Angeles CV, Wong SL, Karakousis G. The Landmark Series: Randomized Trials Examining Surgical Margins for Cutaneous Melanoma. Ann Surg Oncol 2020; 27(1):3–12.
3. Cosimi AB, Sober AJ, Mihm MC, et al. Conservative surgical management of superficially invasive cutaneous melanoma. Cancer 1984;53(6):1256–9.
4. Balch CM, Murad TM, Soong SJ, et al. Tumor thickness as a guide to surgical management of clinical stage I melanoma patients. Cancer 1979;43(3):883–8.
5. Day CL, Mihm MC, Sober AJ, et al. Narrower margins for clinical stage I malignant melanoma. N Engl J Med 1982;306(8):479–82.
6. Veronesi U, Cascinelli N, Adamus J, et al. Thin stage I primary cutaneous malignant melanoma. Comparison of excision with margins of 1 or 3 cm. N Engl J Med 1988;318(18):1159–62.
7. Veronesi U, Cascinelli N. Narrow excision (1-cm margin). A safe procedure for thin cutaneous melanoma. Arch Surg 1991;126(4):438–41.
8. Balch CM, Soong S, Ross MI, et al. Long-term results of a multi-institutional randomized trial comparing prognostic factors and surgical results for intermediate

thickness melanomas (1.0 to 4.0 mm). Intergroup Melanoma Surgical Trial. Ann Surg Oncol 2000;7(2):87–97.

9. Karakousis CP, Balch CM, Urist MM, et al. Local recurrence in malignant melanoma: long-term results of the multiinstitutional randomized surgical trial. Ann Surg Oncol 1996;3(5):446–52.

10. Balch CM, Urist MM, Karakousis CP, et al. Efficacy of 2-cm surgical margins for intermediate-thickness melanomas (1 to 4 mm). Results of a multi-institutional randomized surgical trial. Ann Surg 1993;218(3):262–7 [discussion: 267–9].

11. Cohn-Cedermark G, Rutqvist LE, Andersson R, et al. Long term results of a randomized study by the Swedish Melanoma Study Group on 2-cm versus 5-cm resection margins for patients with cutaneous melanoma with a tumor thickness of 0.8-2.0 mm. Cancer 2000;89(7):1495–501.

12. Ringborg U, Andersson R, Eldh J, et al. Resection margins of 2 versus 5 cm for cutaneous malignant melanoma with a tumor thickness of 0.8 to 2.0 mm: randomized study by the Swedish Melanoma Study Group. Cancer 1996;77(9):1809–14.

13. Utjés D, Malmstedt J, Teras J, et al. 2-cm versus 4-cm surgical excision margins for primary cutaneous melanoma thicker than 2 mm: long-term follow-up of a multicentre, randomised trial. Lancet 2019;394(10197):471–7.

14. Gillgren P, Drzewiecki KT, Niin M, et al. 2-cm versus 4-cm surgical excision margins for primary cutaneous melanoma thicker than 2 mm: a randomised, multicentre trial. Lancet 2011;378(9803):1635–42.

15. Khayat D, Rixe O, Martin G, et al. Surgical margins in cutaneous melanoma (2 cm versus 5 cm for lesions measuring less than 2.1-mm thick). Cancer 2003;97(8): 1941–6.

16. Thomas JM, Newton-Bishop J, A'Hern R, et al. Excision margins in high-risk malignant melanoma. N Engl J Med 2004;350(8):757–66.

17. Hayes AJ, Maynard L, Coombes G, et al. Wide versus narrow excision margins for high-risk, primary cutaneous melanomas: long-term follow-up of survival in a randomised trial. Lancet Oncol 2016;17(2):184–92.

18. Cascinelli N, Morabito A, Santinami M, et al. Immediate or delayed dissection of regional nodes in patients with melanoma of the trunk: a randomised trial. WHO Melanoma Programme. Lancet 1998;351(9105):793–6.

19. Balch CM, Soong SJ, Bartolucci AA, et al. Efficacy of an elective regional lymph node dissection of 1 to 4 mm thick melanomas for patients 60 years of age and younger. Ann Surg 1996;224(3):255–63 [discussion: 263–6].

20. Veronesi U, Adamus J, Bandiera DC, et al. Delayed regional lymph node dissection in stage I melanoma of the skin of the lower extremities. Cancer 1982;49(11): 2420–30.

21. Bello DM, Faries MB. The Landmark Series: MSLT-1, MSLT-2 and DeCOG (Management of Lymph Nodes). Ann Surg Oncol 2020;27(1):15–21.

22. Morton DL, Thompson JF, Cochran AJ, et al. Sentinel-node biopsy or nodal observation in melanoma. N Engl J Med 2006;355(13):1307–17.

23. Morton DL, Thompson JF, Cochran AJ, et al. Final trial report of sentinel-node biopsy versus nodal observation in melanoma. N Engl J Med 2014;370(7):599–609.

24. Leiter U, Stadler R, Mauch C, et al. Complete lymph node dissection versus no dissection in patients with sentinel lymph node biopsy positive melanoma (DeCOG-SLT): a multicentre, randomised, phase 3 trial. Lancet Oncol 2016;17(6): 757–67.

25. Ariyan C, Brady MS, Gönen M, et al. Positive nonsentinel node status predicts mortality in patients with cutaneous melanoma. Ann Surg Oncol 2009;16(1): 186–90.

26. Faries MB, Thompson JF, Cochran AJ, et al. Completion Dissection or Observation for Sentinel-Node Metastasis in Melanoma. N Engl J Med 2017;376(23): 2211–22.
27. Pucci C, Martinelli C, Ciofani G. Innovative approaches for cancer treatment: current perspectives and new challenges. Ecancermedicalscience 2019;13:961.
28. Ascierto PA, Kirkwood JM, Grob JJ, et al. The role of BRAF V600 mutation in melanoma. J Transl Med 2012;10:85.
29. Bhatia P, Friedlander P, Zakaria EA, et al. Impact of BRAF mutation status in the prognosis of cutaneous melanoma: an area of ongoing research. Ann Transl Med 2015;3(2):24.
30. Sahni S, Valecha G, Sahni A. Role of Anti-PD-1 Antibodies in Advanced Melanoma: The Era of Immunotherapy. Cureus 2018;10(12):e3700.
31. Eroglu Z, Ribas A. Combination therapy with BRAF and MEK inhibitors for melanoma: latest evidence and place in therapy. Ther Adv Med Oncol 2016;8(1): 48–56.
32. Chapman PB, Hauschild A, Robert C, et al. Improved survival with vemurafenib in melanoma with BRAF V600E mutation. N Engl J Med 2011;364(26):2507–16.
33. Ascierto PA, Minor D, Ribas A, et al. Phase II trial (BREAK-2) of the BRAF inhibitor dabrafenib (GSK2118436) in patients with metastatic melanoma. J Clin Oncol 2013;31(26):3205–11.
34. Hauschild A, Grob JJ, Demidov LV, et al. Dabrafenib in BRAF-mutated metastatic melanoma: a multicentre, open-label, phase 3 randomised controlled trial. Lancet 2012;380(9839):358–65.
35. Sosman JA, Kim KB, Schuchter L, et al. Survival in BRAF V600-mutant advanced melanoma treated with vemurafenib. N Engl J Med 2012;366(8):707–14.
36. Maio M, Lewis K, Demidov L, et al. Adjuvant vemurafenib in resected, BRAF. Lancet Oncol 2018;19(4):510–20.
37. Long GV, Hauschild A, Santinami M, et al. Adjuvant Dabrafenib plus Trametinib in Stage III BRAF-Mutated Melanoma. N Engl J Med 2017;377(19):1813–23.
38. Eggermont AM, Chiarion-Sileni V, Grob JJ, et al. Adjuvant ipilimumab versus placebo after complete resection of high-risk stage III melanoma (EORTC 18071): a randomised, double-blind, phase 3 trial. Lancet Oncol 2015;16(5):522–30.
39. Eggermont AMM, Blank CU, Mandalà M, et al. Adjuvant pembrolizumab versus placebo in resected stage III melanoma (EORTC 1325-MG/KEYNOTE-054): distant metastasis-free survival results from a double-blind, randomised, controlled, phase 3 trial. Lancet Oncol 2021;22(5):643–54.
40. Weber J, Mandala M, Del Vecchio M, et al. Adjuvant Nivolumab versus Ipilimumab in Resected Stage III or IV Melanoma. N Engl J Med 2017;377(19):1824–35.
41. Luke JJ, Rutkowski P, Queirolo P, et al. Pembrolizumab versus placebo as adjuvant therapy in completely resected stage IIB or IIC melanoma (KEYNOTE-716): a randomised, double-blind, phase 3 trial. Lancet 2022;399(10336):1718–29.
42. Grossman K, Othus M, Pratel S, et al. Final analysis of overall survival (OS) and relapse-free-survival (RFS) in the intergroup S1404 phase III randomized trial comparing either high-dose interferon (HDI) or ipilimumab to pemnbrolizumab in patients with high-risk resected melanoma. J Clin Oncol 2021;9501.
43. Grossmann KF, Othus M, Patel SP, et al. Adjuvant Pembrolizumab versus IFNα2b or Ipilimumab in Resected High-Risk Melanoma. Cancer Discov 2022;12(3): 644–53.
44. Moncrieff MD, Gyorki D, Saw R, et al. 1 Versus 2-cm Excision Margins for pT2-pT4 Primary Cutaneous Melanoma (MelMarT): A Feasibility Study. Ann Surg Oncol 2018;25(9):2541–9.

45. Coit D, Ariyan C. MelMART Trial: It's Now or Never. Ann Surg Oncol 2018;25(9): 2493–5.
46. Bristol Myers Squibb. Press release: Bristol-Myers Squibb announces update on CheckMate-915 for Opdivo (nivolumab) plus Yervoy (ipilimumab) versus Opdivo alone in patients with resected high-risk melanoma and PD-L1 <1%. November 20th 2019. Available at: https://news.bms.com/news/details/2019/Bristol-Myers-Squibb-Announces-Update-on-CheckMate–915-for-Opdivo-nivolumab-Plus-Yervoy-ipilimumab-Versus-Opdivo-Alone-in-Patients-with-Resected-High-Risk-Melanoma-and-PD-L1-1/default.aspx.
47. Neoadjuvant Ipilimumab Plus Nivolumab Versus Standard Adjuvant Nivolumab in Macroscopic Stage III Melanoma (NADINA). 2021. Available at: https://clinicaltrials.gov/ct2/show/NCT04949113.
48. A Study to Compare the Administration of Pembrolizumab After Surgery Versus Administration Both Before and After Surgery for High-Risk Melanoma. 2018. Available at: https://clinicaltrials.gov/ct2/show/NCT03698019.
49.. Wilson M, Geskin LJ, Carvajal RD, et al. Adjuvant nivolumab in high-risk stage IIb/IIc melanoma patients: Results from investigator initiated clinical trial. J Clin Oncol 2021;39(15_suppl).

The Perioperative and Operative Management of Esophageal and Gastric Cancer

Amn Siddiqi, MBBS[a], Fabian M. Johnston, MD, MHS, FSSO[b],*

KEYWORDS

- Gastric cancer • Esophageal cancer • Esophagogastric cancer • RAMIE
- D1 versus D2 lymphadenectomy • CRS + HIPEC • FLOT • CROSS

KEY POINTS

- D2 lymphadenectomy shows a better prognosis in patients with advanced gastric cancer, whereas D1 lymphadenectomy portends better overall- and disease-free survival in patients over 70 or in those with early-stage gastric cancer.
- Endoscopic mucosal resection/endoscopic mucosal dissection provides an alternative to surgical resection for the management of T1 cancer while maintaining therapeutic oncologic standards.
- Cytoreductive surgery + heated intraperitoneal chemotherapy offers prophylactic, therapeutic, and palliative management for peritoneal carcinomatosis.
- Early trials exploring the utility of targeted therapy during the perioperative period have shown promising results.

INTRODUCTION

In 2020, 604,000 new cases of esophageal cancer and more than 1 million new cases of gastric cancer were diagnosed globally.[1] Gastric and esophageal cancer account for the fourth and seventh highest causes of cancer mortality worldwide, with the highest incidence rates found in East Asia.[2] These malignancies often present with vague symptoms in their early stages and, as a result, are diagnosed late in their course. In fact, studies suggest that only 30% of esophageal tumors are limited to the primary site at the time of presentation, and more than half of patients with gastric cancer in the United States have metastasis at the time of diagnosis.[3,4]

The last 40 years have seen significant strides in the diagnosis and management of esophageal and gastric cancers. Technical advancements in endoscopic

[a] Department of Surgery, Johns Hopkins University School of Medicine, 600 North Wolfe Street, Baltimore, MD 21287, USA; [b] Division of Gastrointestinal Surgical Oncology, Johns Hopkins University, 600 North Wolfe Street, Baltimore, MD 21287, USA
* Corresponding author.
E-mail address: fjohnst4@jhmi.edu

Surg Oncol Clin N Am 32 (2023) 65–81
https://doi.org/10.1016/j.soc.2022.07.006
1055-3207/23/© 2022 Elsevier Inc. All rights reserved.

surgonc.theclinics.com

procedures, minimally invasive surgical techniques, and robotic surgery have led to higher rates of curative resections and improved survival outcomes. Peritoneal disease, previously terminal, is now managed using cytoreductive surgery (CRS) with heated intraperitoneal chemotherapy (HIPEC) in select cases. Radiation and chemotherapy regimens are constantly improving, and investigations in targeted and immune therapy are currently underway. Despite this progress, the overall 5-year survival rate for gastric cancer is 28.4%, whereas for esophageal cancer it remains a dismal 14.3% to 18%.[5–7]

PATHOGENESIS AND CLASSIFICATION

Squamous cell carcinoma (SCC) and adenocarcinoma (AC) account for the two most commonly diagnosed esophageal cancers. The major risk factors for developing SCC are tobacco and alcohol use, achalasia, and nutritional deficiencies.[1,5] Before 1990, SCC was the predominant histologic type worldwide. Today, the rate of esophageal SCC has declined in high income countries, attributable to a decrease in tobacco and alcohol use, whereas the rate of esophageal AC has almost doubled from 35% to 65%.[8] This trend is observed in conjunction with rising obesity, increased diagnoses of gastroesophageal reflux disease (GERD) and Barrett's Esophagus; all of which are known risk factors of the disease.[9–11]

Gastric cancer is most commonly caused by chronic inflammation of the gastric lining. H. Pylori atrophic gastritis is particularly associated with its development.[12] Other risk factors include a high intake of salty and smoked foods, cigarette smoking, and low socio-economic status. AC makes up 95% of all gastric malignancies.[13] In 1965, Lauren classified gastric ACs into 2 broad histologic subtypes: well-differentiated intestinal subtype and poorly differentiated diffuse subtype.[14] This is still the most common classification system used today.[15]

ACs in the esophagogastric junction (EGJ) share characteristics with both esophageal and gastric ACs. The anatomic location of these tumors within the EGJ is significant in guiding management and is classified best by the Siewert classification.[16] Siewert type 1 tumors arise from an area of intestinal metaplasia of the distal esophagus, infiltrating the EGJ from above. Type 2 tumors are true carcinomas of the EGJ, arising from the gastric cardia. Siewert type 3 tumors are subcardial gastric tumors which infiltrate the EGJ from below.

DIAGNOSIS AND STAGING

Esophageal cancer is often asymptomatic in its early stages. Its diagnosis is most commonly preceded by progressive dysphagia and unintentional weight loss.[5,11] Chest pain, odynophagia, dyspepsia, hemoptysis, hematemesis, and hoarseness may occur late in disease progression. Similarly, signs and symptoms associated with gastric cancer are vague, nonspecific, and usually appear once the cancer has spread. If present, these include nausea, emesis, early satiety, weight loss and epigastric pain. Physical examination may reveal an abdominal mass, Virchow's node (left supraclavicular lymphadenopathy), Sister Mary Joseph's node (umbilical nodule), or Bulmer's shelf (tumor deposit anterior to the rectum, palpable on a digital rectal examination). Patients with suspicious findings must be investigated thoroughly.

The gold standard for diagnosing esophageal and gastric cancer is an upper gastrointestinal endoscopy. This allows a thorough visualization of the mucosa, localization of the tumor, and biopsy of suspicious lesions.[5,17,18] Studies suggest that six to eight biopsies should be obtained to ensure an adequate sample for histologic and molecular analysis. Adding brushings to the sample can increase its sensitivity to almost 100%.[3,19]

Once cancer has been diagnosed, proper disease staging is crucial to guide therapy. The American Joint Committee on Cancer and International Union Against Cancer (AJCC/UICC) staging system uses the traditional tumor/node/metastasis (TNM) classification to stage cancer.[20] Its most recent update saw notable changes: first, junctional tumors with epicenters within the proximal 2 cm of the gastric cardia (Siewert types 1 and 2) are classified as esophageal cancers, whereas those with epicenters distal to the cardia (Siewert type 3) are classified as gastric cancers. Second, the TNM framework has been adapted to now include clinical staging (cTNM) and postneoadjuvant staging (ypTNM). As a result, disease prognosis is more specific to each patient's treatment history, allowing for a more tailored management approach.

Several diagnostic modalities are used to inform staging. Endoscopic ultrasound (EUS) is the indicated modality to determine cT stage. It provides a detailed view of the layers of the gastrointestinal wall and determines the depth of tumor invasion with an accuracy of 71% to 92% for esophageal cancer and 80% for gastric cancer.[21–25] Its ability to discern between T1a and T1b, however, is limited.[26,27] A more accurate staging of the superficial layers can be performed using endoscopic mucosal resection (EMR) and endoscopic mucosal dissection (ESD) (see Multidisciplinary Treatment). EUS has also shown utility in evaluating cN in esophageal cancer. It can assess the size, shape and echogenicity pattern of regional lymph nodes with a sensitivity of 85%.[22] Fine-needle aspiration (EUS-FNA) increases the sensitivity and specificity to 97% and 96%, respectively, and is strongly recommended.[5] However, the usefulness of EUS in assessing cN for gastric cancer is limited (83% sensitivity and 67% specificity) due to the difficulty of identifying distant positive nodes.[28,29]

Cross-sectional imaging using computed tomography (CT) and PET compliment EUS by evaluating locoregional disease and distant metastasis. Fluorodeoxyglucose (FDG) PET/CT in combination evaluates the presence of distant metastasis with a sensitivity and specificity of 83.3% and 98.4%, respectively. FDG-PET/CT continues to be the mainstay of diagnosing metastatic burden which is pivotal when deciding between curative versus palliative surgery.

Some studies suggest that as many as 30% of patients with junctional and gastric AC have the peritoneal disease at the time of diagnosis.[30] The presence of peritoneal disease constitutes stage IV disease and alters management from curative-intent surgical resection to systemic therapy instead.[31] Cross-sectional imaging provides limited yield in identifying peritoneal involvement and therefore, diagnostic laparoscopy is critical to evaluate the peritoneal surface for disease, biopsy suspicious lesions, and obtain peritoneal washings for cytology.

MULTIDISCIPLINARY TREATMENT
Surgical Management

Complete surgical resection remains the only opportunity for cure in both esophageal and gastric cancer. The goal of resection is to gain maximum locoregional control of the cancer, while minimizing tissue and function loss.

Esophagectomy is the definitive treatment for patients with esophageal cancer staged cT1,N+ and cT2-4a.[32] The two most common approaches are transthoracic esophagectomy (TTE) and transhiatal esophagectomy (THE). Historically, TTE has been the operation of choice. It comprises combined laparotomy and right thoracotomy, whereas THE involves a midline laparotomy and left cervical incision.[33] Omloo and colleagues[34] conducted a randomized control trial comparing oncologic outcomes in patients who underwent a TTE to those who underwent a THE for ACs of the mid/distal esophagus. They found that patients in the TTE group had a 5-year overall survival benefit of 14%. Hulcher and colleagues[35] conducted a similar trial with 220 patients and observed a trend toward improved overall and disease-free survival at 5 years after TTE. Theoretically, TTE permits more thorough visualization and exposure of the thoracic esophagus than THE, which should allow wider excision of the tumor and more extensive lymph node dissection.[33,34,36,37] It should be noted, however, that the transhiatal approach is associated with lower morbidity and mortality rates, and can be suitable for patients with significant comorbidities.[38] A recent metanalysis also observed benefit in using the transhiatal approach to resect Seiwert type 3 junctional cancer; however, its long-term outcomes still need to be explored.[38]

Lymphadenectomy is critical for successful disease resection and oncologic staging. Literature shows that a higher lymph node yield is associated with increased overall survival after esophagectomy.[39,40] Furthermore, a study following 616 cancer patients after esophagectomy observed that more extensive lymph node resection did not decrease a patient's short- or long-term health-related quality of life.[41] Currently, the National Comprehensive Cancer Network (NCCN) guidelines recommend that at least 15 lymph nodes be submitted for histopathologic evaluation and adequate staging.[42]

Gastrectomy with lymphadenectomy is the recommended management for gastric cancer stages T1b-T3. The type of gastrectomy (total, subtotal and distal) largely depends on the tumor size and location. Regardless of the type of surgery, the critical aspects of an effective oncologic resection are negative margins and sufficient clearance of nodal disease. Retrospective data from patients undergoing curative intent gastrectomy suggests that margins of 2 to 6 cm decrease the likelihood of an R1 resection (microscopically positive margins).[43] Currently, the NCCN recommends at least 4 cm gross margins.[44]

Optimal lymphadenectomy in the setting of gastric cancer has been a focus of debate for the last few decades. Studies comparing D1 (perigastric lymph nodes only), D2 (perigastric and celiac lymph nodes) and D3 (perigastric, celiac, and para-arotic lymph nodes) lymphadenectomies display varying results. The Dutch D1D2 trial followed patients who underwent gastrectomy for gastric cancer over 15 years and found that D2 lymphadenectomy is associated with lower locoregional recurrence and gastric cancer-related death than D1 lymphadenectomy.[45] The D2 procedure was also associated with higher morbidity, mortality, and reoperation rates; however, the resection has since evolved to eliminate routine splenectomy which may lower complication rates. The Italian Gastric Cancer Study Group conducted a similar trial, but found that after 15 years of follow-up there was no significant difference in the overall- and disease-free survival between the D1 and D2 groups.[46] However, when accounting for disease stage and patient age, they observed that disease free survival was significantly higher after D2 in patients with advanced disease (pT >1, N+), whereas overall survival and disease free survival were better after D1 in patients above 70 years or those with early stage cancer. This evidence highlights the importance of accurate preoperative staging to perform an adequate surgical resection while minimizing patient morbidity and mortality. The Japanese Clinical Oncology Group (JCOG) compared D2 and D3 lymphadenectomy and found no difference in 5-year recurrence-free and overall survival.[47] In fact, D3 lymphadenectomy was associated with more complications. A Cochrane systematic review comparing the outcomes of all three procedures in patient with gastric cancer concluded that D2 lymphadenopathy was associated with a better disease specific survival than D1; however, it was also associated with higher postoperative mortality rates.[48] Disease free survival and overall survival were comparable between both groups. Although currently, no specific approach is considered standard, D2 lymphadenectomy has become the staple in Western countries. Ultimately, the NCCN recommends procurement of a minimum of 15 lymph nodes for optimal oncologic outcomes.[44]

Minimally invasive surgery and robotic surgery

Minimally invasive esophagectomy (MIE) using scoping techniques was first introduced in the 1990s. Studies comparing MIE to open esophagectomy (OE) show that MIE is associated with less blood loss, lower pain scores, shorter hospitalization, fewer pulmonary complications, and overall lower morbidity than OE, without compromising lymph node yield and overall survival.[49–53] Most notably, the TIME trial randomized 115 patients to undergo either OE or MIE.[54] At 3 years of follow-up, the MIE group displayed an overall-survival benefit of 10.1% and a disease-free survival benefit of 5.1%. Even though these findings were not statistically significant, they prove that MIE presents suitable alternative to OE which maintains oncologic standards.

In 2003, the advent of robot-assisted MIE (RAMIE) provided surgeons an even better overview and reach of the thoracic inlet. Patients with extensive locoregional disease of the upper third of the esophagus, who were previously deemed inoperable due to difficult access, can now be surgically managed using RAMIE. Sluis and colleagues[55] conducted the ROBOT trial comparing RAMIE to OE. They found that patients who underwent RAMIE had significantly fewer pulmonary and cardiac complications than those who underwent OE (32% vs 58%, $P = .005$; and 22% vs 47%, $P = .006$, respectively). Functional recovery at post op day 14 was also significantly better in the RAMIE group than the OE group (70% vs 51%, $P = .038$), whereas oncologic outcomes were similar. An R0 resection was achieved in 93% of RAMIE patients and 96% of OE patients ($P = .35$) and there was no difference in median disease-free survival ($P = .983$). Currently, trials are underway to compare RAMIE to MIE for patients with resectable esophageal cancer.[56] Early results show that RAMIE can achieve a shorter operative duration and better lymph node dissection; however, long-term follow-up is required to compare meaningful oncologic outcomes.

Similarly, data from trials comparing laparoscopic gastrectomy (LG) to open gastrectomy (OG) show comparable overall survival and cancer specific survival rates in both groups.[57–59] Additional benefits of LG include reduced blood loss, shorter time to resumption of oral intake, and shorter hospitalization. A recent metanalysis comparing robotic gastrectomy (RG) to LG concluded that RG for gastric cancer seems to be safe and feasible alternative associated with a higher rate of lymph node retrieval and better short term surgical outcomes.[60] Further follow-up is required to explore its long-term outcomes.

Endoscopic mucosal resection and endoscopic submucosal dissection

Although surgical resection remains the management of choice for T1b + tumors, advancements in endoscopic techniques have made EMR and ESD an increasingly used alternative to treat T1a N0 esophageal and gastric cancer. Studies comparing endoscopic resection to surgical resection have reported similar survival outcomes, with endoscopic resection portending a better quality of life.[61–64] In the Eastern hemisphere, endoscopic resection is now the standard treatment for Tis and T1a lesions.[65,66]

Before undergoing EMR/ESD, the lesion must be evaluated by an expert endoscopist using high-resolution white light endoscopy or magnified endoscopy. Chromoendoscopy using dyes (eg, Lugol, acetate) is helpful in detecting and delineating the tumor.[67] The degree of dysplasia should be confirmed by direct sampling of visible lesions.

EMR consists of three steps: marking, lifting, and cutting. A submucosal injection of saline lifts the lesion along with the surrounding mucosa which is then removed using a snare. In ESD, an electrocautery knife is used to make a circumferential cut around the lesion, followed by dissection of the submucosal layer from the proper muscle layer using pressurized water jets or a series of incisions.[65,68] A metanalysis comparing the two concluded that ESD achieved a significantly higher rate of en bloc resections (97.1% vs 49.3%) and pathologically curative resections (92.3% vs 52.7%). Local recurrence after ESD was found to be 0.3%, as opposed to 11.5% after EMR.

The choice of using EMR or ESD for esophageal cancer largely depends on the size of the tumor, circumferential involvement of the esophagus, degree of dysplasia, and level of operator expertise. In general, superficial lesions up to 2 cm in size, which involve less than 2/3 of the esophageal circumference and that can be easily lifted, may be approached using EMR.[65,67–70] T1 tumors that do not fit these criteria should be approached via ESD. Endoscopic resection is considered curative if the specimen margins are free from tumor (R0), the depth of invasion is less than 500 μm beneath the muscularis mucosa, the tumor is not mucinous or poorly differentiated, and there is no lymphovascular invasion (LVI).[65]

For gastric cancer, the Japanese Gastric Cancer Association recommends EMR or ESD for T1a, intestinal-type ACs, without ulcerations and with a diameter less than or equal to 2 cm.[66] Lesions without ulcerations that are greater than 2 cm in diameter, and lesions with ulcerations less than 3 cm in diameter should be resected using ESD and not EMR. If these tumors are resected en bloc and have negative margins with no LVI, patients should be followed with annual endoscopy and surveillance for metastatic disease. If these criteria are not met, subsequent management depends on the depth of invasion and amount of undifferentiated tumor, and ranges from repeat endoscopy to gastrectomy with lymphadenectomy.

Adverse events for both EMR and ESD include bleeding, perforation, and stricture formation, with higher risk attributed to ESD because of its steeper learning curve and longer procedure time. It should be noted, however, that these risks are inversely proportional to operator experience. Therefore, it is recommended that ESD be performed by experienced endoscopists at high-volume, tertiary centers.[67]

Cytoreductive surgery and heated intraperitoneal chemotherapy

Peritoneal carcinomatosis (PC) is a common sequalae of esophageal and gastric cancer, associated with high recurrence rates and a dismal median survival of less than 1 year.[71] For this reason, standard practice supports the use of palliative management such as systemic therapy, chemoradiation, and best supportive care, as opposed to surgical resection. Unfortunately, evidence shows that these strategies only increase median overall survival by 4 to 7 months.[72] An explanation for such poor response may be that the blood peritoneal barrier may not allow adequate penetration of chemotherapeutic drugs into the peritoneal cavity, and although some may enter, an effective drug concentration cannot be maintained long enough.[73] One strategy to combat this limitation is to use HIPEC.

The utility of CRS and HIPEC in esophageal and gastric cancer is being explored in three capacities: a potential prophylactic option to prevent the development of PC, a therapeutic modality along with CRS in patients with established PC, and a palliative measure in patients with extensive PC. The CYTO-CHIP study, published in 2018, used propensity score matching to compare overall survival and recurrence-free survival between CRS + HIPEC and CRS only (CRSa).[74] Results showed that

CRS + HIPEC dramatically improved the median overall survival from 12.1 months to 18.8 months. Overall survival at 3 and 5 years, and recurrence-free survival were also significantly higher (P = .005, P = .001, respectively). Granieri and colleagues[75] published a metanalysis encompassing 12 randomized control trials investigating HIPEC + CRS in patients with advanced gastric cancer. Results showed significantly improved overall-survival at 1 and 3 years (P<.001), and higher disease-free survival at 1, 2, and 3 years of follow-up (P = .017, P = .0001, P = .005, respectively). More recently, Zhang and colleagues[73] conducted a metanalysis to assess the efficacy and safety of HIPEC in patients with advanced gastric cancer, specific to the presence or absence of PC. Among patients without PC, the HIPEC group showed significantly higher overall survival rates at 1 and 3 years (P = .004, P<.00001), as well as a significant reduction in disease recurrence (P<.00001). Patients with PC who underwent HIPEC saw in increase in overall median survival time of 4.67 months compared with the control. Overall-survival at 1, 2 and 3 years had also significantly increased. This metanalysis provides evidence favoring the use of HIPEC in prophylactic, therapeutic, and palliative capacities.

There are multiple ongoing prospective trails exploring the utility of CRS + HIPEC in patients with PC from gastric and EGJ cancer. The GASTRICHIP study (NCT01882933) is randomizing patients to receive either HIPEC + D2 resection + perioperative chemotherapy or D2 resection + perioperative chemotherapy.[76] The PERIOSCOPE-II trial (NCT03348150) aims to compare CRS + HIPEC to systemic chemotherapy in patients with PC from gastric cancer.[77] The phase 3 CHIMERA trial (NCT04597294) is comparing FLOT + HIPEC to FLOT + surgery to evaluate the efficacy of HIPEC in patients with advanced gastric cancer.[78] The PREVENT trial (NCT04447352) is a phase 3 randomized control trial exploring the use of preventive HIPEC + perioperative FLOT versus FLOT alone for diffuse type gastric and junctional cancer.[79] Diffuse type gastric cancer is associated with a higher risk of PC than intestinal gastric cancer. If this intervention proves effective, it could potentially result in a new standard of therapy for diffuse type gastric cancer.

Chemotherapy

Although the optimal perioperative chemotherapy regimen is yet to be established, current evidence favors its use in improving both surgical outcomes and overall survival and recurrence. The largest randomized control trial investigating the effect of chemotherapy in patients with resectable esophageal cancer was conducted by the United Kingdom Medical Research Council Esophageal Cancer (OE02) in 2002.[80] 802 patients were randomized to either receive chemotherapy comprising cisplatin and fluorouracil followed by surgery, or to undergo surgery alone. Few patients experienced toxic effects and the chemotherapy group saw a substantial improvement in dysphagia before surgery. An R0 (microscopically negative) resection was achieved in 60% of the chemotherapy group compared with 54% in the surgery alone group (P<0·0001), and survival rates at 5 years of follow-up were higher in the chemotherapy group (23.0%) compared with the surgery alone group (17.1%) (HR 0.84).[81] The US Radiation Therapy Oncology group conducted a similar trial with 440 patients.[82] Results failed to show an overall survival benefit; however, a metanalysis which included data from both studies indicated a 2-year absolute survival benefit of 7% in patients receiving neoadjuvant chemotherapy.[83]

In 2006, the landmark MAGIC trial compared perioperative chemotherapy to surgery alone in patients with resectable esophageal, junctional, and gastric AC.[84] The intervention group received three preoperative and three postoperative cycles of epirubicin, cisplatin and fluorouracil (ECF). This regimen proved effective in reducing tumor size and significantly improved progression free (HR 0.66, $P<.001$) and overall survival (HR 0.75. $P = .009$). The results of this study cemented the role of perioperative chemotherapy in managing esophageal and gastric cancer.

The French FNCLCC trial compared the efficacy of perioperative chemotherapy using fluorouracil and cisplatin to surgery alone.[85] Although the trial was ended early due to poor accrual, the chemotherapy group displayed better overall ($P = .02$) and disease-free survival ($P = .01$) at 5 years. The curative resection rate also improved significantly from 73% to 83% ($P = .04$).

The German FLOT4-AIO phase 3 randomized control trial compared perioperative chemotherapy with docetaxel, oxaliplatin, fluorouracil, and leucovorin (FLOT) to ECF or ECX (EC and capecitabine) in patients with resectable gastric and junctional cancer.[86] Patients in the FLOT group showed higher rates of complete pathologic regression, progression free survival, and overall survival. These findings have led to a dramatic shift in the chemotherapeutic treatment of gastric cancer. Currently, perioperative FLOT is the preferred chemotherapeutic regimen recommended by the NCCN for AC of the esophagus and stomach.[42,44]

Chemoradiotherapy

The importance of adjuvant chemoradiotherapy (XRT) in treating EGJ and gastric cancer was established by the Southwest Oncology Group's Intergroup-0116 trial (SWOG 9008).[87] At 10 years of follow-up, patients who underwent postoperative chemoradiation showed exceptional overall (HR $= 1.32$, $P = .004$) and disease-free survival (HR $= 1.51$, $P<.001$), compared with those who underwent observation. These promising results have since prompted further investigation into the use of perioperative XRT in treating esophageal and gastric cancer.

The CROSS Trial was a landmark multicenter randomized control trial that investigated the effect of XRT followed by surgery to surgery alone in the management of esophageal and junctional cancer.[88] The intervention group received carboplatin and paclitaxel for 5 weeks with concurrent radiotherapy before surgery. Not only did the median overall survival rate in increase from 24.0 to 49.4 months ($P = .003$), the rate of R0 resections improved dramatically from 69% to 92% ($P<.001$), with 29% of patients in the XRT group showing complete pathologic resection (ypT0N0). Furthermore, locoregional recurrence reduced from 34% in the surgery alone group to 14% in the XRT group ($P<.001$) and PC from 14% to 4% ($P<.001$). At 10 years, the overall survival benefit was 13%.[89]

Although multiple studies have established the benefit of chemotherapy and trimodal therapy compared with surgery alone management, literature comparing XRT to chemotherapy is sparse and presents mixed results. The CRITICS Trial, reported in 2018, compared perioperative chemoradiation comprising epirubicin, cisplatin or oxaliplatin, and capecitabine to postoperative chemoradiation for gastric cancer. Results showed no overall difference in survival between the two groups.[90] The study did make note of poor postoperative compliance to treatment, and so the subsequent CRITICS-II trial (NCT02931890), currently underway, aims to optimize preoperative treatment by comparing preoperative chemotherapy, chemotherapy followed by XRT, and XRT only.[91]

The ARTIST trial, reported in 2018, compared postoperative chemotherapy with capecitabine and cisplatin to capecitabine with concurrent radiotherapy in patients with curatively resected gastric cancer who underwent D2 lymphadenectomy.[92] Results concluded that the addition of radiation therapy had no significant effect on overall disease-free survival. However, patients with regional lymph node metastasis at the time of surgery showed superior disease-free survival after undergoing XRT ($P = .0365$). The ARTIST-II trial, published in 2020, compared three adjuvant regimens: S-1 only, S-1 and oxaliplatin (SOX), and SOX with concurrent XRT (SOXRT).[93] Estimated 3-year disease-free survival rates were 64.8%, 74.3%, and 72.8%, respectively. Although both the SOX and SOXRT groups showed improved disease-free survival compared with the S-1 only group, there was no significant difference between disease free survival in SOX and SOXRT ($P = .074$).

The ongoing Australasian Gastro-Intestinal Trials Group's TOPGEAR trial (NCT01924819) randomized patients with gastric cancer to receive either perioperative ECF, or perioperative ECF with preoperative radiation therapy.[94] Interim results show safe utility of the XRT regimen without a significant increase in toxicity and morbidity.[95] The study is estimated to be complete in 2026.

With regard to esophageal cancer, current evidence comparing XRT to chemotherapy is severely lacking. Many randomized control trials have been initiated to explore this subject; however, it will take several years to obtain meaningful results. The ongoing ESOPEC trial (NCT02509286) aims to compare perioperative chemotherapy using the FLOT protocol to XRT using the CROSS protocol.[96] The Neo-AEGIS trial (NCT01726452) is randomizing patients with esophageal and EGJ cancer (cT2-3, N0-3, M0) to receive either the CROSS or MAGIC regimen.[97] Its aim is to compare overall survival, disease-free survival, recurrence rates, pathologic response rates, toxicity, tumor regression, in-hospital complications, and health related quality of life.

Targeted Therapy

Efforts to understand the genetic drivers of neoplasia have driven the development of monoclonal antibodies tailored to target specific cell receptors and their signaling pathways at the molecular level. Both esophageal and gastric cancer share common growth factor receptors which when targeted, display promising results in inhibiting cancer growth and inducing tumor cell apoptosis.

The expression of the human epidermal growth factor receptor, HER-2, is well recorded in esophageal and gastric cancer.[98,99] The phase 3 randomized control ToGA trial compared trastuzumab (anti-HER2 monoclonal antibody) + chemotherapy to chemotherapy alone in patients with gastric and EGJ cancer. Disease-free and overall survival were better in the trastuzumab + chemotherapy group.[100] Similarly, RTOG-1010 randomized patients with HER-2 positive esophageal cancer to receive perioperative XRT with or without trastuzumab.[101] Even though no additional benefit was seen, adding trastuzumab did not increase the rate of toxicity and should be studied further. Currently, NCCN guidelines for both cancers include trastuzumab as part of first-line systemic therapy.[42,44]

Tumor angiogenesis regulated via the vascular endothelial growth factor (VEGF) pathway also plays an important role in cancer development. The REGARD trial compared ramucirumab (anti-VEGFR monoclonal antibody) monotherapy with a placebo in patients with gastric cancer and found that ramucirumab was associated with a higher median overall survival.[102] The RAINBOW trial showed that gastric cancer patients receiving ramucirumab in combination with paclitaxel had a significantly better progression-free and overall survival as opposed to those who received paclitaxel alone.[103]

Although evidence supports the use of targeted therapy in patients with advanced cancer, the question remains whether or not this modality can offer benefit during the perioperative period. Phase 2 RAMSES/FLOT7 trial (NCT02661971) randomized 180 patients with gastric and EGJ cancer to receive perioperative FLOT with or without ramucirumab.[104] The addition of ramucirumab improved R0 resection rates from

83% to 97% (P = .0049). Similarly, PETRARCA, a phase 2/3 trial compared trastuzumab and pertuzumab with FLOT to FLOT alone in patients with resectable HER2+ junctional cancer.[105] Although the trial ended prematurely, results showed that combination therapy significantly improved complete pathologic resection rates.

Therapeutic strategies geared toward immune checkpoint inhibition have shown significant potential in preventing evasion of apoptosis by cancer cells. In particular, drugs that target programmed cell death protein and its ligand (PD-1/PD-L1), such as nivolumab (anti-PD-1 monoclonal antibody) and pembrolizumab (anti-PD-1 monoclonal antibody), have shown great efficacy in patients who have advanced esophageal and gastric cancer.[106–108] Their usefulness within the perioperative timeframe is yet to be explored.

SUMMARY

Optimal perioperative and operative management of esophageal and gastric cancer requires a multidisciplinary approach to treatment. Evolution in surgical techniques has ushered an exciting era of endoscopic and robotic resections, which show promising results as therapeutic modalities at par with current standards. The use of CRS and HIPEC in a prophylactic or therapeutic capacity may provide new treatment opportunities for patients for whom palliation is the only current option. Improvements in perioperative chemotherapy and radiation therapy not only show a benefit in survival rates, but may also be effective in downsizing unresectable tumors so that they may be operable. Moving forward, applying principles of targeted therapy to management during the perioperative period may set a new and improved standard for survival outcomes.

CLINICS CARE POINTS

- An Upper GI endoscopy with biopsies is the gold standard for diagnosing gastric and esophageal cancer. Once diagnosed, the cancer should be staged using EUS as well as cross sectional imaging modalities.
- Experienced endoscopists at high volume tertiary centers should consider performing enoscopic mucosal resection or endoscopic submucosal dissection for patients with Tis and T1a disease.
- RAMIE allows better overview and reach of the thoracic inlet than OE, making it more suitable in patients with extensive disease of the upper third of the esophagus.
- Consider using HIPEC for prophylaxis, therapy, and palliation of advanced disease.
- Evidence supports the use of chemotherapy and radiotherapy during the perioperative period. Involving a multidisciplinary team of surgeons, oncologists and radiologists early in patient management is recommended.

DISCLOSURE

The authors have nothing to disclose.

REFERENCES

1. Sung H, Ferlay J, Siegel RL, et al. Global Cancer Statistics 2020: GLOBOCAN Estimates of Incidence and Mortality Worldwide for 36 Cancers in 185 Countries. CA Cancer J Clin 2021;71(3):209–49.

2. Machlowska J, Baj J, Sitarz M, et al. Gastric Cancer : Epidemiology , Risk Factors , Classification , Genomic Characteristics and Treatment Strategies. Int J Mol Sci 2020;21(11):4012.
3. Iriarte F, Su S, Petrov Rv, et al. Surgical Management of Early Esophageal Cancer. Surg Clin North Am 2021;101(3):427–41.
4. Leake PA, Cardoso R, Seevaratnam R, et al. A systematic review of the accuracy and indications for diagnostic laparoscopy prior to curative-intent resection of gastric cancer. Gastric Cancer 2012;15(SUPPL.1):38–47.
5. Alsop BR, Sharma P. Esophageal Cancer. Gastroenterol Clin North Am 2016; 45(3):399–412.
6. He H, Chen N, Hou Y, et al. Trends in the incidence and survival of patients with esophageal cancer: A SEER database analysis. Thorac Cancer 2020;11(5): 1121.
7. Thrift AP, Nguyen TH. Gastric Cancer Epidemiology. Gastrointest Endosc Clin North Am 2021;31(3):425–39.
8. Trivers KF, Sabatino SA, Stewart SL. Trends in esophageal cancer incidence by histology, United States, 1998-2003. Int J Cancer 2008;123(6):1422–8.
9. Avgerinos KI, Spyrou N, Mantzoros CS, et al. Obesity and cancer risk: Emerging biological mechanisms and perspectives. Metab Clin Exp 2019;92:121–35.
10. Coleman HG, Xie SH, Lagergren J. The Epidemiology of Esophageal Adenocarcinoma. Gastroenterology 2018;154(2):390–405.
11. Esophageal Cancer - American Family Physician. Available at: https://www.aafp. org/afp/2017/0101/p22.html. Accessed April 2, 2022.
12. Karimi P, Islami F, Anandasabapathy S, et al. Gastric Cancer: Descriptive Epidemiology, Risk Factors, Screening, and Prevention. Cancer Epidemiol Biomarkers Prev 2014. https://doi.org/10.1158/1055-9965.EPI-13-1057.
13. Rawla P, Barsouk A. Epidemiology of gastric cancer: global trends, risk factors and prevention. Gastroenterol Rev 2019;14(1).
14. Lauren P. The two histological main types of gastric carcinoma: diffuse and so-called intestinal-type carcinoma. Acta Pathol Microbiol Scand 1965;1(64): 31–49.
15. Berlth F, Bollschweiler E, Drebber U, et al. Pathohistological classification systems in gastric cancer: Diagnostic relevance and prognostic value. World J Gastroenterol 2014;20:5679–84.
16. Rü Diger Siewert J, Feith M, Werner M, et al. Adenocarcinoma of the Esophagogastric Junction Results of Surgical Therapy Based on Anatomical/Topographic Classification in 1,002 Consecutive Patients. Ann Surg 2000;232(3):353–61.
17. Shahbaz Sarwar CM, Luketich JD, Landreneau RJ, et al. Esophageal cancer: An update. Int J Surg 2010;8(6):417–22.
18. di Pietro M, Canto MI, Fitzgerald RC. Endoscopic Management of Early Adenocarcinoma and Squamous Cell Carcinoma of the Esophagus: Screening, Diagnosis, and Therapy. Gastroenterology 2018;154(2):421–36.
19. Graham DY, Schwartz JT, Cain GD, et al. Prospective evaluation of biopsy number in the diagnosis of esophageal and gastric carcinoma. Gastroenterology 1982;82(2):228–31.
20. AJCC Cancer Staging Manual Eighth Edition. Available at: www.cancerstaging. org. Accessed April 20, 2022.
21. Rice TW, Ishwaran H, Ferguson MK, et al. Cancer of the Esophagus and Esophagogastric Junction: An Eighth Edition Staging Primer. J Thorac Oncol 2017; 12(1):36–42.

22. Betancourt-Cuellar SL, Benveniste MFK, Palacio DP, et al. Esophageal Cancer: Tumor-Node-Metastasis Staging. Radiol Clin North Am 2021;59(2):219–29.
23. Krill T, Baliss M, Roark R, et al. Accuracy of endoscopic ultrasound in esophageal cancer staging. J Thorac Dis 2019;11:S1602–9.
24. Hong SJ, Kim TJ, Nam KB, et al. New TNM staging system for esophageal cancer: What chest radiologists need to know. Radiographics 2014;34(6):1722–40.
25. Chen Z da, Zhang PF, Xi HQ, et al. Recent Advances in the Diagnosis, Staging, Treatment, and Prognosis of Advanced Gastric Cancer: A Literature Review. Front Med 2021;8:744839.
26. Van Zoonen M, Van Oijen MGH, Van Leeuwen MS, et al. Low impact of staging EUS for determining surgical resectability in esophageal cancer. Surg Endosc 2012. https://doi.org/10.1007/s00464-012-2254-z.
27. Shah PM, Gerdes H. Endoscopic options for early stage esophageal cancer. J Gastrointest Oncol 2015;6(1):20–30.
28. Spolverato G, Ejaz A, Kim Y, et al. Use of endoscopic ultrasound in the preoperative staging of gastric cancer: a multi-institutional study of the US gastric cancer collaborative. J Am Coll Surg 2015;220(1):48–56.
29. Fairweather M, Jajoo K, Sainani N, et al. Accuracy of EUS and CT imaging in preoperative gastric cancer staging. J Surg Oncol 2015;111(8):1016–20.
30. Sarela AI, Lefkowitz R, Brennan MF, et al. Selection of patients with gastric adenocarcinoma for laparoscopic staging. Am J Surg 2006;191(1):134–8.
31. American Joint Comission on Cancer. AJCC Cancer Staging Manual. In: Amin MB, Edge SB, Greene FL, et al, editors. AJCC cancer staging Manual. 8ht edition. Chicago, IL: Springer International Publishing; 2017. p. 185–202.
32. Borggreve AS, Kingma BF, Domrachev SA, et al. Surgical treatment of esophageal cancer in the era of multimodality management. Ann N Y Acad Sci; 2018. https://doi.org/10.1111/nyas.13677.
33. Barreto JC, Posner MC. Transhiatal versus transthoracic esophagectomy for esophageal cancer. World J Gastroenterol 2010;16(30):3804.
34. Omloo JMT, Lagarde SM, Hulscher JBF, et al. Extended transthoracic resection compared with limited transhiatal resection for adenocarcinoma of the mid/distal esophagus: five-year survival of a randomized clinical trial. Ann Surg 2007;246(6):992–1000.
35. Hulscher JBF, van Sandick JW, de Boer AGEM, et al. Extended transthoracic resection compared with limited transhiatal resection for adenocarcinoma of the esophagus. N Engl J Med 2002;347(21):1662–9.
36. Johansson J, DeMeester TR, Hagen JA, et al. En bloc vs transhiatal esophagectomy for stage T3 N1 adenocarcinoma of the distal esophagus. Arch Surg 2004;139(6):627–33.
37. Takahashi C, Shridhar R, Huston J, et al. Comparative outcomes of transthoracic versus transhiatal esophagectomy. Surgery 2021;170(1):263–70.
38. Wei MT, Zhang YC, Deng XB, et al. Transthoracic vs transhiatal surgery for cancer of the esophagogastric junction: A meta-analysis META-ANALYSIS. World J Gastroenterol 2014;20(29):10183–92.
39. Visser E, Markar SR, Ruurda JP, et al. Prognostic Value of Lymph Node Yield on Overall Survival in Esophageal Cancer Patients: A Systematic Review and Meta-analysis. Ann Surg 2019;269(2):261–8.
40. Peyre CG, Hagen JA, DeMeester SR, et al. Predicting systemic disease in patients with esophageal cancer after esophagectomy a multinational study on the significance of the number of involved lymph nodes. Ann Surg 2008;248(6):979–84.

41. Schandl A, Johar A, Lagergren J, et al. Lymphadenectomy and health-related quality of life after oesophageal cancer surgery: a nationwide, population-based cohort study. BMJ Open 2016. https://doi.org/10.1136/bmjopen-2016-012624.

42. National Comprehensive Cancer Network. Esophageal and Esophagogastric Junction Cancers (Version 2.2022). 2022. Available at: https://www.nccn.org/professionals/physician_gls/pdf/gastric.pdf. Accessed May 9, 2022.

43. Johnston FM, Beckman M. Updates on Management of Gastric Cancer. Curr Oncol Rep 2019;21(8). https://doi.org/10.1007/s11912-019-0820-4.

44. National Comprehensive Cancer Network. Gastric Cancer (Version 2.2022). Available at: https://www.nccn.org/professionals/physician_gls/pdf/gastric.pdf. Accessed May 9, 2022.

45. Songun I, Putter H, Kranenbarg EMK, et al. Surgical treatment of gastric cancer: 15-year follow-up results of the randomised nationwide Dutch D1D2 trial. Lancet Oncol 2010;11(5):439–49.

46. Degiuli M, Reddavid R, Tomatis M, et al. D2 dissection improves disease-specific survival in advanced gastric cancer patients: 15-year follow-up results of the Italian Gastric Cancer Study Group D1 versus D2 randomised controlled trial. Eur J Cancer 2021;150:10–22.

47. Fujimura T, Nakamura K, Oyama K, et al. Selective lymphadenectomy of para-aortic lymph nodes for advanced gastric cancer. Oncol Rep 2009;22(3):509–14.

48. Mocellin S, Mcculloch P, Kazi H, et al. Extent of lymph node dissection for adenocarcinoma of the stomach. Cochrane Database Syst Rev 2015;2015(8). https://doi.org/10.1002/14651858.CD001964.PUB4/MEDIA/CDSR/CD001964/IMAGE_N/NCD001964-CMP-002-02.PNG.

49. Biere SSAY, van Berge Henegouwen MI, Maas KW, et al. Minimally invasive versus open oesophagectomy for patients with oesophageal cancer: a multi-centre, open-label, randomised controlled trial. Lancet 2012;379(9829):1887–92.

50. Sgourakis G, Gockel I, Radtke A, et al. Minimally invasive versus open esoph-agectomy: meta-analysis of outcomes. Dig Dis Sci 2010;55(11):3031–40.

51. Smithers BM, Gotley DC, Martin I, et al. Comparison of the Outcomes Between Open and Minimally Invasive Esophagectomy. Ann Surg 2007;245(2):232.

52. Sakamoto T, Fujiogi M, Matsui H, et al. Comparing Perioperative Mortality and Morbidity of Minimally Invasive Esophagectomy Versus Open Esophagectomy for Esophageal Cancer: A Nationwide Retrospective Analysis. Ann Surg 2021;274(2):324–30.

53. Yibulayin W, Abulizi S, Lv H, et al. Minimally invasive oesophagectomy versus open esophagectomy for resectable esophageal cancer: a meta-analysis. World J Surg Oncol 2016;14(1). https://doi.org/10.1186/S12957-016-1062-7.

54. Straatman J, van der Wielen N, Cuesta MA, et al. Minimally Invasive Versus Open Esophageal Resection: Three-year Follow-up of the Previously Reported Randomized Controlled Trial: the TIME Trial. Ann Surg 2017;266(2):232–6.

55. van der Sluis PC, van der Horst S, May AM, et al. Robot-assisted Minimally Inva-sive Thoracolaparoscopic Esophagectomy Versus Open Transthoracic Esopha-gectomy for Resectable Esophageal Cancer: A Randomized Controlled Trial. Ann Surg 2019;269(4):621–30.

56. Yang Y, Li B, Yi J, et al. Robot-assisted Versus Conventional Minimally Invasive Esophagectomy for Resectable Esophageal Squamous Cell Carcinoma: Early Results of a Multicenter Randomized Controlled Trial: The RAMIE Trial. Ann Surg 2022;275(4):646–53.

57. Huang C, Liu H, Hu Y, et al. Laparoscopic vs Open Distal Gastrectomy for Locally Advanced Gastric Cancer: Five-Year Outcomes From the CLASS-01 Randomized Clinical Trial. JAMA Surg 2022;157(1):9–17.

58. Kim HH, Han SU, Kim MC, et al. Effect of Laparoscopic Distal Gastrectomy vs Open Distal Gastrectomy on Long-term Survival Among Patients With Stage I Gastric Cancer: The KLASS-01 Randomized Clinical Trial. JAMA Oncol 2019; 5(4):506–13.

59. Huscher CGS, Mingoli A, Sgarzini G, et al. Laparoscopic versus open subtotal gastrectomy for distal gastric cancer: five-year results of a randomized prospective trial. Ann Surg 2005;241(2):232–7.

60. Guerrini GP, Esposito G, Magistri P, et al. Robotic versus laparoscopic gastrectomy for gastric cancer: The largest meta-analysis. Int J Surg 2020;82:210–28.

61. Gong EJ, Kim H, Ahn JY, et al. Comparison of long-term outcomes of endoscopic submucosal dissection and surgery for esophagogastric junction adenocarcinoma. Gastric Cancer 2017. https://doi.org/10.1007/s10120-016-0679-0.

62. Kim GH, Jung HY. Endoscopic Resection of Gastric Cancer. Gastrointest Endosc Clin North Am 2021;31(3):563–79.

63. Quero G, Fiorillo C, Longo F, et al. Propensity score-matched comparison of short- and long-term outcomes between surgery and endoscopic submucosal dissection (ESD) for intestinal type early gastric cancer (EGC) of the middle and lower third of the stomach: a European tertiary referral center experience. Surg Endosc 2021;35(6):2592–600.

64. Choi IJ, Lee JH, Kim Y il, et al. Long-term outcome comparison of endoscopic resection and surgery in early gastric cancer meeting the absolute indication for endoscopic resection. Gastrointest Endosc 2015;81(2):333–41.e1.

65. Ahmed Y, Othman M. EMR/ESD: Techniques, Complications, and Evidence. Curr Gastroenterol Rep 2020. https://doi.org/10.1007/s11894-020-00777-z.

66. Japanese Gastric Cancer Association. Japanese gastric cancer treatment guidelines 2018 (5th edition) Preface to the English version. Gastric Cancer 2021. https://doi.org/10.1007/s10120-020-01042-y.

67. Pimentel-Nunes P, Dinis-Ribeiro M, Ponchon T, et al. Endoscopic submucosal dissection: European Society of Gastrointestinal Endoscopy (ESGE) Guideline. Endoscopy 2015;47:829–54.

68. Wang J, Zhang XH, Ge J, et al. Endoscopic submucosal dissection vs endoscopic mucosal resection for colorectal tumors: A meta-analysis. World J Gastroenterol 2014;20(25):8282–7.

69. Draganov Pv, Wang AY, Othman MO, et al. AGA Institute Clinical Practice Update: Endoscopic Submucosal Dissection in the United States. Clin Gastroenterol Hepatol 2019;17(1):16–25.e1.

70. Ishihara R, Arima M, Iizuka T, et al. Endoscopic submucosal dissection/endoscopic mucosal resection guidelines for esophageal cancer. Dig Endosc 2020. https://doi.org/10.1111/den.13654.

71. Seshadri RA, Glehen O. Cytoreductive surgery and hyperthermic intraperitoneal chemotherapy in gastric cancer. World J Gastroenterol 2016;22(3):1114.

72. Wagner AD, Syn NLX, Moehler M, et al. Chemotherapy for advanced gastric cancer. Cochrane Database Syst Rev 2017;2017(8). https://doi.org/10.1002/14651858.CD004064.PUB4/MEDIA/CDSR/CD004064/IMAGE_N/NCD004064-CMP-010-06.PNG.

73. Zhang JF, Lv L, Zhao S, et al. Hyperthermic Intraperitoneal Chemotherapy (HIPEC) Combined with Surgery: A 12-Year Meta-Analysis of this Promising

Treatment Strategy for Advanced Gastric Cancer at Different Stages. Ann Surg Oncol 2022;29(5):3170–86.

74. Bonnot PE, Piessen G, Kepenekian V, et al. Cytoreductive Surgery With or Without Hyperthermic Intraperitoneal Chemotherapy for Gastric Cancer With Peritoneal Metastases (CYTO-CHIP study): A Propensity Score Analysis. J Clin Oncol 2019;37(23):2028–40.

75. Granieri S, Bonomi A, Frassini S, et al. Prognostic impact of cytoreductive surgery (CRS) with hyperthermic intraperitoneal chemotherapy (HIPEC) in gastric cancer patients: A meta-analysis of randomized controlled trials. Eur J Surg Oncol 2021;47(11):2757–67.

76. Glehen O, Passot G, Villeneuve L, et al. GASTRICHIP: D2 resection and hyperthermic intraperitoneal chemotherapy in locally advanced gastric carcinoma: a randomized and multicenter phase III study. BMC Cancer 2014;14(1).

77. Koemans WJ, van der Kaaij RT, Boot H, et al. Cytoreductive surgery and hyperthermic intraperitoneal chemotherapy versus palliative systemic chemotherapy in stomach cancer patients with peritoneal dissemination, the study protocol of a multicentre randomised controlled trial (PERISCOPE II). BMC Cancer 2019; 19(1). https://doi.org/10.1186/S12885-019-5640-2.

78. Prophylactic Preoperative HIPEC in Advanced Gastric Cancer at High Risk of Peritoneal Recurrence - Full Text View - ClinicalTrials.gov. Available at: https:// clinicaltrials.gov/ct2/show/NCT04597294?term=HIPEC&type=Intr&cond= Gastric+Cancer&draw=2&rank=1. Accessed May 9, 2022.

79. Götze TO, Piso P, Lorenzen S, et al. Preventive HIPEC in combination with perioperative FLOT versus FLOT alone for resectable diffuse type gastric and gastroesophageal junction type II/III adenocarcinoma - the phase III "PREVENT"- (FLOT9) trial of the AIO/CAOGI/ACO. BMC Cancer 2021;21(1). https:// doi.org/10.1186/S12885-021-08872-8.

80. Girling DJ, Bancewicz J, Clark PI, et al. Surgical resection with or without preoperative chemotherapy in oesophageal cancer: a randomised controlled trial. Lancet 2002;359(9319):1727–33.

81. Allum WH, Stenning SP, Bancewicz J, et al. Long-term results of a randomized trial of surgery with or without preoperative chemotherapy in esophageal cancer. J Clin Oncol 2009;27(30):5062–7.

82. Avid D, Elsen PK, Obert R, et al. Chemotherapy Followed by Surgery Compared with Surgery Alone for Localized Esophageal Cancer. N Engl J Med 2009; 339(27):1979–84.

83. Gebski V, Burmeister B, Smithers BM, et al. Survival benefits from neoadjuvant chemoradiotherapy or chemotherapy in oesophageal carcinoma: a meta-analysis. Lancet Oncol 2007;8(3):226–34.

84. Cunningham D, Allum WH, Stenning SP, et al. Perioperative Chemotherapy versus Surgery Alone for Resectable Gastroesophageal Cancer From the Departments of Medicine (D. Vol 355.; 2006. Available at: www.nejm.org. Accessed April 20, 2022.

85. Ychou M, Boige V, Pignon JP, et al. Perioperative chemotherapy compared with surgery alone for resectable gastroesophageal adenocarcinoma: An FNCLCC and FFCD multicenter phase III trial. J Clin Oncol 2011;29(13):1715–21.

86. Al-Batran SE, Homann N, Pauligk C, et al. Perioperative chemotherapy with fluorouracil plus leucovorin, oxaliplatin, and docetaxel versus fluorouracil or capecitabine plus cisplatin and epirubicin for locally advanced, resectable gastric or gastro-oesophageal junction adenocarcinoma (FLOT4): a randomised, phase 2/3 trial. Lancet 2019;393(10184):1948–57.

87. Macdonald JS, Benedetti J, Smalley S, et al. Chemoradiation of resected gastric cancer: A 10-year follow-up of the phase III trial INT0116 (SWOG 9008). Am J Clin Oncol 2009;27(15_suppl):4515.

88. van Hagen P, Hulshof MCCM, van Lanschot JJB, et al. Preoperative Chemoradiotherapy for Esophageal or Junctional Cancer. N Engl J Med 2012;366(22): 2074–84.

89. Eyck BM, van Lanschot JJB, Hulshof MCCM, et al. Ten-Year Outcome of Neoadjuvant Chemoradiotherapy Plus Surgery for Esophageal Cancer: The Randomized Controlled CROSS Trial. J Clin Oncol 2021;39(18):1995–2004.

90. Cats A, Jansen EPM, van Grieken NCT, et al. Chemotherapy versus chemoradiotherapy after surgery and preoperative chemotherapy for resectable gastric cancer (CRITICS): an international, open-label, randomised phase 3 trial. Lancet Oncol 2018;19(5):616–28.

91. Slagter AE, Jansen EPM, van Laarhoven HWM, et al. CRITICS-II: a multicentre randomised phase II trial of neo-adjuvant chemotherapy followed by surgery versus neo-adjuvant chemotherapy and subsequent chemoradiotherapy followed by surgery versus neo-adjuvant chemoradiotherapy followed by surgery in resectable gastric cancer. BMC Cancer 2018;18(1). https://doi.org/10.1186/S12885-018-4770-2.

92. Lee J, Lim DH, Kim S, et al. Phase III trial comparing capecitabine plus cisplatin versus capecitabine plus cisplatin with concurrent capecitabine radiotherapy in completely resected gastric cancer with D2 lymph node dissection: the ARTIST trial. J Clin Oncol 2012;30(3):268–73.

93. Park SH, Lim DH, Sohn TS, et al. A randomized phase III trial comparing adjuvant single-agent S1, S-1 with oxaliplatin, and postoperative chemoradiation with S-1 and oxaliplatin in patients with node-positive gastric cancer after D2 resection: the ARTIST 2 trial. Ann Oncol 2021;32(3):368–74.

94. Leong T, Smithers BM, Michael M, et al. TOPGEAR: a randomised phase III trial of perioperative ECF chemotherapy versus preoperative chemoradiation plus perioperative ECF chemotherapy for resectable gastric cancer (an international, intergroup trial of the AGITG/TROG/EORTC/NCIC CTG). BMC Cancer 2015;15(1).

95. Leong T, Smithers BM, Haustermans K, et al. TOPGEAR: A Randomized, Phase III Trial of Perioperative ECF Chemotherapy with or Without Preoperative Chemoradiation for Resectable Gastric Cancer: Interim Results from an International, Intergroup Trial of the AGITG, TROG, EORTC and CCTG. Ann Surg Oncol 2017;24(8):2252–8.

96. Hoeppner J, Lordick F, Brunner T, et al. ESOPEC: prospective randomized controlled multicenter phase III trial comparing perioperative chemotherapy (FLOT protocol) to neoadjuvant chemoradiation (CROSS protocol) in patients with adenocarcinoma of the esophagus (NCT02509286). BMC Cancer 2016; 16(1). https://doi.org/10.1186/S12885-016-2564-Y.

97. Reynolds Jv, Preston SR, O'Neill B, et al. ICORG 10-14: NEOadjuvant trial in Adenocarcinoma of the oEsophagus and oesophagoGastric junction International Study (Neo-AEGIS). BMC Cancer 2017;17(1). https://doi.org/10.1186/S12885-017-3386-2.

98. Gravalos C, Jimeno A. HER2 in gastric cancer: a new prognostic factor and a novel therapeutic target. Ann Oncol 2008;19(9):1523–9.

99. Gerson JN, Skariah S, Denlinger CS, et al. Perspectives of HER2-targeting in gastric and esophageal cancer. Expert Opin Investig Drugs 2017;26(5):531–40.

100. Bang YJ, van Cutsem E, Feyereislova A, et al. Trastuzumab in combination with chemotherapy versus chemotherapy alone for treatment of HER2-positive advanced gastric or gastro-oesophageal junction cancer (ToGA): a phase 3, open-label, randomised controlled trial. Lancet 2010;376(9742):687–97.
101. Safran HP, Winter K, Ilson DH, et al. Trastuzumab with trimodality treatment for oesophageal adenocarcinoma with HER2 overexpression (NRG Oncology/RTOG 1010): a multicentre, randomised, phase 3 trial. Lancet Oncol 2022; 23(2):259–69.
102. Fuchs CS, Tomasek J, Yong CJ, et al. Ramucirumab monotherapy for previously treated advanced gastric or gastro-oesophageal junction adenocarcinoma (RE-GARD): an international, randomised, multicentre, placebo-controlled, phase 3 trial. Lancet 2014;383(9911):31–9.
103. Wilke H, Muro K, van Cutsem E, et al. Ramucirumab plus paclitaxel versus placebo plus paclitaxel in patients with previously treated advanced gastric or gastro-oesophageal junction adenocarcinoma (RAINBOW): a double-blind, randomised phase 3 trial. Lancet Oncol 2014;15(11):1224–35.
104. Al-Batran SE, Hofheinz RD, Schmalenberg H, et al. Perioperative ramucirumab in combination with FLOT versus FLOT alone for resectable esophagogastric adenocarcinoma (RAMSES/FLOT7): Results of the phase II-portion—A multi-center, randomized phase II/III trial of the German AIO and Italian GOIM. Am J Clin Oncol 2020;38(15_suppl):4501.
105. Hofheinz RD, Haag GM, Ettrich TJ, et al. Perioperative trastuzumab and pertuzumab in combination with FLOT versus FLOT alone for HER2-positive resectable esophagogastric adenocarcinoma: Final results of the PETRARCA multicenter randomized phase II trial of the AIO. Am J Clin Oncol 2020; 38(15_suppl):4502.
106. Kojima T, Shah MA, Muro K, et al. Randomized Phase III KEYNOTE-181 Study of Pembrolizumab Versus Chemotherapy in Advanced Esophageal Cancer. J Clin Oncol 2020;38(35):4138–48.
107. Chin K, Kato K, Cho BC, et al. Three-year follow-up of ATTRACTION-3: A phase III study of nivolumab (Nivo) in patients with advanced esophageal squamous cell carcinoma (ESCC) that is refractory or intolerant to previous chemotherapy. Am J Clin Oncol 2021;39(3_suppl):204.
108. Kang YK, Boku N, Satoh T, et al. Nivolumab in patients with advanced gastric or gastro-oesophageal junction cancer refractory to, or intolerant of, at least two previous chemotherapy regimens (ONO-4538-12, ATTRACTION-2): a randomised, double-blind, placebo-controlled, phase 3 trial. Lancet 2017; 390(10111):2461–71.

Past, Present, and Future Management of Localized Biliary Tract Malignancies

Janet Li, MD[a], Flavio G. Rocha, MD[b], Skye C. Mayo, MD, MPH[c],*

KEYWORDS

- Biliary tract cancer • Cholangiocarcinoma • Gallbladder cancer • Clinical trials
- Liver resection

KEY POINTS

- Evaluation of patients with potentially resectable biliary tract cancer includes multiphasic liver imaging to assess both extent of disease (eg, multifocality and lymph nodes) and the relationship to vascular and biliary structures that will determine surgical options.
- Next-generation sequencing of biopsy specimens is recommended given targetable mutations found in upwards of 35% of patients with intrahepatic cholangiocarcinoma (fibroblast growth factor receptor 2 and isocitrate dehydrogenase 1), hilar cholangiocarcinoma (ERBB2), and gallbladder cancer (ERBB2).
- The goals of resection for patients with biliary tract cancer include a margin-negative resection, portal lymphadenectomy, and biliary reconstruction, if needed, with a sufficient liver remnant volume to avoid post-hepatectomy liver failure.
- Adjuvant capecitabine for 6 months is the current standard of care for patients with biliary tract cancers resected with curative intent; additional regimens including gemcitabine with cisplatin are being evaluated in ongoing randomized trials.
- There are several trials evaluating the role of neoadjuvant, peri-operative, and combinatorial approaches including cytotoxic chemotherapy combined with targeted inhibitors and liver-directed therapy including hepatic arterial infusion.

[a] Division of Surgical Oncology, Department of Surgery, Oregon Health & Science University, 3181 Southwest. Sam Jackson Park Road, Mail Code L-619, Portland, OR 97239, USA; [b] Department of Surgery, Knight Cancer Institute at Oregon Health & Science University, 3181 Southwest Sam Jackson Park Road, Mail Code L-619, Portland, OR 97239, USA; [c] Division of Surgical Oncology, Department of Surgery, Knight Cancer Institute at Oregon Health & Science University, 3181 Southwest Sam Jackson Park Road, Mail Code L-619, Portland, OR 97239, USA
* Corresponding author.
E-mail address: mayos@ohsu.edu
Twitter: @JanetLiMD (J.L.); @FlavioRochaMD (F.G.R.); @drymtn (S.C.M.)

Surg Oncol Clin N Am 32 (2023) 83–99
https://doi.org/10.1016/j.soc.2022.07.007
1055-3207/23/© 2022 Elsevier Inc. All rights reserved.
surgonc.theclinics.com

Abbreviations	
BTC	Biliary Tract Cancer
GBC	Gallbladdder cancer
iCCA	Intrahepatic cholangiocarcinoma
NGS	Next generation sequencing
pCCA	perihilar cholangiocarcinoma

INTRODUCTION

Patients diagnosed with biliary tract cancers (BTC) present a significant clinical management challenge. These aggressive cancers are often diagnosed at an advanced stage and consequentially carry a poor prognosis. Surgical resection of BTC remains the only curative treatment of patients. Biliary tract malignancies are rising in incidence worldwide and are projected to increase over the next several decades.[1] Given their rarity, the 4 distinct cancers that comprise BTC, are often grouped together for the purposes of clinical trials. However, there has been significant progress in the last decade toward understanding the unique genetic underpinnings of each of these tumor sites. Recently, it has been recommended that all patients with a newly diagnosed BTC have a next-generation sequencing (NGS) evaluation if there is enough available tissue as this can inform future treatment options.[2] Neoadjuvant and peri-operative clinical trials have recently been completed and those with distinct genetic drivers are planned. In this article, the researchers review data defining the evolving operative management strategy for 3 of the BTCs: gallbladder cancer (GBC), intrahepatic cholangiocarcinoma (iCCA), and perihilar cholangiocarcinoma (pCCA) (**Fig. 1**). Where possible for this group of rare cancers, the researchers have included relevant clinical trials, meta-analyses, systematic reviews, high-quality single and multi-institutional experiences, and referenced consensus recommendations from the most recent version of the National Comprehensive Cancer Network (NCCN) Guidelines for Hepatobiliary Cancers.[3]

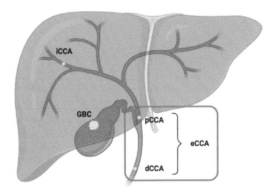

Fig. 1. Schematic of the anatomic subgroups of biliary tract cancers. Extrahepatic cholangiocarcinoma includes the 2 subcategories of perihilar cholangiocarcinoma and distal cholangiocarcinoma, dCCA, eCCA, GBC, iCCA, and pCCA. (*From* Rizzo A, Tavolari S, Ricci AD, Frega G, Palloni A, Relli V, Salati M, Fenocchio E, Massa A, Aglietta M, Brandi G. Molecular Features and Targeted Therapies in Extrahepatic Cholangiocarcinoma: Promises and Failures. Cancers. 2020; 12(11):3256. https://doi.org/10.3390/cancers12113256.)

BACKGROUND
Gallbladder Cancer

GBC is the most common malignancy of the biliary tract.[4] Unfortunately, upwards of 90% of patients with GBC present with advanced disease that is not amenable to surgical resection,[4] which is reflective of the poor overall survival that is less than 5% at 5 years.[5] GBC can be discovered incidentally after cholecystectomy or on imaging review of a suspected gallbladder mass. The NCCN Guidelines for Hepatobiliary Cancers differentiates pre-operative recommendations for GBC depending on the patient presentation.[3] Worldwide, approximately 30% of patients have GBC incidentally discovered on final surgical pathology after cholecystectomy with this number approaching an estimated 60% of patients in the United States.[6-8]

Intrahepatic Cholangiocarcinoma

iCCA is the third most common BTC in the United States with approximately 4000 cases reported each year.[9] Worldwide, the incidence of iCCA has been increasing and is the second most common primary liver cancer, after hepatocellular carcinoma.[10] In the United States, the incidence of iCCA has increased more than 150% between 1975 and 1999.[10] Patients presenting with iCCA discovered on cross-sectional imaging often have a delay to diagnosis given the rarity of this cancer and the difficulties after biopsy in distinguishing it from hepatocellular carcinoma or metastatic disease.

Peri-Hilar Cholangiocarcinoma

pCCA, also called a Klastkin tumor,[11] is the most common of the BTCs, comprising approximately 60% of the BTCs diagnosed each year in the United States with upwards of 7000 cases diagnosed each year in North America.[9] It remains one of the most challenging of the BTCs to diagnose, evaluate for surgical resection, and to ultimately resect given that a biliary reconstruction must be coupled with a liver resection in a setting often complicated by biliary obstruction requiring endoscopic or percutaneous biliary drainage. Endoluminal brushings or clamshell biopsies of the biliary stricture can provide a tissue diagnosis but are not always diagnostic or possible.

PRE-OPERATIVE EVALUATION

For all BTCs, tumor markers (eg, carcinoembryonic antigen, AFP, and CA19-9) and complete staging imaging should be obtained at baseline. Imaging should include a chest computed tomography (CT), and a multiphasic liver CT with intravenous (IV) contrast or contrast-enhanced MRI with magnetic resonance cholangiopancreatography (MRCP). This imaging should be reviewed to determine the extent of liver disease, relation of the cancer to intrahepatic biliary and vascular structures, extrahepatic disease, suspicious nodal disease, and intrahepatic multi-focality.[3] Suspicious nodal disease can often be sampled with endoscopic ultrasound with fine-needle aspiration. Any tissue biopsies that are obtained should be sent for NGS to assess for actionable driver mutations.

Gallbladder Cancer

For patients with GBC, the operative report from the cholecystectomy should be evaluated for other concerning sites of potential disease spread, integrity of the cholecystectomy specimen, and if there was any evidence of bile spillage or incomplete cholecystectomy as part of the operation.[12] Similarly, the pathology report should

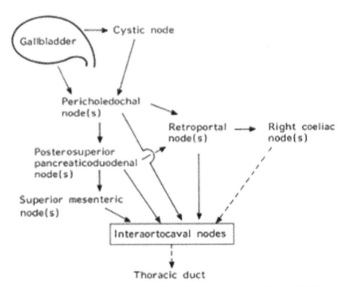

Fig. 2. The topographic location of the regional lymph nodes of the gallbladder. The head of the pancreas is raised medially to expose posteriorly located lymph nodes. The Arabic numerals indicate each group of lymph nodes: 1, cystic (duct) node; 2, pericholedochal nodes; 3, postero-superior pancreaticoduodenal nodes; 4, retroportal nodes; 5, right celiac nodes; 6, superior mesenteric nodes; 7, interaortocaval nodes. Ao, aorta; IMA, inferior mesenteric artery; IVC, inferior vena cava; LRV, left renal vein; RRV, right renal vein; SMA, superior mesenteric artery. (*From* Shirai Y, Yoshida K, Tsukada K, Ohtani T, Muto T. Identification of the regional lymphatic system of the gallbladder by vital staining. Br J Surg. 1992 Jul;79(7):659-62. https://doi.org/10.1002/bjs.1800790721. PMID: 1643479.)

be examined for presence of the cystic lymph node, margin status of the cystic duct, and the AJCC T stage of the cancer, which in the 8th edition also includes either the T2a or T2b designation to indicate the peritoneal side versus parenchymal location of the GBC. Currently, re-resection is recommended for patients with incidentally discovered lesions with a T stage of T1b or greater, with fewer resections possible due to distant disease spread and involvement of adjacent structures in T3 and T4 GBC. Lymphatic spread most commonly extends to the porta hepatis, left gastric, and aorto-caval nodal basins (**Fig. 2**).[13] Nodal disease beyond the hepatoduodenal ligament is generally deemed outside of the regional nodal distribution and associated with worse outcomes.

Intrahepatic Cholangiocarcinoma

Pre-operative biopsy is not required in patients with suspected iCCA before considering resection if the high-quality imaging has features that are radiographically consistent with iCCA. Nodal drainage patterns for iCCA are important to consider for left-sided tumors as drainage may take one of two possible drainage pathways with nodal disease spreading to the celiac axis, beyond what many would initially consider outside of the regional nodal basin for a cancer of the liver (**Fig. 3**).[14]

Peri-Hilar Cholangiocarcinoma

For patients with suspected pCCA, an evaluation with an MRI with MRCP is preferred when evaluating the degree of bile duct involvement. Biliary decompression can be

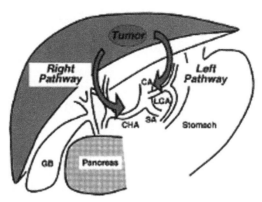

Fig. 3. Schematic of 2 possible drainage pathways. Two lymphatic pathways from the hepatic left lobe are shown: the right pathway through the hepatoduodenal ligament and the left pathway through the lesser omentum to the cardiac portion of the stomach and the gastric lesser curvature. CA, celiac artery; CHA, common hepatic artery; GB, gallbladder; LGA, left gastric artery; SA, splenic artery. (*From* Okami J, Dono K, Sakon M, Tsujie M, Hayashi N, Fujiwara Y, Nagano H, Umeshita K, Nakamori S, Monden M. Patterns of regional lymph node involvement in intrahepatic cholangiocarcinoma of the left lobe. J Gastrointest Surg. 2003 Nov;7(7):850-6. https://doi.org/10.1007/s11605-003-0029-5. PMID: 14592657.)

achieved with endoscopic retrograde cholangiopancreatography (ERCP) or percutaneous transhepatic cholangiography (PTC) and subsequent biliary stenting. The imaging obtained from an ERCP along with cholangioscopy or a PTC can help determine the extent of biliary involvement and classify the patient according to the Bismuth–Corlette classification system (**Fig. 4**).[15] The relationship of the pCCA to the hepatic arterial and portal venous structures is essential to determine on pre-operative imaging as this will dictate the options for surgical resection and reconstruction (eg, involvement of the right hepatic artery in a Type IIIb pCCA). A percutaneous or transabdominal pre-operative biopsy should be obtained only after the patient is assessed by a multi-disciplinary tumor board to determine whether the disease is resectable and bilio-enteric reconstruction is possible or potential candidacy for orthotopic liver transplantation.

EXTENT OF SURGICAL RESECTION
Gallbladder Cancer

Given that many patients with GBC have early nodal spread and peritoneal disease, both the NCCN Guidelines[3] as well as the Americas Hepato-Pancreato-Biliary Association expert consensus statement support a staging laparoscopy before proceeding to hepatic resection.[13,16] A prospective study of 409 patients with primary GBC who underwent staging laparoscopy found disseminated disease in 23% and was estimated to obviate a nontherapeutic laparotomy in 56% (95 of 170) of patients with ultimately unresectable disease.[17]

For patients with a suspicious mass found intra-operatively or on pre-operative imaging, guidelines support a radical cholecystectomy with en bloc hepatic resection and portal lymphadenectomy.[3] The liver resection is performed to the extent needed obtain margins clear of disease, which usually consists of resection of a portion of segments IVB and V. There has been a trend away from the initial treatment of GBC with an extended hepatic resection (eg, right trisectionectomy) in all cases to a more

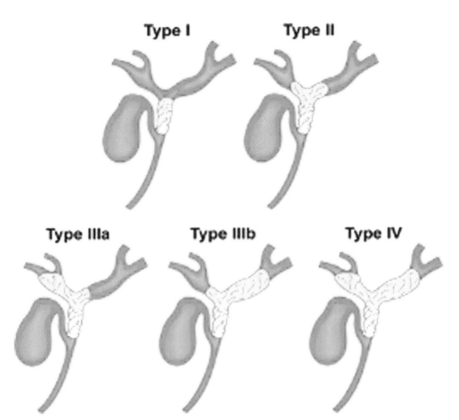

Fig. 4. The Bismuth–Corlette classification of perihilar cholangiocarcinoma. Type I tumors are below the confluence. Type II tumors involve the confluence of the left and right hepatic ducts. Type IIIa and IIIb tumors involve the confluence and the right and left hepatic ducts, respectively. Type IV tumors involve the confluence and extend into the second-order ducts on both sides. (Kimberly M. Brown, David A. Geller, Proximal Biliary Tumors, Surgical Clinics of North America, 94 (2), 2014, 311-323, https://doi.org/10.1016/j.suc.2013.12.003.)

localized resection. The goal remains achieving negative hepatic and biliary margins while reducing morbidity.

For patients with incidentally discovered GBC on pathologic review of the cholecystectomy specimen, the additional information of T stage dictates the recommended surgical treatment. For patients who underwent a simple cholecystectomy and were found to have a T1a GBC incidentally, no additional resection or treatment is recommended.[13] For patients with incidental GBC stage T1b or greater, the recommendation is for re-operation with a hepatic resection of segments IVB and V, portal lymphadenectomy, and bile duct resection if a positive cystic margin is encountered.[13] In a retrospective study, re-resection was associated with increased survival for T2 and T3 disease with a difference in 5-year survival from 15% to 41% compared with patients not treated with re-resection ($P = .0001$); 56% of patients had residual disease at the time of re-resection.[18] Importantly, the re-resections in this study included resection of the cystic plate, resection of segments IVB and V, and patients treated with a more extended hepatic resections with no difference in survival between the different extent of hepatic re-resections.[18] These results were confirmed review of more than 4000 patients with GBC in a large Japanese registry demonstrating no difference in survival between patients who were treated with gallbladder fossa resection compared with resection of segment IVB/V or a major hepatectomy.[19] The only factors that were associated with a worse disease-specific survival were a higher T stage, higher N stage, poor differentiation, and involvement of the common bile duct.[20]

For patients who underwent initial laparoscopic cholecystectomy, there has been a historical practice of resecting the extraction port sites given the risk of malignant port site seeding. However, routine resection of port sites not been shown to be associated with an improvement in survival or disease recurrence.[21]

For complete staging of patients with GBC, the AJCC 8th edition recommends the portal lymphadenectomy should include at least 6 lymph nodes in the porta hepatis, gastrohepatic ligament, and retroduodenal regions.[22] When less than 3 lymph nodes were retrieved, only 22% of patients were found to have nodal metastases compared with 40% of patients when 3 or more lymph nodes were retrieved (see **Fig. 2**).[23] The underdiagnosis of GBC nodal metastases leads to a stage migration where patients deemed N0 with less than 6 lymph nodes retrieved had a worse disease-specific survival compared with patients deemed N0 with 6 or more lymph nodes retrieved.[23]

Intrahepatic Cholangiocarcinoma

Surgical treatment of patients with iCCA begins with a diagnostic laparoscopy to rule out disseminated disease followed by margin-negative hepatic resection with regional lymphadenectomy.[13] The goal of the hepatic resection is to achieve negative margins leaving adequate remnant liver volume. This can be accomplished with parenchymal sparing, segmental resections, or may require a major hepatic resection potentially with portal vein embolization of the standardized future liver remnant volume is calculated to be less than an acceptable threshold. An international multi-institutional database including 449 patients treated with surgical resection for iCCA was analyzed for prognostic factors associated with survival.[24] Positive margin status, multifocal disease, and vascular invasion were all independently associated with decreased survival.[24] Among all patients with an R0 resection, a margin ≥ 1 cm was associated with improved recurrence-free and overall survival when compared with patients with an R0 resection <1 cm.[25]

Patients with iCCA who are resected with curative intent have metastatic nodal disease upwards of 30%.[24] Resection of at least 6 lymph nodes with the portal lymphadenectomy has been demonstrated to most accurately stage patients with resected iCCA.[26,27] Similar to patients with GBC, a portal lymphadenectomy for iCCA involves clearing the porta hepatis of lymphatic tissue including all tissue down to and along the common hepatic artery (station 8) and within the hepatoduodenal ligament (station 12).[13] However, the location of the iCCA within the liver is associated with specific lymphatic drainage patterns. Patients with a left-sided iCCA can have lymphatic drainage to nodal stations around the gastric cardia or along the lesser curve of the stomach in 54% of patients.[14] Lymphatic drainage in patients with right-sided iCCA can be to the retropancreatic region (see **Fig. 3**).[14]

Peri-Hilar Cholangiocarcinoma

Surgical resection of pCCA requires careful pre-operative planning given the central anatomic nature of the lesions and the potential for both portal venous and hepatic arterial vascular involvement within the porta hepatis. The overarching goal of the operation is a margin-negative resection of both the proximal and distal bile ducts to include the ipsilateral hemi-liver often with the caudate, a portal lymphadenectomy, and biliary reconstruction with a Roux-en-Y hepaticojejunostomy to the uninvolved hepatic ducts. Because a major hepatectomy is often required, it is important to assess the patient's liver for underlying fibrosis, steatosis, or portal hypertension as this may influence a patient's operative candidacy. In addition, before an operation, it is essential to achieve complete biliary drainage and to determine objectively whether there will be sufficient volume of the future liver remnant. The presence of underlying liver disease, biliary drainage, and remnant liver volume will impact the ability of the liver to hypertrophy after major hepatectomy and the subsequent risk of post-hepatectomy liver failure. The Bismuth–Corlette classification (see **Fig. 4**) influences the overall operative approach to patients with pCCA. In general, Types I and II are treated with complete extrahepatic biliary tree resection and ipsilateral hepatectomy of the side with the closest surgical margin ± caudate resection; importantly, the side chosen may be reflective of the ability of biliary reconstruction due to cancer involvement or anomalous biliary anatomy precluding/complicating reconstruction on one side versus another. For example, the right hepatic duct is often much shorter length and with a shorter extrahepatic course with earlier division into secondary biliary radicles (anterior and posterior sectoral ducts), whereas the left hepatic duct has a much longer course and length before draining segments in the left liver and caudate. Type IIIa pCCA are most often treated with a right hepatectomy, whereas Type IIIb are often approached with a left hepatectomy; both ± caudate resection. Type IV pCCA are the least likely types to be resected and often involve a right or left extended hepatic resection with biliary reconstruction to second order biliary radicles. In a retrospective study of 225 patients with pCCA, those with an R0 resection had a survival of 42 months compared with 21 months for patients having an R1 resection ($P < .0075$).[28] Of note, caudate lobe resections are often recommended to increase the likelihood of an R0 resection with the anatomic rationale that 44% of caudate bile ducts drain into the confluence of the right and left hepatic ducts.[29] A retrospective study of 159 patients with pCCA who underwent a major hepatectomy with or without caudate lobe resection showed that 62% of patients who had caudate lobe preservation had a positive resection margin compared with 29% of patients who had caudate lobe resection ($P < .001$).[30] In a meta-analysis of 8 studies including 1350 patients with pCCA, caudate lobe resection was associated with improved overall survival without a statistically significant difference in post-operative morbidity and mortality.[31]

GENETIC LANDSCAPE OF BILIARY TRACT CANCERS

It is now recognized that GBC, iCCA, and pCCA have distinct molecular aberrations that likely explain the varied sensitivities seen in treatment responses born out in clinical trials that historically included all BTCs.[32] As demonstrated in **Fig. 5**, NGS techniques of BTCs have revealed fibroblast growth factor receptor (FGFR) alterations or isocitrate dehydrogenase mutations (IDH) present in upwards of 20%, epidermal growth factor receptor tyrosine-protein kinase erbB-2 (ERBB2; previously HER-2) amplification in 10% to 15%, and high microsatellite instability or mismatch repair deficiency occurring in less than 5% of patients.[32] These alterations tend to be mutually exclusive.[33] Specifically, iCCA are characterized by actionable alterations in IDH1 (15%–20%) or fibroblast growth factor receptor 2 (FGFR2; 20%) targetable by small molecule or protein kinase inhibitors. In cancers where ERBB2 amplification is present such as GBC and pCCA, they may be amenable to treatment with novel tyrosine kinase inhibitors potentially combined with monoclonal antibodies (**Table 1**).[33] Several recent trials targeting patients with BTC with alterations in IDH1, FGFR2, and ERBB2 have now established the respective inhibitors as second-line therapy.[34,35] Current trials are evaluating FGFR2 inhibitors as first-line therapy in patients with advanced BTC with FGFR2 fusion-positive disease.[36] Combinatorial therapy using cytotoxic

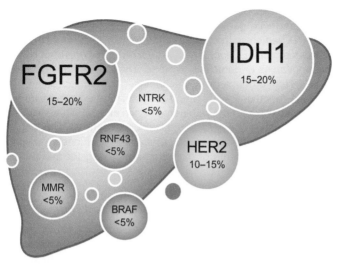

Fig. 5. Current overview of "Precision Medicine" in biliary tract cancers. FGFR2 and IDH1 are the best understood targets to date. Other targets are being investigated, but are less prevalent. Size of spheres is proportional to number of patients with biliary tract cancer likely to harbor these targetable alterations (approximate percentages extracted and adapted from **Fig. 1** are provided). Empty spheres represent other potential targets with lower prevalence in biliary tract cancers: FGFR2; HER2, human epidermal growth factor receptor 2; IDH1; NTRK, neurotropic tyrosine kinase; MMR, mismatch repair deficiency (for the purpose of this figure, this also includes microsatellite instability). (*From* Lamarca A, Barriuso J, McNamara MG, Valle JW. Molecular targeted therapies: Ready for "prime time" in biliary tract cancer. J Hepatol. 2020 Jul;73(1):170-185. https://doi.org/10.1016/j.jhep.2020.03.007. Epub 2020 Mar 12. PMID: 32171892.)

regimens in combination with inhibitors targeted to these molecular drivers are being developed in the neo-adjuvant, peri-operative, and adjuvant settings for patients with resectable biliary tract malignancies.

ADJVUANT THERAPY TRIALS

The BTC discussed in this article all have a high risk of recurrence even after a margin-negative resection. Two years after surgical resection with curative intent, 66% of GBC,[37] 68% pCCA,[37] and 84% of iCCA had recurrent disease.[38] Consequently, there has been great interest in establishing an adjuvant therapy regimen. However, because of the rarity of BTC and the limited number of patients who are surgical candidates (<20%), trials have historically included patients with GBC, iCCA, and pCCA (as well as distal CCA and ampullary cancer) often grouped all together to achieve sufficient statistically power to assess primary outcomes. The reseachers reviewed the landmark adjuvant therapy trials with attention to disease-specific subgroup analysis if available. Before reviewing the true adjuvant trials, the authors discussed the ABC-02 trial for patients with advanced BTC that formed a foundation for studying this disease and influenced the subsequent adjuvant regimens trialed over the next decade.

ABC-02: Gemcitabine with or Without Cisplatin in Treating Patients with Unresectable Locally Advanced or Metastatic Cholangiocarcinoma or Other Biliary Tract Tumors

The ABC-02 was the landmark phase III trial published in 2010 demonstrating improved overall survival with the systemic cytotoxic doublet of gemcitabine plus cisplatin as compared with gemcitabine alone (NCT00262769).[39] This trial included 410 patients from 37 centers in the United Kingdom with locally advanced or metastatic cholangiocarcinoma or GBC (*not an adjuvant trial*) who were randomized to receive cisplatin plus gemcitabine or gemcitabine alone. The trial demonstrated that patients treated with the systemic doublet of gemcitabine–cisplatin had an improved overall survival (11.7 vs 8.1 months, $P < .001$) and progression-free survival (8 vs 5 months, $P < .001$) compared with treatment with gemcitabine alone.[39] There was no difference in adverse events. Although the ABC-02 trial included patients with locally advanced or metastatic cholangiocarcinoma or GBC, these data have been extrapolated to the adjuvant setting with components of this regimen forming the basis of subsequent adjuvant trials for patients with BTC.

PRODIGE-12/ACCORD-18: Gemcitabine Hydrochloride and Oxaliplatin or Observation in Treating Patients with Biliary Tract Cancer that Has Been Removed by Surgery

With new enthusiasm for gemcitabine-based therapies following the results of ABC-02, PRODIGE-12/ACCORD-18 (NCT01313377) published in 2019 was a phase III multicenter trial in France that compared 12 cycles of adjuvant gemcitabine and oxaliplatin to surveillance alone in 196 patients with resected BTC (46% iCCA, 20% GBC, and 8% pCCA).[40] The study was powered to detect a difference in median relapse-free survival of 18 months in the surveillance arm compared with 30 months in the gemcitabine and oxaliplatin arm. Ultimately, there was no difference observed in relapse-free survival, quality of life, and overall survival between the 2 treatment arms.[40] The study has been criticized for the statistical parameters used to determine effect size that may have ultimately led to the study not being adequately powered to detect a smaller but potentially important clinical difference between the 2 groups. Nonetheless, the doublet of gemcitabine–oxaliplatin remains a treatment option and continues to be incorporated into clinical trial design for patients with advanced BTC.

BILCAP: Capecitabine or Observation After Surgery in Treating Patients with Biliary Tract Cancer

The multicenter phase III BILCAP trial United Kingdom included 447 patients from the United Kingdom with cholangiocarcinoma (19% iCCA, 29% pCCA, and 35% distal CCA) or GBC (18%) who underwent resection with curative intent and then randomized to 8 cycles of adjuvant capecitabine or surveillance (NCT00363584).[41] The trial was powered to detect a difference in overall survival from 20% to 32% with the primary endpoint as overall survival in the intent-to-treat population and overall survival as a secondary endpoint in the per-protocol population. When the trial was reported in 2017 it did not meet its primary endpoint in the intention-to-treat population ($P = .09$). However, in the per-protocol analysis, there was a significant overall survival benefit in the group treated with capecitabine (53 vs 36 months, adjusted hazard ratio [HR] 0.75, 95% CI 0.58–0.97; $P=.028$).[41] Currently, adjuvant capecitabine is the adjuvant standard of care for patients with BTC resected with curative intent.

BCAT: The Bile Duct Cancer Adjuvant Trial

The BCAT was a phase III multicenter trial in Japan published in 2018 randomized 226 patients with extrahepatic cholangiocarcinoma (hilar 45% and distal 55%) who had undergone resection and then were to receive 6 cycles of gemcitabine compared with surveillance alone (UMIN 000000820).[42] There was no difference observed in overall survival (62.3 vs 63.8 months) or relapse-free survival among the 2 groups (36 vs 39.9 months).[42]

Table 1
Therapeutic targets and approach to molecular profiling in biliary tract cancers

	Frequency*	Targeted agents	Molecular test
IDH1	13% of intrahepatic cholangiocarcinoma cases[100,117]	Ivosidenib	Tumour next-generation DNA sequencing or targeted sequencing for hotspot mutations in coding region of IDH1
FGFR pathway	20% of intrahepatic cholangiocarcinoma cases[121]	Erdafitinib;[122] futibatinib;[121] infigratinib;[123] pemigatinib[101]	Tumour next-generation DNA sequencing including FGFR2 intronic region, targeted RNAseq, or FISH testing for FGFR2 translocation
BRAF	5% of intrahepatic cholangiocarcinoma cases[114,116]	Dabrafenib plus trametinib;[124] vemurafenib[125]	Tumour next-generation DNA sequencing or targeted sequencing for hotspot mutations in coding region of BRAF
MSI-high or MMR deficiency	2% of biliary tract cancer cases[126]	Pembrolizumab[126]	Multiple testing modalities available: PCR, immunohistochemistry, or tumour next-generation DNA sequencing
ERBB2 (HER2)	15–20% gallbladder cancer and extrahepatic cholangiocarcinoma cases[114,116]	..	Multiple testing modalities available including immunohistochemistry and FISH for expression and amplification, tumour next-generation DNA sequencing for mutations
NTRK	Rare	Entrectinib;[127] larotrectenib[128]	Tumour next-generation DNA sequencing including NTRK intronic region or targeted RNAseq, or FISH testing for NTRK translocation

IDH1=isocitrate dehydrogenase-1. FGFR=fibroblast growth factor receptor-2. FISH=fluorescent in-situ hybridisation. BRAF=activating serine threonine-protein kinase B-raf kinase. MSI=microsatellite instability. MMR=mismatch repair. ERBB2=receptor tyrosine-protein kinase erbB-2. NTRK=neurotrophic receptor tyrosine kinase. *All percentages are approximations.

Reprinted with permission from Elsevier. The Lancet, Vol 397, Issue 10272, 2021, p.428-444, Juan W Valle et al., "Biliary tract cancer", https://doi.org/10.1016/S0140-6736(21)00153-7.

S0809: The Adjuvant Capecitabine and Gemcitabine Followed by Radiotherapy and Concurrent Capecitabine in Extrahepatic Cholangiocarcinoma and Gallbladder Carcinoma

The S0809 (NCT00789958) cooperative group trial run through SWOG evaluated the impact of chemoradiation in the adjuvant setting to improve overall survival possibly by decreasing locoregional recurrence.[43] This study reported in 2015 was a single-arm, phase II multicenter trial of 79 patients with extrahepatic cholangiocarcinoma (pCCA or distal CCA) or GBC who underwent surgical resection with curative intent having stage pT2-4, node-positive, or positive resection margins. Patients were given 4 cycles of gemcitabine and capecitabine and then concurrent capecitabine with radiotherapy to the regional lymphatics and tumor bed. The overall survival was 67% in the R0 group and 60% in the R1 group. Local recurrence at 2 years was 9% in the R0 group and 16% in the R1 group. This trial has not been expanded to a phase III randomized design but does remain a treatment option at many cancer centers for patients meeting the pathologic criteria who have excellent performance status.

Prospective Randomized Controlled Trial Comparing Adjuvant Chemotherapy Versus No Chemotherapy for Patients with Carcinoma of Gallbladder Undergoing Curative Resection

In a single-center open-label phase III trial (NCT02778308) reported in 2022, 100 patients with GBC who had undergone R0 resection were randomized to surveillance alone or 6 cycles of adjuvant gemcitabine and cisplatin.[44] There was no statistical difference in recurrence (44% vs 56%; P=.23), disease-free survival (DFS), or overall survival between the 2 arms.[44]

ASCOT: The Adjuvant S-1 for Cholangiocarcinoma Trial (JCOG1202)

Reported in 2022, ASCOT (JCOG1202) was an open-label, multicenter, randomized phase III trial of 440 patients treated with adjuvant S-1 (oral fluoropyrimidine derivative) for up to 24 weeks compared with surveillance alone (UMIN000011688).[45] The study was powered to detect a 10% improvement in the 3-year overall survival in the S-1 adjuvant arm compared with surveillance alone. Similar to the ABC-02 trial, the JCOG1202 trial included patients with ampullary adenocarcinoma (17%), extrahepatic CCA (56%), GBC (15%), and iCCA (13%). Patients randomized to adjuvant S-1 had improved overall survival compared with surveillance at 3 years (77% vs 68%, HR 0.694; 95% CI, 0.514–0.935; P = .008). However, there was no difference in relapse-free survival at 3 years between the 2 arms.[46]

ACTICCA-1: Adjuvant Chemotherapy with Gemcitabine and Cisplatin Compared with Observation after Curative Intent Resection of Cholangiocarcinoma and Muscle Invasive Gallbladder Carcinoma

When the ACTICCA-1 trial opened in 2014, it was a randomized, multicenter, multinational phase III trial of patients with resected GBC or CCA comparing adjuvant therapy with gemcitabine and cisplatin or surveillance alone (NCT02170090). However, when BILCAP was reported in 2017, adjuvant capecitabine become the new monotherapy standard of care for patients with resected BTCs and the control arm was changed from observation to adjuvant capecitabine for 24 weeks with study enrollment increased from 450 to 781 in 2017. The study is powered to detect an increase in DFS at 2 years from 40% to 55% in cholangiocarcinoma and 35% to 55% in GBC. The primary endpoint is DFS and secondary endpoints were overall survival, safety and tolerability of chemotherapy, quality of life, and patterns of disease recurrence. The trial is still accruing patients with an expected study completion date of 2024.[47]

Peri-operative clinical trials

Gallbladder cancer: optimal peri-operative therapy for incidental gallbladder cancer (OPT-IN). Given the high-risk of recurrent disease in patients undergoing resection for GBC, there has been growing interest in the peri-operative treatment of patients with incidentally discovered GBC. In 2020, the National Clinical Trials Network opened the EA2197 "Optimal Peri-operative Therapy for Incidental Gallbladder Cancer (OPT-IN)" (NCT04559139). OPT-IN is a phase II/III peri-operative trial randomized for patients with histologically confirmed stage T2 or T3 incidental GBC found during or after elective cholecystectomy. The patients must not have metastatic or advanced loco-regional disease. The trial design includes 186 patients randomized 2:1 to receive neoadjuvant therapy with 4 cycles of gemcitabine and cisplatin, followed by resection, followed by an additional 4 cycles of gemcitabine–cisplatin or upfront re-resection followed by 8 cycles of adjuvant gemcitabine–cisplatin. The primary endpoint is overall survival. The trial is currently accruing patients with an estimated study completion date of September 2023.[48]

Neoadjuvant clinical trials

Intrahepatic cholangiocarcinoma: a single-arm feasibility study of gemcitabine, cisplatin, and nab-paclitaxel as neoadjuvant therapy for resectable oncologically high-risk intrahepatic cholangiocarcinoma. The results of the phase II trial "A Single-Arm Feasibility Study of Gemcitabine, Cisplatin, and Nab-Paclitaxel as Neoadjuvant Therapy for Resectable Oncologically High-Risk Intrahepatic Cholangiocarcinoma (NEO-GAP)" were just reported at ASCO 2022 after the trial completed accrual of 30 patients over 3 years from 2018 to 2021 (NCT03579771).[49] This single-arm trial used the triplet of gemcitabine, cisplatin, and nab-paclitaxel (GAP) as neoadjuvant therapy for high-risk but resectable iCCA based on encouraging results from the recently completed S1815 trial that randomized patients with advanced BTC to gemcitabine–cisplatin versus GAP (NCT03768414). "High-risk" iCCA was defined as T stage greater or equal to Ib, solitary lesion greater than 5 cm in size, multi-focal intrahepatic tumors, presence of major vascular invasion, or suspicious or involved regional lymph nodes. After treatment with up to 4 cycles of neoadjuvant GAP, patients underwent standard of care hepatectomy with portal lymphadenectomy. The primary objective of the trial was feasibility and the secondary objectives include radiographic response rate, R0 resection rate, recurrence-free survival, and overall survival. Overall, 23 (77%) patients completed all neoadjuvant GAP treatment and underwent surgical resection. Partial response was seen in 23% with the disease control rate of 90% with the trial meeting its primary objective of feasibility.[49]

Liver-directed therapy trials

Intrahepatic cholangiocarcinoma: hepatic arterial infusion with floxuridine and dexamethasone combined with systemic gemcitabine and oxaliplatin in patients with unresectable intrahepatic cholangiocarcinoma. The use of hepatic arterial infusion (HAI) of floxuridine has been studied in combination with systemic gemcitabine and oxaliplatin in patients with unresectable liver-dominant iCCA.[50] In a single-arm phase II clinical trial reported in 2020 (NCT01862315), 38 patients were treated with HAI floxuridine/dexamethasone and concurrent systemic gemcitabine plus oxaliplatin with the primary endpoint of progression-free survival of 80% at 6 months. The median PFS was 11.8 months (one-sided 90% CI, 11.1) with a 6-month PFS rate of 84.1% (90% CI, 74.8% to infinity). Overall, 58% of patients achieved a partial radiographic response with 13% of patients (*n* = 4) were converted from initially unresectable to resectable status and treated with hepatic resecton.[50] The results of this trial have led to a multicenter phase II trial recently open to accrual now randomizing 164 patients with unresectable iCCA to systemic chemotherapy with gemcitabine and oxaliplatin or to combinatorial therapy with systemic gemcitabine–oxaliplatin plus HAI floxuridine/dexamethasone (NCT04891289). The trial is powered on the primary outcome of progression-free survival with study completion anticipated in 2024.

SUMMARY

The group of biliary tract malignancies covered in this article—including GBC, iCCA, and pCCA—often present at an advanced stage with metastatic or unresectable disease. Patients are rarely cured without a having margin-negative surgical resection that is now often accompanied by a portal lymphadenectomy for staging. Although biliary malignancies have historically been grouped together in clinical trials, they are genetically heterogenous with distinct mutational drivers rendering them sensitive to specific targeted therapies. Adjuvant therapy for patients BTC resected with curative intent is capecitabine for 24 weeks (8 cycles) based on the BILCAP trial.[41] Several disease-specific neoadjuvant and peri-operative trials are underway with the potential to incorporate combinatorial therapy with cytotoxic and targeted inhibitors. Integrating liver-directed therapy with HAI and combined with systemic therapy can control hepatic disease and facilitate conversion to resection in 10% of patients with initially unresectable iCCA. As our understanding of the unique biology driving the family of biliary tract malignancies continues to evolve, we anticipate an ongoing evolution of a personalized therapy approach rendering more patients these rare cancers candidates for surgical resection and ultimately cure of their disease.

CLINICS CARE POINTS

- Pre-operative contrast-enhanced liver MRI can detect intrahepatic disease multifocality and staging laparoscopy can detect radiographically occult metastatic disease—both modalities can help select patients most likely to benefit from resection with curative intent.

- Next-generation sequencing can detect mutational drivers in upwards of 30% of patients with biliary tract cancers and should be ordered as the standard of care on pre-operative biopsies or the surgical resection specimen to fully inform treatment and potential clinical trial options.

- Similar to other disease sites, systemic treatment of biliary tract cancers is evolving from single agent adjuvant cytotoxic chemotherapy regimens into multi-agent therapies with cytotoxic and targeted agents delivered in the neoadjuvant and peri-operative setting.

DISCLOSURE

The authors have nothing to disclose.

REFERENCES

1. Siegel RL, Miller KD, Fuchs HE, et al. Cancer statistics, 2022. CA Cancer J Clin 2022;72(1):7–33.
2. Mosele F, Stefanovska B, Lusque A, et al. Outcome and molecular landscape of patients with PIK3CA-mutated metastatic breast cancer. Ann Oncol 2020;31(3):377–86.
3. National Comprehensive Cancer Network. Hepatobiliary Cancers.(Version 1.2022). Available at: https://www.nccn.org/professionals/physician_gls/pdf/hepatobiliary.pdf. Accessed May 23, 2022.
4. Hundal R, Shaffer EA. Gallbladder cancer: epidemiology and outcome. Clin Epidemiol 2014;6:99–109.
5. Henley SJ, Weir HK, Jim MA, et al. Gallbladder Cancer Incidence and Mortality, United States 1999-2011. Cancer Epidemiol biomarkers Prev 2015;24(9):1319–26.
6. Varshney S, Butturini G, Gupta R. Incidental carcinoma of the gallbladder. Eur J Surg Oncol 2002;28(1):4–10.
7. Duffy A, Capanu M, Abou-Alfa GK, et al. Gallbladder cancer (GBC): 10-year experience at Memorial Sloan-Kettering Cancer Centre (MSKCC). J Surg Oncol 2008;98(7):485–9.
8. Misra MC, Guleria S. Management of cancer gallbladder found as a surprise on a resected gallbladder specimen. J Surg Oncol 2006;93(8):690–8.
9. Patel N, Benipal B. Incidence of Cholangiocarcinoma in the USA from 2001 to 2015: A US Cancer Statistics Analysis of 50 States. Cureus 2019;11(1):e3962.
10. Shaib YH, Davila JA, McGlynn K, et al. Rising incidence of intrahepatic cholangiocarcinoma in the United States: a true increase? J Hepatol 2004;40(3):472–7.

11. Klatskin G. Adenocarcinoma of the Hepatic Duct at Its Bifurcation within the Porta Hepatis. An Unusual Tumor with Distinctive Clinical and Pathological Features. Am J Med 1965;38:241–56.
12. Sutton TL, Walker BS, Radu S, et al. Degree of biliary tract violation during treatment of gallbladder adenocarcinoma is independently associated with development of peritoneal carcinomatosis. J Surg Oncol 2021;124(4):581–8.
13. Benson AB, D'Angelica MI, Abbott DE, et al. Hepatobiliary Cancers, Version 2.2021, NCCN Clinical Practice Guidelines in Oncology. J Natl Compr Canc Netw 2021;19(5):541–65.
14. Okami J, Dono K, Sakon M, et al. Patterns of regional lymph node involvement in intrahepatic cholangiocarcinoma of the left lobe. J Gastrointest Surg 2003;7(7): 850–6.
15. Bismuth H, Nakache R, Diamond T. Management strategies in resection for hilar cholangiocarcinoma. Ann Surg 1992;215(1):31–8.
16. Aloia TA, Jarufe N, Javle M, et al. Gallbladder cancer: expert consensus statement. HPB (Oxford) 2015;17(8):681–90.
17. Agarwal AK, Kalayarasan R, Javed A, et al. The role of staging laparoscopy in primary gall bladder cancer–an analysis of 409 patients: a prospective study to evaluate the role of staging laparoscopy in the management of gallbladder cancer. Ann Surg 2013;258(2):318–23.
18. Fuks D, Regimbeau JM, Le Treut YP, et al. Incidental gallbladder cancer by the AFC-GBC-2009 Study Group. World J Surg 2011;35(8):1887–97.
19. Araida T, Higuchi R, Hamano M, et al. Hepatic resection in 485 R0 pT2 and pT3 cases of advanced carcinoma of the gallbladder: results of a Japanese Society of Biliary Surgery survey–a multicenter study. J Hepatobiliary Pancreat Surg 2009; 16(2):204–15.
20. D'Angelica M, Dalal KM, DeMatteo RP, et al. Analysis of the extent of resection for adenocarcinoma of the gallbladder. Ann Surg Oncol 2009;16(4):806–16.
21. Maker AV, Butte JM, Oxenberg J, et al. Is port site resection necessary in the surgical management of gallbladder cancer? Ann Surg Oncol 2012;19(2):409–17.
22. Edge SBMB, Frederick LG. American Joint Committee on cancer (AJCC) staging Handbook: from the AJCC cancer staging Manual. 8th edition. Cham, Switzerland: American Cancer Society; 2016.
23. Ito H, Ito K, D'Angelica M, et al. Accurate staging for gallbladder cancer: implications for surgical therapy and pathological assessment. Ann Surg 2011; 254(2):320–5.
24. de Jong MC, Nathan H, Sotiropoulos GC, et al. Intrahepatic cholangiocarcinoma: an international multi-institutional analysis of prognostic factors and lymph node assessment. J Clin Oncol 2011;29(23):3140–5.
25. Spolverato G, Yakoob MY, Kim Y, et al. The Impact of Surgical Margin Status on Long-Term Outcome After Resection for Intrahepatic Cholangiocarcinoma. Ann Surg Oncol 2015;22(12):4020–8.
26. Zhang XF, Pawlik TM. Response to the Comment on "Number and Station of Lymph Node Metastasis After Curative-intent Resection of Intrahepatic Cholangiocarcinoma Impact Prognosis. Ann Surg 2021;274(6):e743.
27. Zhang XF, Xue F, Dong DH, et al. Number and Station of Lymph Node Metastasis After Curative-intent Resection of Intrahepatic Cholangiocarcinoma Impact Prognosis. Ann Surg 2021;274(6):e1187–95.
28. Jarnagin WR, Fong Y, DeMatteo RP, et al. Staging, resectability, and outcome in 225 patients with hilar cholangiocarcinoma. Ann Surg 2001;234(4):507–17 [discussion: 517–9].

29. Jain V, Krishnamurthy G, Kumar H, et al. Anatomical Basis of Routine Caudate Lobe Resections in Hilar Cholangiocarcinoma. J Gastrointest Surg 2021;25(8): 2114–5.

30. Wahab MA, Sultan AM, Salah T, et al. Caudate lobe resection with major hepatectomy for central cholangiocarcinoma: is it of value? Hepatogastroenterology 2012;59(114):321–4.

31. Birgin E, Rasbach E, Reissfelder C, et al. A systematic review and meta-analysis of caudate lobectomy for treatment of hilar cholangiocarcinoma. Eur J Surg Oncol 2020;46(5):747–53.

32. Lamarca A, Barriuso J, McNamara MG, et al. Molecular targeted therapies: Ready for "prime time" in biliary tract cancer. J Hepatol 2020;73(1):170–85.

33. Valle JW, Kelley RK, Nervi B, et al. Biliary tract cancer. Lancet 2021;397(10272): 428–44.

34. Zhu AX, Macarulla T, Javle MM, et al. Final Overall Survival Efficacy Results of Ivosidenib for Patients With Advanced Cholangiocarcinoma With IDH1 Mutation: The Phase 3 Randomized Clinical ClarIDHy Trial. JAMA Oncol 2021;7(11):1669–77.

35. Abou-Alfa GK, Sahai V, Hollebecque A, et al. Pemigatinib for previously treated, locally advanced or metastatic cholangiocarcinoma: a multicentre, open-label, phase 2 study. Lancet Oncol 2020;21(5):671–84.

36. Bekaii-Saab TS, Valle JW, Van Cutsem E, et al. FIGHT-302: first-line pemigatinib vs gemcitabine plus cisplatin for advanced cholangiocarcinoma with FGFR2 rearrangements. Future Oncol 2020;16(30):2385–99.

37. Jarnagin WR, Ruo L, Little SA, et al. Patterns of initial disease recurrence after resection of gallbladder carcinoma and hilar cholangiocarcinoma: implications for adjuvant therapeutic strategies. Cancer 2003;98(8):1689–700.

38. Doussot A, Gonen M, Wiggers JK, et al. Recurrence Patterns and Disease-Free Survival after Resection of Intrahepatic Cholangiocarcinoma: Preoperative and Postoperative Prognostic Models. J Am Coll Surg 2016;223(3):493–505 e2.

39. Valle J, Wasan H, Palmer DH, et al. Cisplatin plus gemcitabine versus gemcitabine for biliary tract cancer. N Engl J Med 2010;362(14):1273–81.

40. Edeline J, Benabdelghani M, Bertaut A, et al. Gemcitabine and Oxaliplatin Chemotherapy or Surveillance in Resected Biliary Tract Cancer (PRODIGE 12-ACCORD 18-UNICANCER GI): A Randomized Phase III Study. J Clin Oncol 2019;37(8):658–67.

41. Primrose JN, Fox RP, Palmer DH, et al. Capecitabine compared with observation in resected biliary tract cancer (BILCAP): a randomised, controlled, multicentre, phase 3 study. Lancet Oncol 2019;20(5):663–73.

42. Ebata T, Hirano S, Konishi M, et al. Randomized clinical trial of adjuvant gemcitabine chemotherapy versus observation in resected bile duct cancer. Br J Surg 2018;105(3):192–202.

43. Ben-Josef E, Guthrie KA, El-Khoueiry AB, et al. SWOG S0809: A Phase II Intergroup Trial of Adjuvant Capecitabine and Gemcitabine Followed by Radiotherapy and Concurrent Capecitabine in Extrahepatic Cholangiocarcinoma and Gallbladder Carcinoma. J Clin Oncol 2015;33(24):2617–22.

44. Saluja SS, Nekarakanti PK, Mishra PK, et al. Prospective Randomized Controlled Trial Comparing Adjuvant Chemotherapy vs. No Chemotherapy for Patients with Carcinoma of Gallbladder Undergoing Curative Resection. J Gastrointest Surg 2022;26(2):398–407.

45. Nakachi K, Konishi M, Ikeda M, et al. A randomized Phase III trial of adjuvant S-1 therapy vs. observation alone in resected biliary tract cancer: Japan Clinical

Oncology Group Study (JCOG1202, ASCOT). Jpn J Clin Oncol 2018;48(4): 392–5.

46. Ikeda M, Nakachi K, Konishi M, et al. Adjuvant S-1 versus observation in curatively resected biliary tract cancer: A phase III trial (JCOG1202: ASCOT). J Clin Oncol 2022;40(suppl 4). https://doi.org/10.1200/JCO.2022.40.4_suppl.382):382.

47. Deutsche Krebshilfe E.V. BGCRUAG-ITGDHC, (DHCG) CCG. Adjuvant Chemotherapy With Gemcitabine and Cisplatin Compared to Standard of Care After CurativeIntent Resection of Biliary Tract Cancer (ACTICCA-1). Available at: https://www.clinicaltrials.gov/ct2/show/NCT02170090. Accessed April 20, 2022.

48. SK M. Comparison of Chemotherapy Before and After Surgery Versus After Surgery Alone for the Treatment of Gallbladder Cancer (OPT-IN EA2197). Available at: https://clinicaltrials.gov/ct2/show/NCT04559139. Accessed April 20, 2022.

49. Maithel SK, Javle MM, Mahipal A, et al. NEO-GAP: A phase II single-arm prospective feasibility study of neoadjuvant gemcitabine/cisplatin/nab-paclitaxel for resectable high-risk intrahepatic cholangiocarcinoma. J Clin Oncol 2022;(16_suppl):4097.

50. Cercek A, Boerner T, Tan BR, et al. Assessment of Hepatic Arterial Infusion of Floxuridine in Combination With Systemic Gemcitabine and Oxaliplatin in Patients With Unresectable Intrahepatic Cholangiocarcinoma: A Phase 2 Clinical Trial. JAMA Oncol 2020;6(1):60–7.

An Overview of Clinical Trials in the Treatment of Resectable Hepatocellular Carcinoma

Nicole M. Nevarez, MD*, Gloria Y. Chang, MD,
Adam C. Yopp, MD

KEYWORDS

- Hepatocellular carcinoma • Liver cancer • Clinical trials

KEY POINTS

- Extensive research has been conducted to identify therapeutic strategies using many different modalities to complement curative HCC therapy (resection, ablation, or transplantation).
- There are currently no adjuvant or neoadjuvant therapy options with sufficient data to be implemented as the standard of care.
- The results of numerous ongoing randomized clinical trials evaluating immunotherapy options are eagerly awaited.

INTRODUCTION

Hepatocellular carcinoma (HCC) has the seventh highest incidence and is the third most common cause of cancer-related mortality worldwide.[1] Most commonly found in a background of underlying chronic liver disease with concomitant cirrhosis, overall prognosis is dependent on tumor stage, patient functional status, and degree of hepatic dysfunction.[2] The concomitant liver dysfunction and tumor burden influence the HCC treatment paradigm and ultimately long-term survival. A multidisciplinary treatment approach encompassing specialists along the cancer care continuum is paramount to ensure appropriate HCC treatment decisions.[3]

Currently, the only curative therapeutic options for HCC are hepatic transplantation, partial hepatectomy, and hepatic tumor ablation. Although liver transplantation not only treats the HCC tumor but also the underlying cirrhotic liver, the majority of

Supported with funding by: 1R01MD012565-01 (A.C. Yopp and N.M. Nevarez).
Department of Surgery, Division of Surgical Oncology, University of Texas Southwestern Medical Center, 5323 Harry Hines Boulevard, Dallas, TX 75390, USA
* Corresponding author.
E-mail address: nicole.nevarez@phhs.org

Surg Oncol Clin N Am 32 (2023) 101–117
https://doi.org/10.1016/j.soc.2022.07.008
1055-3207/23/

surgonc.theclinics.com

patients presenting with HCC fail to meet the criteria for liver transplantation either due to size of tumor, number of tumors, or macrovascular invasion.[4] Additionally, the shortage of organs makes this option challenging. In the setting of preserved liver function, hepatic tumor ablation and partial hepatectomy are equivalent in outcomes with the suitability of ablation dependent on smaller tumors, typically less than 2 cm.[5] Despite 5-year survival rates following surgical resection approaching 60%, less than 40% of patients newly diagnosed with HCC are suitable for partial hepatectomy due to advanced tumor biology and low HCC screening rates.[6–9] As such, numerous investigators through clinical trials, either surgical or nonsurgical therapy based, have attempted to improve overall survival by reducing rates of recurrence.

The goals of this review are to describe the existing clinical trials that have been conducted assessing surgical technique in partial hepatectomy and adjuvant and neoadjuvant therapies for HCC and to use this information to formulate evidence-based treatment plans for resectable HCC to reduce the risk of recurrence and improve survival.

CLINICAL TRIALS IN THE SURGICAL TECHNIQUE FOR HEPATECTOMY
Anatomic and Nonanatomic Approaches to Partial Hepatectomy

Curative therapy for HCC remains hepatic resection, liver transplantation, and ablation. However, even with hepatic resection, recurrence rates of HCC remain high, with reports of recurrence in 50% in the first 3 years and up to 70% during the first 5 years.[6] The goal of curative hepatic resection involves obtaining negative resection margins while preserving sufficient liver volume thus avoiding postoperative liver failure. This is often challenging because those with HCC frequently have underlying liver disease. The 2 primary surgical techniques for curative resection of HCC are anatomic resection (AR) and nonanatomic resection (NAR).

AR, as first described by Makuuchi in 1985, the primary tumor, the parenchyma of the segment or subsegment wherein the tumor resides, and its associated portal venous tributaries are resected together thus the tumor free margin is not contingent on cut liver surface.[10] NAR relies on the removal of the tumor using a parenchymal preserving method independent of segmental or lobar anatomy, with the cut liver surface providing the tumor-free margin. Because NAR typically involves less extensive liver resection, it confers the theoretical benefit of decreased risk of postoperative liver failure secondary to insufficient future liver remnant.

From a technical perspective, one of 2 main surgical approaches is used to accomplish AR: (1) ultrasound-guided transection or (2) Glissonean pedicle transection. With ultrasound-guided transection, indigo carmine dye is injected into the portal vein under ultrasound guidance while the hepatic artery is occluded at the hilum. A line of demarcation becomes visible along the liver surface and the blue stained parenchyma is used as a guide as dissection is carried out starting from the liver surface moving inward toward the portal pedicle.[10] Indocyanine green fluorescent dye can be used in lieu of indigo carmine, particularly in settings in which ultrasound liver mapping is difficult, as may be the case due to portal hypertension from cirrhosis.[11]

Glissonean pedicle transection was initially described by Couinaud for anatomic left hepatectomy in 1985.[12] Takasaki described a modified method in 1998 using a Glissonean pedicle tree classification in which the liver is divided into 3 hepatic segments (not including the caudate): right, middle, and left.[13] The structures within the hepatoduodenal ligament (artery, portal vein, and bile duct) continue to travel together in their branching pattern within the same fibrous sheath. The main pedicle, formed by the hepatoduodenal ligament, divides at the hilum into right and left primary branches, then into secondary branches as right, middle, and left branches, which supply the corresponding right (Couinaud segments 6 and 7), middle (Couinaud segments 5 and 8), and left hepatic segments (Couinaud segments 2, 3, and 4). The right hepatic vein courses between the right and middle segments, making up the right interseg-mental plane, whereas the middle hepatic vein runs between the middle and left he-patic segments to make up the left intersegmental plane. Subsequent division of the right, middle, and left branches lead to the tertiary branches that supply the small-est segmental unit, termed "cone unit." With the Glissonean pedicle transection tech-nique, the pedicle corresponding to the tumor-containing hepatic segment is first ligated and transected, and then the liver parenchyma is dissected along the interseg-mental plane, following the trunk of the hepatic vein.

Because HCC tends to invade portal venous branches, HCC tumor cells are theo-rized to disseminate via the portal venous system, leading to intrahepatic metasta-ses.[6] Because AR removes the tumor-containing liver segment along with its portal vein tributaries, AR in theory should reduce micrometastatic disease and therefore local recurrence (LR) of HCC after hepatic resection. However, despite this potential benefit, there is a lack of consensus in the literature regarding the superiority of AR over NAR.

Current literature comparing AR and NAR approaches in patients with HCC largely relies on retrospective studies with heterogeneous patient populations. As such, mul-tiple systemic reviews and meta-analyses have been conducted in an attempt to consolidate patient data and reach a consensus about which surgical approach is associated with improved outcome measures (**Table 1**). Surprisingly, despite many of the studies including cases from the same retrospective studies, conclusions

Table 1
Summary of meta-analyses comparing anatomic vs nonanatomic resection in hepatocellular carcinoma patients

Reference	Extent of Resection	Number of Patients	Outcome
Zhou et al,[15] 2011	AR	1577	5-y OS: 66.8%
	NAR	1340	55.5%
Ye et al,[16] 2012	AR	810	5-y OS OR: 1.24
	NAR	766	
Cucchetti et al,[17] 2012	AR	4012	Pooled 5-y OS: 62.0%
	NAR	5024	54.4%
Feng et al,[18] 2017	AR	52	Median OS: 210 wk
	NAR	53	150 wk
Huang [19] 2017	AR	1626	5-y OS: 69%
	NAR	1503	56%
TaN et al,[20] 2017	AR	4576	5-y OS: 64.9%
	NAR	5640	61.1%
Moris et al,[21] 2018	AR	6839	5-y OS HR: 0.88
	NAR	5590	
Famularo et al,[22] 2021	AR	1776	5-y RR: 0.89
	NAR	1669	
Sun et al, 2022	AR	449	5-y OS RR: 0.76
	NAR	488	

vary between the studies depending on the variables and outcome measures that were included in the meta-analyses.[14–23]

There is only one published randomized controlled trial comparing AR and NAR for HCC resection. In 2017, Feng and colleagues[18] published a single institution, prospective clinical trial in China where 105 patients with confirmed, localized HCC were randomized to AR or NAR. The primary endpoint was 2-year LR rate, which was defined as recurrence occurring in the same hepatic section as that of the resected primary tumor. Tumor recurrence in liver parenchyma outside the original primary tumor-containing segment was defined as distant recurrence, whereas recurrence outside the liver was deemed extrahepatic recurrence.

The AR group had a significantly lower 2-year LR at 30% compared with 59% for the NAR group. Total LR rates were 42% and 68% for the AR and NAR groups, respectively. No significant differences were found between the 2 groups for perioperative outcomes or postoperative complications. There was also no significant difference in overall survival nor overall recurrence rate, which was defined as the combined rates of local, distant, and extrahepatic recurrences. The authors concluded that their results suggest a benefit of AR in reducing LR rates, thus supporting the hypothesis of dissemination of micrometastases via portal blood.

This study was limited, however, by the narrow scope of the primary endpoint and their definition of LR. In limiting LR to only the same segment as that of the primary tumor, recurrent disease elsewhere in the liver or extrahepatically are effectively censored. When they are accounted for, as measured by overall recurrence, there is no significant difference between the 2 groups. The study population was also limited to HCC patients classified as Child-Pugh A with only about half of the patient population carrying a diagnosis of liver cirrhosis. Furthermore, the majority of their study population had chronic liver disease attributed to viral hepatitis B (HBV). These population characteristics make their findings difficult to apply in settings in patients with severe liver dysfunction, cirrhosis, or other causes of chronic liver disease.

Although AR theoretically provides the benefit of preventing further dissemination of micrometastatic disease via the portal venous system, it remains a challenging operation with the risk of considerable morbidity and mortality, particularly with patients with severe liver dysfunction or borderline future liver remnants. NAR, however, mitigates the risk of postoperative liver failure by allowing for a parenchymal-sparing approach. The current evidence supporting the superiority of AR over NAR remains mixed due to heterogeneous study populations, narrow endpoints, and limited clinical trials.

Anterior and Conventional Approaches to Right Hepatectomy

When right hepatectomy is required for HCC, 2 main surgical approaches are used: a conventional approach (CA) and an anterior approach (AA). The CA involves complete mobilization of the right liver and vascular inflow and outflow control before performing parenchymal transection. With AA, vascular inflow control is obtained, parenchymal transection is completed, vascular outflow control is then obtained, and finally liver mobilization is performed removing the specimen.

With CA, vascular inflow control at the portal pedicle is first obtained with hilar dissection and isolation of the right hepatic artery and right portal vein. The right lobe of the liver is then dissected away from its attachments and moved away from the retrohepatic space to expose the inferior vena cava (IVC). During this maneuver, the right lobe is rotated anteriorly and to the left, resulting in twisting of the hepatoduodenal ligament. Once the anterior surface of the IVC is exposed, small caval venous branches are ligated and divided; the right hepatic vein is similarly isolated, ligated, and divided. Only after vascular inflow and outflow control has been attained and the right lobe of the liver has been completely mobilized is the hepatic parenchymal transection performed.

Although advances in surgical technique and anesthetic management during major hepatic resections have improved over the years, a CA during right hepatectomy remains a major surgery with several disadvantages. Particularly when right-sided tumors are large in size, the mobilization and obtaining of access to the right hepatic vein can be made more difficult with the limited space. Additionally, during mobilization, the hepatic vein and caval branches are at risk of avulsion and the rotation of the mobilized lobe twists the hepatoduodenal ligament, which can result in ischemic injury to the liver remnant.[24] Finally, mobilization can lead to iatrogenic tumor rupture and spillage of cancer cells contributing to postoperative HCC recurrence.

AA was introduced in 1996 by Lai and colleagues[25] as an alternative technique to the CA because vascular inflow is similarly first controlled with hilar dissection. The hepatic parenchyma is then transected starting on the anterior surface of the liver and moving toward the hepatic hilum. Once parenchymal transection is complete and the anterior surface of the IVC is exposed, venous outflow control is obtained by division and ligation of small caval veins and the right hepatic vein. Liver mobilization is then performed, only after inflow and outflow control and parenchymal transection is complete.

Although AA mitigates the risks of the aforementioned disadvantages presented with CA, the surgeon may still encounter the right or middle hepatic vein during deep parenchymal transection. Vascular injury at this stage can lead to massive bleeding that is difficult to control without a mobilized right liver and vascular control of the right hepatic vein. Belghiti and colleagues[26] expanded on the aforementioned through the utilization of the liver hanging maneuver in which a retrohepatic tunnel in an avascular space between the liver and IVC is created. A tape or Penrose tube is passed through this tunnel and utilized to suspend the liver away from the vena cava, thereby improving exposure and creating a straight transection plane. Although this modification of AA may decrease the risk of massive bleeding from the hepatic veins, there still remains the risk of increased intraoperative blood loss due to the blind passage of an instrument just anterior to the IVC placing the venous drainage of the caudate lobe at risk of being injured.

Liu and colleagues[27] performed the first prospective randomized controlled trial comparing AA technique with the CA on operative and survival outcomes for large HCC. One hundred twenty patients with right-sided liver HCC greater than or equal to 5 cm were randomized to curative major right hepatic resection via AA or CA. Although there was no significant difference between the 2 groups for overall operative blood loss, patients undergoing AA had a significantly decreased rate of major operative blood loss (defined as $\geq$ 2 L) and a corresponding decreased blood transfusion requirement compared with the CA group. No significant differences were found between the 2 groups in hospital or operative morbidity and duration of hospital stay. On survival analysis, although there was no significant difference in median disease-free survival between the 2 groups, patients undergoing AA had significantly improved overall survival with a median of greater than 68.1 months compared with the CA group (22.6 months, $P < .001$).

Because venous outflow remains intact at the time of liver mobilization, there is a theoretical increased risk of tumor cell dissemination into the systemic circulation with the CA. In their trial, Liu and colleagues measured plasma albumin-mRNA at various stages to reflect the circulation of liver cells during surgery. The AA group was found to have significantly lower plasma albumin-mRNA levels both before parenchymal transection and at the end of surgery after tumor removal compared with the CA group, thus supporting the notion that liver mobilization with intact venous outflow may lead to spillage of tumor cells into the venous system.

On multivariate analysis, tumor stage, AA resection, and resection margin were found to independently affect the overall survival. They concluded that the AA technique leads to improved operative and survival outcomes and propose it as the preferred technique for major right hepatic resection.

Liu and colleagues[27] findings demonstrated the benefit of the AA technique over CA for fewer major blood loss events and transfusion requirements and improved the overall survival. The findings of subsequent retrospective studies further substantiated these results.[28,29] Although AA technique may confer these benefits, there remains the difficult-to-control scenario of encountering massive bleeding from right hepatic vein or middle hepatic vein injury during deep parenchymal transection. Previous studies have demonstrated infrahepatic IVC clamping as a safe and effective method of reducing blood loss during hepatectomy.[30,31] In 2015, Zhou and colleagues[32] performed a prospective randomized controlled trial to evaluate the effect of combined AA right hepatectomy and infrahepatic IVC clamping on intraoperative blood loss with large HCC. A total of 101 patients with large right HCC eligible for right hepatectomy were randomized to undergo AA with infrahepatic clamping or AA alone. The group that underwent AA with infrahepatic clamping had significantly less total blood loss and blood loss during liver transection with a corresponding decrease in blood transfusion requirements compared to the AA alone group. There were no significant differences in severity of postoperative complications. There were no reported IVC clamping-associated morbidities and renal function was preserved in the AA with infrahepatic clamping group.

In both aforementioned RCTs, the study population was composed of patients with large HCC (>5 cm) undergoing right hepatectomy. Although their findings demonstrate improved operative outcomes and overall survival for this specific cohort of patients, the applicability of these findings to other populations remains unclear. In 2012, Capussotti and colleagues[33] performed a randomized clinical trial with 65 patients with primary or metastatic liver tumors of any size eligible for right hepatectomy. Patients were randomized to AA or CA with the aim of evaluating if routine application of AA right hepatectomy was associated with decreased intraoperative blood loss. They found no significant differences in overall blood loss, blood loss during parenchymal transection, and perioperative transfusion rates between the 2 groups. Parenchymal transection time was longer in the AA group but morbidity and mortality rates were similar. The authors concluded that AA for routine right hepatectomy compared with CA does not lead to improved early postoperative outcome, specifically overall blood loss, bleeding during parenchymal transection, and perioperative transfusion requirement. Notably, Capussotti's series was composed of a relatively heterogenous population with a variety of tumor pathologies, lesion median size smaller than that reported in other studies, and a low rate of cirrhotic patients. These factors may be important contributors to the mitigation of the potential benefits of AA on operative outcomes.

CLINICAL TRIALS IN ADJUVANT THERAPY FOR HEPATOCELLULAR CARCINOMA
Antiviral Therapy

Because many patients with HCC have underlying chronic liver disease from HBV and viral hepatitis C (HCV), some of the first therapies that were investigated centered around controlling viral hepatitis. Researchers hypothesized that HBV antiviral treatment will mitigate the progression of chronic liver disease and prevent intrahepatic recurrence of HCC after resection thereby improving overall survival. Many of these studies used interferon (IFN) as antiviral therapy but with mixed results. Chen and colleagues[34] enrolled 268 patients who were either hepatitis B surface antigen seropositive or hepatitis C antibody seropositive and randomized them to IFNα-2b or control. After median follow-up of 63.8 months, recurrence-free survival and overall survival were no different between the 2 groups. The 1-year, 3-year, and 5-year recurrence-free survival rates were 72.2%, 53.1%, 42.7% and 74.7%, 55.3%, 45.5% for the IFNα-2b and control groups, respectively (P = .829). The 1-year, 3-year, and 5-year overall survival rates were 96.2%, 84.1%, 75.4% and 95.6%, 83.7%, 72.5% for the IFNα-2b and control groups, respectively (P = .863). Notably, many patients in the treatment arm underwent dose reductions or withdrew from therapy due to adverse effects. In contrast to the findings of Chen and colleagues, Kubo and colleagues[35] found that adjuvant IFNα benefited patients with HCV-related HCC by improving cumulative survival rate over the control group (P = .041). Lo and colleagues investigated the role of adjuvant IFNα following curative HCC resection. There was no difference in the 1-year and 5-year survival rates between the control group and the IFNα group (85% and 61% versus 97% and 79%, P = .137). However, on subanalysis of stage III/IVA HCC tumors, IFNα prevented early recurrence and improved the 5-year overall survival from 24% to 68% (P = .038).[36] With regard to recurrence, both Kubo and colleagues[37] and Ikeda and colleagues[38] performed a small, randomized, controlled trials including HCV-related HCC patients, which showed that the recurrence rate was lower with IFNα over the control group.

In addition to IFN, many studies have investigated the role of nucleotide/nucleoside analogs as adjuvant antiviral therapy after surgical resection for HCC. Huang and colleagues[39] performed a randomized controlled trial of 200 patients with HBV who underwent curative resection for HCC and randomized them to adjuvant adefovir or no antiviral treatment. The 1-year, 3-year, and 5-year recurrence-free survival and overall survival rates for the antiviral group were significantly improved over the control group at 85.0%, 50.3%, 46.1% and 96.0%, 77.6%, 63.1% versus 84.0%, 37.9%, 27.1% and 94.0%, 67.4%, 41.5%, respectively (recurrence-free survival [RFS] P = .026 and overall survival [OS] P = .001). This recurrence and survival benefit was sustained with the use of telbivudine even when patients with low preoperative HBV-DNA levels were analyzed in another trial by Huang and colleagues.[40] Similar to the previous studies with adefovir and telbivudine, antiviral treatment with lamivudine compared with controls resulted in significantly decreased HCC recurrence and HCC-related death (hazard ratio [HR] 0.48, 95% CI 0.32–0.70 and HR 0.26, 95% CI 0.14–0.50).[41]

Brachytherapy

Little is known about the role of brachytherapy in HCC. The therapy is now largely abandoned with only one randomized clinical trial by Chen and colleagues in 2013.[42] In their study, 68 patients were randomized to either ^{125}iodine or placebo seed implantation after curative hepatectomy in Child's A patients with HCC. After median follow-up of 47.6 months, the time to recurrence was 60.0 months in the ^{125}iodine brachytherapy group versus 36.7 months in the control group (P = .008), which was the primary endpoint. The mean overall survival was 63.6 months versus 38.9 months in the ^{125}iodine and control group, respectively (P = .026). The 1-year, 3-year, and 5-year overall survival rates were 94.12%, 73.53%, and 55.88% for the ^{125}iodine brachytherapy group and 88.24%, 52.94%, and 29.41% for the control group (P = .026). More trials investigating brachytherapy are needed to confirm its survival benefits in HCC.

Systemic Chemotherapy

Sorafenib was the mainstay of treatment in advanced HCC for more than a decade before the pivotal trial of atezolizumab/bevacizumab.[43] Due to its benefit in advanced HCC, there was some thought that this drug may prevent recurrence and provide a survival benefit as an adjuvant treatment in patients undergoing resection for HCC. The STORM trial, a phase III, randomized, double-blind, placebo-controlled trial, compared adjuvant sorafenib to placebo in 1114 patients with HCC after surgical resection or local ablation.[44] Patients were stratified based on treatment modality, geography, Child's classification, and recurrence risk. There was no significant difference between the sorafenib and control groups in recurrence-free survival (HR 0.940, 95% CI 0.780–1.134, $P = .26$), time to recurrence (HR 0.891, 95% CI 0.735–1.081, $P = .12$), or overall survival (HR 0.995, 95% CI 0.761–1.300, $P = .48$).

Another chemotherapy regimen that has been studied is tegafur/uracil, a fluorinated pyrimidine. Previous studies indicated that there was a correlation between dihydropyrimidine dehydrogenase (DPD) and thymidylate synthase (TS) messenger RNA levels in HCC tumors and the antitumor effects of 5-fluorouracil.[45] In the study by Ishizuka and colleagues,[46] 117 patients who underwent a surgical resection for HCC were randomized to either adjuvant tegafur/uracil or surgery only. There was no difference in 1-year and 3-year recurrence-free survival rates between the tegafur/uracil group and the control group (87% and 27.5% versus 58.5% and 25.4%, $P = .16$) or 3-year and 5-year overall survival rates (89.3% and 64.3% versus 75.9% and 62.2%, $P = .29$). Only an overall survival benefit was identified in patients who received tegafur/uracil and had low TS and low DPD in their tumors ($P = .04$) but there was no difference in recurrence-free survival. In addition to not being an effective adjuvant therapy after resection of HCC, tegafur/uracil is not very well tolerated because more than half of the treatment arm in this study discontinued use due to adverse effects.

Finally, the only other systemic chemotherapeutic regimen that has been studied in the adjuvant setting is capecitabine due to effectiveness in other cancer types and previous studies showing its increased concentration in liver tissue in murine models.[47–49] Using this rationale, Xia and colleagues[50] conducted a randomized controlled trial, which enrolled 60 patients to either capecitabine or control after surgical resection for HCC. Although there was no difference in 5-year overall survival between the 2 arms, the capecitabine arm had significantly longer time to recurrence at 40.0 months compared with the control arm at 20.0 ($P = .046$). Moreover, in contrast to tegafur/uracil mentioned previously, capecitabine was rather well tolerated with mild adverse effects.

Immunotherapy

Immunotherapy has played a role in advanced HCC for many years now; however, little is known about the role of immunotherapy as adjuvant therapy after surgery or ablation.[51–56] The NIVOLVE trial, a phase II prospective multicenter single-arm trial, examined the safety and efficacy of adjuvant nivolumab after surgical resection or radiofrequency ablation.[57] The 1-year recurrence-free survival was 78.6% with a median recurrence-free survival of 26.3 months. Kudo and colleagues also concluded that copy number gains in the WNT/beta-catenin-related genes, activation of the WNT/beta-catenin pathway, presence of Foxp3+ cells, and low numbers of CD8+ tumor infiltrating lymphocytes may be markers for recurrence after surgical resection or radiofrequency ablation with adjuvant nivolumab. The results of ongoing clinical trials, including CheckMate 9DX investigating adjuvant nivolumab (NCT03383458),

IMBrave050 investigating adjuvant bevacizumab and atezolizumab (NCT04102098), KEYNOTE-937 investigating adjuvant pembrolizumab (NCT03867084), and EMERALD-2 investigating durvalumab with or without bevacizumab (NCT03847428) after surgical resection or ablation of HCC in patients that are high-risk for recurrence, are eagerly awaited.[58,59]

Another type of immunotherapy that gained traction was autologous cytokine-induced killer cells given in the adjuvant setting. Studies by Takayama and colleagues,[60] Hui and colleagues,[61] and Lee and colleagues[62] all performed randomized trials of "adoptive immunotherapy" versus control after curative treatment (surgical resection, radiofrequency ablation, or percutaneous ethanol injection) for HCC. Their protocols involved harvesting peripheral blood mononuclear cells from patients and treating the cells in vitro with interleukin-2 and a monoclonal antibody to CD3 to stimulate differentiation into cytokine-induced killer (CIK) cells. Hui and colleagues also treated the cells with IFN gamma and had 2 treatment arms (CIK-1 and CIK-2) differing only in the number of times that patients underwent cell transfusions. After in vitro treatment, the cytokine-induced killer cells were then transfused back to the patients in the treatment arm. Survival, either recurrence-free or disease-free depending on the study, was significantly longer in the treatment arms in all 3 studies compared with the control arms (Takayama 3-year: 48% vs 22%, 5-year: 38% vs 22%, $P = .008$; Hui 3-year: CIK-1 31.7% vs CIK-2 30.5% vs control 20.9%, 5-year: 23.3% vs 19.4% vs 11.2%, $P = .001$ [between CIK-1 and control] and $P = .004$ [between CIK-2 and control]; Lee HR 0.63, 95% CI 0.43–0.94, $P = .01$). There were no differences in overall survival in 2 of the studies[60,61]; only Lee and colleagues[62] found a significant overall survival benefit in the immunotherapy arm (HR 0.21, 95% CI 0.06–0.75, $P = .008$).

Transarterial Radioembolization

Transarterial radioembolization (TARE) using [90]yttrium and [131]iodine as an effective treatment modality for HCC was first documented in the 1980s.[63–65] Although [90]yttrium became a mainstay in the treatment algorithm for unresectable HCC, there was much interest in [131]iodine as an adjuvant therapeutic option after resection.[66] At first, the results were promising. The first randomized trial evaluating adjuvant [131]iodine-labeled lipiodol after resection was by Lau and colleagues[67] in 1999 where 43 patients were randomized to surgery then adjuvant [131]iodine lipiodol or surgery alone. The [131]iodine lipiodol group experienced a significantly lower recurrence rate compared with the control group (28.5% vs 59%, $P = .04$), median disease-free survival was 57.2 months in the [131]iodine lipiodol group compared with 13.6 months for the control group ($P = .037$), and a significantly longer 5-year overall survival (86.4 vs 46.3%, $P = .01$). When this same group published a long-term follow-up of their original study, they found that the disease-free and overall survival benefits from adjuvant treatment with [131]iodine lipiodol after surgical resection lasted for about 8 years after randomization but then disappeared.[68]

As researchers continued to study [131]iodine lipiodol for TARE, further studies failed to yield promising results. In 2013, Chung and colleagues[69] enrolled 103 patients after surgical resection and randomized them to either hepatic intra-arterial injection of [131]iodine lipiodol arm or control arm. Recurrence-free survival at 3 and 5 years were 47.6% and 45.0% versus 48.1% and 32.5% for the lipiodol and control, respectively (HR = 0.75, 95% CI 0.46–1.23, $P = .25$). The overall survival at 3 and 5 years were 86.6% and 54.2% and 69.2% and 54.3% for the lipiodol and control arms, respectively (HR 0.88, 95% CI 0.51–1.51, $P = .64$).

To further complicate the use of [131]iodine lipiodol, a subsequent study performed in 2014 by Dumortier and colleagues[70] had mixed results. This group studied 58 patients who underwent curative treatment of HCC and randomized them to [131]iodine lipiodol or unlabeled lipiodol arms. The 2-year intrahepatic recurrence rate was 28% in the [131]iodine lipiodol group and 56% in the unlabeled lipiodol group ($P = .0449$). The 2-year recurrence-free survival was 73% in the [131]iodine lipiodol group and 45% in the unlabeled lipiodol group ($P = .0259$). However, the overall survival was not statistically significantly different between the [131]iodine and unlabeled lipiodol groups ($P = .9378$).

Transarterial Chemoembolization

Similar to TARE, transarterial chemoembolization (TACE) has remained an important treatment modality in unresectable HCC. As such, investigators were eager to test its use in resectable HCC. In 2009, Zhong and colleagues[71] conducted a prospective, randomized trial where they enrolled 115 patients with stage IIIA HCC (according to the International Union Against Cancer, sixth edition)[72] or HCC complicated by portal venous tumor thrombus (PVTT) to either hepatectomy with adjuvant TACE (using epirubicin) or hepatectomy alone. The 1-year, 3-year, and 5-year overall survival for the adjuvant TACE arm were 80.7%, 33.3%, 22.8% compared with 56.5%, 19.4%, 17.5% for the control arm ($P = .048$). The 1-year, 3-year, and 5-year disease-free survival for the adjuvant TACE arm were 29.7%, 9.3%, 9.3% versus 14.0%, 3.5%, 1.7% for the control arm ($P = .004$). Similarly, Wang and colleagues[73] performed the same study protocol except using adriamycin but with a different patient population: patients with HBV-related HCC in China. Again, adjuvant TACE significantly increased 3-year recurrence-free survival and 3-year overall survival compared with the control group (56.0% vs 42.1%, $P = .01$ and 85.2% vs 77.4%, $P = .04$). Although these initial results of TACE as an adjuvant therapeutic option seemed to show a survival benefit, studies that are more modern show otherwise.

In 2020, Hirokawa and colleagues[74] performed a prospective randomized controlled trial of hepatectomy and adjuvant transarterial infusion (TAI; 2 doses: cisplatin alone then cisplatin with lipiodol) versus hepatectomy alone in 114 patients. There were no significant differences in disease-free survival or overall survival between the 2 groups. Specifically, the 1-year, 3-year, and 5-year disease-free survival 82%, 55%, and 40% in the TAI group and 75%, 48%, and 35% in the control group ($P = .441$). Furthermore, the 1-year, 3-year, and 5-year overall survival were 94%, 87%, and 67% in the TAI group and 89%, 80%, and 67% in the control group ($P = .830$). Currently, adjuvant TACE is not part of the standard of care after resection and more studies are needed to elucidate whether patients truly benefit.

Transarterial infusion therapy

As previously mentioned, trials studying [131]iodine in TARE as an adjuvant therapy for HCC produced unclear results with regard to survival benefit. As such, Li and colleagues[75] performed a randomized, controlled phase II trial of adjuvant transarterial [131]iodine-labeled metuximab, a monoclonal antibody to CD147 expressed by HCC tumor cells, after hepatectomy in patients with HCC. The 1-year, 3-year, and 5-year recurrence-free survivals were 80.0%, 64.0%, and 43.8% in the treatment group compared with 56.3%, 31.0%, and 21.0% in the control group, respectively ($P = .0029$). The 1-year, 3-year, and 5-year overall survivals were 97.4%, 76.9%, and 61.3% in the treatment group compared to 82.1%, 50.0%, and 35.9% in the control group ($P = <.001$). Although these transarterial infusion therapies are more recent advances in adjuvant therapy in HCC, they may hold more promise than the other treatment modalities in this review.

Due to the success in treating colorectal cancer liver metastases, another transarterial infusion therapy that has been studied in HCC is transarterial chemotherapy (without embolization like in TACE/TARE). Li and colleagues[76] performed a phase III, prospective randomized controlled trial investigating the role of adjuvant transarterial infusion chemotherapy with folinic acid, leucovorin, 5-fluorouracil, and oxaliplatin (FOLFOX) after hepatectomy. This group enrolled and randomized 127 patients with HCC with microvascular invasion to either adjuvant transarterial FOLFOX or control. The 6-month, 12-month, and 18-month overall survival for the adjuvant FOLFOX group were significantly improved at 100.0%, 97.7%, and 97.7% versus 94.5%, 89.6%, and 78.5% for the control group (P = .037). The 6-month, 12-month, and 18-month disease-free survival for the adjuvant FOLFOX group were also significantly improved compared with the control group at 84.7%, 61.8%, and 58.7%, versus 62.9%, 48.1%, and 38.6%, respectively (P = .023).

Radiotherapy

Although radiotherapy (RT) plays a role in intermediate stage HCC, the role of RT in the treatment of resectable HCC is unclear as the only 2 randomized trials that have studied adjuvant RT after partial hepatectomy in HCC have conflicting results. The first study by Yu and colleagues[77] enrolled and randomized 119 patients to either adjuvant three-dimensional conformal RT or control. No significant differences between the adjuvant RT group and the control group were found in 1-year, 3-year, or 5-year recurrence-free survival (78.1%, 56.5%, 36.9% vs 72.4%, 40.1%, 16.0%, respectively; P = .06) or overall survival (96.2%, 72.6%, 48.4%, vs 89.6%, 74.5%, 37.2%, respectively; P = .48). However, Sun and colleagues[78] who studied 52 patients with HCC complicated by PVTT randomized to either adjuvant intensity-modulated RT or control after partial hepatectomy with thrombectomy found that the 1-year, 2-year, and 3-year overall survival rates were significantly improved in the adjuvant intensity-modulated RT group compared to the control group (76.9%, 19.2%, 11.5% vs 26.9%, 11.5%, 0%, respectively; P = .005). To further complicate the conflicting results of RT as a therapeutic modality in HCC, these 2 studies had extremely high-risk patient populations for recurrence: those with narrow margins (<1 cm) and those with PVTT.

CLINICAL TRIALS IN NEOADJUVANT THERAPY FOR HCC
Transarterial Chemoembolization

Zhou and colleagues[79] randomized 108 patients with resectable HCC to either preoperative TACE followed by surgery versus surgery alone. The 1-year, 3-year, and 5-year disease-free survival rates were 48.9%, 25.5%, and 12.8% for the preoperative TACE group compared with 39.2%, 21.4%, and 8.9% for the control group (P = .372). Additionally, the 1-year, 3-year, and 5-year overall survival rates were 73.1%, 40.4%, and 30.7% for the preoperative TACE group and 69.6%, 32.1%, and 21.1% for the control group (P = .679). There was no significant difference in either disease-free survival or overall survival in those patients who received preoperative TACE. For 2 reasons, TACE should not be considered as a neoadjuvant therapy: it does not improve disease-free or overall survival but it also reduces the likelihood of receiving an operation. Almost 10% of the patients randomized to the preoperative TACE group did not undergo surgery.

Immunotherapy

As mentioned previously in this review, immunotherapy is making headway in the treatment of advanced HCC but it is unclear if it has a role in neoadjuvant therapy in resectable HCC.[51–56] There are currently numerous early-phase studies underway. Pinato and colleagues [80,81] are currently conducting PRIME-HCC, a phase Ib trial (NCT03682276), to assess the safety and tolerability of nivolumab/ipilimumab in addition to its effect on the timing of surgery, whereas Kaseb and colleagues are conducting a phase II trial (NCT03222076) assessing the efficacy of perioperative (both before and after surgery) nivolumab/ipilimumab against nivolumab alone.

Other trials involving immunotherapy regimens are NIVOLEP a phase II trial investigating perioperative nivolumab with electroporation (NCT03630640), CaboNivo a phase Ib trial investigating cabozantinib and nivolumab before surgery (NCT03299946), and a phase II trial investigating perioperative pembrolizumab with surgery or ablation (NCT03337841).

Radiotherapy

As with the adjuvant setting, the role of neoadjuvant RT has not been well studied. The study by Wei and colleagues[82] randomized 164 patients with HCC complicated by PVTT to either neoadjuvant three-dimensional conformal RT followed by partial hepatectomy versus hepatectomy alone. The 1-year and 2-year disease-free survival rates for the RT group were 33.0% and 13.3% versus 14.9% and 3.3% for the control group ($P < .001$). The 1-year and 2-year overall survival rates for the RT group were 75.2% and 27.4% compared with 43.1% and 9.4% in the control group ($P < .001$). Although neoadjuvant RT improves the disease-free survival and overall survival in those patients with HCC with PVTT, it is unclear if neoadjuvant RT is beneficial to patients without PVTT.

SUMMARY

Surgical resection for resectable HCC is plagued by a recurrence rate of up to 70% after 5 years. Previous randomized clinical trials have sought ways to improve this high recurrence rate. Surgical technique during partial hepatectomy has been investigated with clinical trials evaluating AR versus NAR and CA versus AA. Adjuvant and neoadjuvant therapy options have also been investigated including TACE, TARE, immunotherapy, systemic chemotherapy, and RT, which are also used in the treatment of intermediate and advanced HCC. In addition, antiviral therapy, brachytherapy, and transarterial infusion therapy have also been investigated but largely abandoned in any stage HCC. Although there are currently no adjuvant or neoadjuvant therapy options with sufficient data to be implemented as the standard of care, numerous randomized clinical trials are currently ongoing, and the results of these are eagerly awaited.

DISCLOSURE

The authors have no commercial or financial conflicts of interest to disclose.

REFERENCES

1. Sung H, Ferlay J, Siegel RL, et al. Global Cancer Statistics 2020: GLOBOCAN estimates of incidence and mortality worldwide for 36 cancers in 185 countries. CA Cancer J Clin 2021;71(3):209–49.

2. Akateh C, Black SM, Conteh L, et al. Neoadjuvant and adjuvant treatment strategies for hepatocellular carcinoma. World J Gastroenterol 2019;25(28):3704–21.

3. Yopp AC, Mansour JC, Beg MS, et al. Establishment of a multidisciplinary hepatocellular carcinoma clinic is associated with improved clinical outcome. Ann Surg Oncol 2014;21(4):1287–95.

4. Mazzaferro V, Regalia E, Doci R, et al. Liver Transplantation for the treatment of small hepatocellular carcinomas in patients with cirrhosis. N Engl J Med 1996; 334(11):693–9.

5. Pompili M, Mirante VG, Rondinara G, et al. Percutaneous ablation procedures in cirrhotic patients with hepatocellular carcinoma submitted to liver transplantation: assessment of efficacy at explant analysis and of safety for tumor recurrence. Liver Transpl 2005;11(9):1117–26.

6. Marubashi S, Gotoh K, Akita H, et al. Anatomical versus non-anatomical resection for hepatocellular carcinoma. Br J Surg 2015;102(7):776–84.

7. Zhu H, Xing H, Yu B, et al. Long-term survival and recurrence after curative resection for hepatocellular carcinoma in patients with chronic hepatitis C virus infection: a multicenter observational study from China. HPB (Oxford) 2020;22(12): 1793–802.

8. Li T, Qin LX, Gong X, et al. Clinical characteristics, outcome, and risk factors for early and late intrahepatic recurrence of female patients after curative resection of hepatocellular carcinoma. Surgery 2014;156(3):651–60.

9. Imamura H, Matsuyama Y, Tanaka E, et al. Risk factors contributing to early and late phase intrahepatic recurrence of hepatocellular carcinoma after hepatectomy. J Hepatol 2003;38(2):200–7.

10. Makuuchi M, Hasegawa H, Yamazaki S. Ultrasonically guided subsegmentectomy. Surg Gynecol Obstet 1985;161:346–50.

11. Aoki T, Murakami M, Yasuda D, et al. Intraoperative fluorescent imaging using indocyanine green for liver mapping and cholangiography. J Hepatobiliary Pancreat Sci 2010;17(5):590–4.

12. Couinaud C. A simplified method for controlled left hepatectomy. Surgery 1985; 97:358–61.

13. Takasaki K. Glissonean pedicle transection method for hepatic resection: a new concept of liver segmentation. J Hepato-Biliary-Pancreatic Surg 1998;5(3): 286–91.

14. Nevarez NM, Yopp AC. Anatomic vs. non-anatomic liver resection for hepatocellular carcinoma: standard of care or unfilled promises? Hepatoma Res 2021. https://doi.org/10.20517/2394-5079.2021.66.

15. Zhou Y, Xu D, Wu L, et al. Meta-analysis of anatomic resection versus nonanatomic resection for hepatocellular carcinoma. Langenbecks Arch Surg 2011; 396(7):1109–17.

16. Ye JZ, Miao ZG, Wu FX, et al. Recurrence after anatomic resection versus nonanatomic resection for hepatocellular carcinoma: a meta-analysis. Asian Pac J Cancer Prev 2012;13(5):1771–7.

17. Cucchetti A, Cescon M, Ercolani G, et al. A comprehensive meta-regression analysis on outcome of anatomic resection versus nonanatomic resection for hepatocellular carcinoma. Ann Surg Oncol 2012;19(12):3697–705.

18. Feng X, Su Y, Zheng S, et al. A double blinded prospective randomized trial comparing the effect of anatomic versus non-anatomic resection on hepatocellular carcinoma recurrence. HPB (Oxford) 2017;19(8):667–74.

19. Huang X, Lu S. A Meta-analysis comparing the effect of anatomical resection vs. non-anatomical resection on the long-term outcomes for patients undergoing hepatic resection for hepatocellular carcinoma. HPB (Oxford) 2017;19(10):843–9.

20. Tan Y, Zhang W, Jiang L, et al. Efficacy and safety of anatomic resection versus nonanatomic resection in patients with hepatocellular carcinoma: A systemic review and meta-analysis. PLoS One 2017;12(10):e0186930.

21. Moris D, Tsilimigras DI, Kostakis ID, et al. Anatomic versus non-anatomic resection for hepatocellular carcinoma: a systematic review and meta-analysis. Eur J Surg Oncol 2018;44(7):927–38.
22. Famularo S, Ceresoli M, Giani A, et al. Is it just a matter of surgical extension to achieve the cure of hepatocarcinoma? A meta-analysis of propensity-matched and randomized studies for anatomic versus parenchyma-sparing liver resection. J Gastrointest Surg 2021;25(1):94–103.
23. Sun Z, Li Z, Shi XL, et al. Anatomic versus non-anatomic resection of hepatocellular carcinoma with microvascular invasion: A systematic review and meta-analysis. Asian J Surg 2021;44(9):1143–50.
24. Ozawa K. Hepatic function and liver resection. J Gastroenterol Hepatol 1990;5(3): 296–309.
25. Lai ECS, Fan S-TF, Lo C-M, et al. Anterior approach for difficult major right hepatectomy. World J Surg 1996;20:314–8.
26. Belghiti J, Guevara OA, Noun R, et al. Liver handing maneuver: a safe approach to right hepatectomy liver mobilization. J Am Coll Surg 2001;193(1):109–11.
27. Liu CL, Fan ST, Cheung ST, et al. Anterior approach versus conventional approach right hepatic resection for large hepatocellular carcinoma: a prospective randomized controlled study. Ann Surg 2006;244(2):194–203.
28. Beppu T, Imai K, Okuda K, et al. Anterior approach for right hepatectomy with hanging maneuver for hepatocellular carcinoma: a multi-institutional propensity score-matching study. J Hepatobiliary Pancreat Sci 2017;24(3):127–36.
29. Chan KM, Wang YC, Wu TH, et al. The preference for anterior approach major hepatectomy: experience over 3 decades and a propensity score-matching analysis in right hepatectomy for hepatocellular carcinoma. Medicine (Baltimore) 2015;94(34):e1385.
30. Otsubo T, Takasaki K, Yamamoto M, et al. Bleeding during hepatectomy can be reduced by clamping the inferior vena cava below the liver. Surgery 2004;135(1): 67–73.
31. Rahbari NN, Koch M, Zimmermann JB, et al. Infrahepatic inferior vena cava clamping for reduction of central venous pressure and blood loss during hepatic resection: a randomized controlled trial. Ann Surg 2011;253(6):1102–10.
32. Zhou YM, Sui CJ, Zhang XF, et al. Anterior approach combined with infrahepatic inferior vena cava clamping right hepatic resection for large hepatocellular carcinoma: a prospective randomized controlled trial. Medicine (Baltimore) 2016; 95(27):e4159.
33. Capussotti L, Ferrero A, Russolillo N, et al. Routine anterior approach during right hepatectomy: results of a prospective randomised controlled trial. J Gastrointest Surg 2012;16(7):1324–32.
34. Chen LT, Chen MF, Li LA, et al. Long-term results of a randomized, observation-controlled, phase III trial of adjuvant interferon Alfa-2b in hepatocellular carcinoma after curative resection. Ann Surg 2012;255(1):8–17.
35. Kubo S, Nishiguchi S, Hirohashi K, et al. Randomized clinical trial of long-term outcome after resection of hepatitis C virus-related hepatocellular carcinoma by postoperative interferon therapy. Br J Surg 2002;89:418–22.
36. Lo CM, Liu CL, Chan SC, et al. A randomized, controlled trial of postoperative adjuvant interferon therapy after resection of hepatocellular carcinoma. Ann Surg 2007;245(6):831–42.
37. Kubo S, Nishiguchi S, Hirohashi K, et al. Effects of Long-Term Postoperative Interferon-Alpha Therapy on Intrahepatic Recurrence after Resection of Hepatitis C Virus–Related Hepatocellular Carcinoma. Ann Intern Med 2001;134(10):963–7.

38. Ikeda K, Arase Y, Saitoh S, et al. Interferon beta prevents recurrence of hepatocellular carcinoma after complete resection or ablation of the primary tumor-A prospective randomized study of hepatitis C virus-related liver cancer. Hepatology 2000;32(2):228–32.

39. Huang G, Lau WY, Wang ZG, et al. Antiviral therapy improves postoperative survival in patients with hepatocellular carcinoma: a randomized controlled trial. Ann Surg 2015;261(1):56–66.

40. Huang G, Li PP, Lau WY, et al. Antiviral therapy reduces hepatocellular carcinoma recurrence in patients with low HBV-DNA levels: a randomized controlled trial. Ann Surg 2018;268(6):943–54.

41. Yin J, LI N, Han Y, et al. Effect of antiviral treatment with nucleotide/nucleoside analogs on postoperative prognosis of hepatitis B virus– related hepatocellular carcinoma: a two-stage longitudinal clinical study. J Clin Oncol 2013;31(29):3647–55.

42. Chen K, Xia Y, Wang H, et al. Adjuvant iodine-125 brachytherapy for hepatocellular carcinoma after complete hepatectomy: a randomized controlled trial. PLoS One 2013;8(2):e57397.

43. Llovet JM, Ricci S, Mazzaferro V, et al. Sorafenib in advanced hepatocellular carcinoma. N Engl J Med 2008;359(4):378–90.

44. Bruix J, Takayama T, Mazzaferro V, et al. Adjuvant sorafenib for hepatocellular carcinoma after resection or ablation (STORM): a phase 3, randomised, double-blind, placebo-controlled trial. Lancet Oncol 2015;16(13):1344–54.

45. Fujiwara H, Terashima M, Irinoda T, et al. Quantitative measurement of thymidylate synthase and dihydropyrimidine dehydrogenase mRNA level in gastric cancer by real-time RT-PCR. Jpn J Cancer Res 2002;93:1342–50.

46. Ishizuka M, Kubota K, Nemoto T, et al. Administration of adjuvant oral tegafur/uracil chemotherapy post hepatocellular carcinoma resection: A randomized controlled trial. Asian J Surg 2016;39(3):149–54.

47. Zhou J, Tang Z, Wu Z. Capecitabine inhibition of recurrence and metastasis after liver cancer resection in nude mice. Chin Med J 2001;39:199–201.

48. Hoff PM, Ansari R, Batist G, et al. Comparison of oral capecitabine versus intravenous fluorouracil plus leucovorin as first-line treatment in 605 patients with metastatic colorectal cancer: results of a randomized phase III study. J Clin Oncol 2001;19(8):2282–92.

49. Zhou J, Tang Z-Y, Fan J, et al. Capecitabine inhibits postoperative recurrence and metastasis after liver cancer resection in nude mice with relation to the expression of platelet-derived endothelial cell growth factor. Clin Cancer Res 2003;9:6030–7.

50. Xia Y, Qiu Y, Li J, et al. Adjuvant therapy with capecitabine postpones recurrence of hepatocellular carcinoma after curative resection: a randomized controlled trial. Ann Surg Oncol 2010;17(12):3137–44.

51. Finn RS, Qin S, Ikeda M, et al. Atezolizumab plus bevacizumab in unresectable hepatocellular carcinoma. N Engl J Med 2020;382(20):1894–905.

52. Finn RS, Ryoo BY, Merle P, et al. Pembrolizumab as second-line therapy in patients with advanced hepatocellular carcinoma in KEYNOTE-240: a randomized, double-blind, phase III trial. J Clin Oncol 2020;38(3):193–202.

53. Zhu AX, Finn RS, Edeline J, et al. Pembrolizumab in patients with advanced hepatocellular carcinoma previously treated with sorafenib (KEYNOTE-224): a non-randomised, open-label phase 2 trial. Lancet Oncol 2018;19(7):940–52.

54. Yau T, Kang YK, Kim TY, et al. Efficacy and safety of nivolumab plus ipilimumab in patients with advanced hepatocellular carcinoma previously treated with

sorafenib: the checkMate 040 randomized clinical trial. JAMA Oncol 2020;6(11): e204564.

55. Yau T, Park J-W, Finn RS, et al. Nivolumab versus sorafenib in advanced hepatocellular carcinoma (CheckMate 459): a randomised, multicentre, open-label, phase 3 trial. Lancet Oncol 2022;23(1):77–90.

56. El-Khoueiry AB, Sangro B, Yau T, et al. Nivolumab in patients with advanced hepatocellular carcinoma (CheckMate 040): an open-label, non-comparative, phase 1/2 dose escalation and expansion trial. Lancet 2017;389(10088): 2492–502.

57. Kudo M, Ueshima K, Nakahira S, et al. Final results of adjuvant nivolumab for hepatocellular carcinoma (HCC) after surgical resection (SR) or radiofrequency ablation (RFA) (NIVOLVE): A phase 2 prospective multicenter single-arm trial and exploratory biomarker analysis. J Clin Oncol 2022;40(4_suppl):416.

58. Hack SP, Spahn J, Chen M, et al. IMbrave 050: a Phase III trial of atezolizumab plus bevacizumab in high-risk hepatocellular carcinoma after curative resection or ablation. Future Oncol 2020;16(15):975–89.

59. Jimenez Exposito MJ, Akce M, Montero Alvarez JL, et al. CA209-9DX: phase III, randomized, double-blind study of adjuvant nivolumab vs placebo for patients with hepatocellular carcinoma (HCC) at high risk of recurrence after curative resection or ablation. Ann Oncol 2018;29:viii267–8. https://doi.org/10.1093/annonc/mdy282.166.

60. Takayama T, Sekine T, Makuuchi M, et al. Adoptive immunotherapy to lower post-surgical recurrence rates of hepatocellular carcinoma: a randomised trial. Lancet 2000;356(9232):802–7.

61. Hui D, Qiang L, Jian W, et al. A randomized, controlled trial of postoperative adjuvant cytokine-induced killer cells immunotherapy after radical resection of hepatocellular carcinoma. Dig Liver Dis 2009;41(1):36–41.

62. Lee JH, Lee JH, Lim YS, et al. Adjuvant immunotherapy with autologous cytokine-induced killer cells for hepatocellular carcinoma. Gastroenterology 2015;148(7): 1383–13891 e6.

63. Yoo HSY, Lee JT, Kim KW, et al. Nodular hepatocellular carcinoma: treatment with subsegmental intraarterial injection of iodine z3 1-labeled iodized Oil. Cancer 1991;68:1878–84.

64. Yumoto Y, Jinno K, Inatsuki S, et al. Treatment of hepatocellular carcinoma by transcatheter hepatic arterial injection of radioactive iodized oil solution. Cancer Chemother Pharmcol 1992;31:S128–36.

65. Mantravadi RVP, Spigos DC, Tan WS, et al. Intraarterial Yttrium 90 in the treatment of hepatic malignancy. Radiology 1982;142:783–6.

66. Partensky C, Sassolas G, Henry L, et al. Intra-arterial iodine 131-labeled lipiodol as adjuvant therapy after curative liver resection for hepatocellular carcinoma. Arch Surg 2000;135:1298–300.

67. Lau WY, Leung TWT, Ho SKW, et al. Adjuvant intra-arterial lipiodol-iodine-131 for resectable hepatocellular carcinoma: a prospective randomised trial. The Lancet 1999;353(9155):797–801. https://doi.org/10.1016/s0140-6736(98)06475-7.

68. Lau WY, Lai EC, Leung TW, et al. Adjuvant intra-arterial iodine-131-labeled lipiodol for resectable hepatocellular carcinoma: a prospective randomized trial-update on 5-year and 10-year survival. Ann Surg 2008;247(1):43–8.

69. Chung AY, Ooi LL, Machin D, et al. Adjuvant hepatic intra-arterial iodine-131-lipiodol following curative resection of hepatocellular carcinoma: a prospective randomized trial. World J Surg 2013;37(6):1356–61.

70. Dumortier J, Decullier E, Hilleret MN, et al. Adjuvant Intraarterial Lipiodol or (1)(3)(1)I-Lipiodol After Curative Treatment of Hepatocellular Carcinoma: A Prospective Randomized Trial. J Nucl Med 2014;55(6):877–83.
71. Zhong C, Guo RP, Li JQ, et al. A randomized controlled trial of hepatectomy with adjuvant transcatheter arterial chemoembolization versus hepatectomy alone for stage III A hepatocellular carcinoma. J Cancer Res Clin Oncol 2009;135(10): 1437–45.
72. (UICC) IUAC. TNM classification of malignant tumors. 6th edition. Hoboken, NJ: Wiley; 2002.
73. Wang Z, Ren Z, Chen Y, et al. Adjuvant transarterial chemoembolization for HBV-related hepatocellular carcinoma after resection: a randomized controlled study. Clin Cancer Res 2018;24(9):2074–81.
74. Hirokawa F, Komeda K, Taniguchi K, et al. Is Postoperative adjuvant transcatheter arterial infusion therapy effective for patients with hepatocellular carcinoma who underwent hepatectomy? A prospective randomized controlled trial. Ann Surg Oncol 2020;27(11):4143–52.
75. Li J, Xing J, Yang Y, et al. Adjuvant 131I-metuximab for hepatocellular carcinoma after liver resection: a randomised, controlled, multicentre, open-label, phase 2 trial. Lancet Gastroenterol Hepatol 2020;5(6):548–60.
76. Li S, Mei J, Wang Q, et al. Postoperative adjuvant transarterial infusion chemotherapy with FOLFOX could improve outcomes of hepatocellular carcinoma patients with microvascular invasion: a preliminary report of a phase III, randomized controlled clinical trial. Ann Surg Oncol 2020;27(13):5183–90.
77. Yu W, Wang W, Rong W, et al. Adjuvant radiotherapy in centrally located hepatocellular carcinomas after hepatectomy with narrow margin (<1 cm): a prospective randomized study. J Am Coll Surg 2014;218(3):381–92.
78. Sun J, Yang L, Shi J, et al. Postoperative adjuvant IMRT for patients with HCC and portal vein tumor thrombus: An open-label randomized controlled trial. Radiother Oncol 2019;140:20–5.
79. Zhou WP, Lai EC, Li AJ, et al. A prospective, randomized, controlled trial of preoperative transarterial chemoembolization for resectable large hepatocellular carcinoma. Ann Surg 2009;249(2):195–202.
80. Pinato DJ, Cortellini A, Sukumaran A, et al. PRIME-HCC: phase Ib study of neoadjuvant ipilimumab and nivolumab prior to liver resection for hepatocellular carcinoma. BMC Cancer 2021;21(1):301.
81. Kaseb AO, Pestana RC, Vence LM, et al. Randomized, open-label, perioperative phase II study evaluating nivolumab alone versus nivolumab plus ipilimumab in patients with resectable HCC. J Clin Oncol 2019;37(4_suppl):185.
82. Wei X, Jiang Y, Zhang X, et al. Neoadjuvant three-dimensional conformal radiotherapy for resectable hepatocellular carcinoma with portal vein tumor thrombus: a randomized, open-label, multicenter controlled study. J Clin Oncol 2019;37(24): 2141–51.

Colorectal Cancer Liver Metastases: Multimodal Therapy

Berk Aykut, MD, Michael E. Lidsky, MD*

KEYWORDS

- Colorectal cancer • Liver metastasis • Chemotherapy • Randomized controlled trial
- Perioperative chemotherapy • Surgery

KEY POINTS

- Colorectal liver metastases (CRLM) are the primary driver of disease-specific mortality for patients with colorectal cancer.
- Surgical metastasectomy with the aim of R0 resection remains the backbone of CRLM therapy and is the only opportunity to achieve a cure. Oncological outcomes of parenchymal-sparing hepatectomy are comparable to more aggressive anatomic resections.
- The role of neoadjuvant chemotherapy for resectable CRLM remains controversial because it may delay surgery and cause hepatotoxicity but without any proven improvement in survival.
- The associating liver partition and portal vein ligation for staged hepatectomy technique may increase resection rates for CRLM, although it remains controversial due to high morbidity and mortality rates.
- Systemic chemotherapy and locoregional therapy such as hepatic artery infusion are promising strategies and have been shown to provide durable disease control and increase resection rates in initially unresectable CRLM.

INTRODUCTION

Public initiatives to reduce the exposure to known risk factors, including smoking, and the uptake of colorectal cancer (CRC) screening programs have led to a steady decline in CRC incidence and mortality rates.[1] However, CRC remains the second most common cancer diagnosis in women and the third most common in men worldwide.[2] Moreover, the incidence of early-onset CRC in patients aged younger than 50 years has been increasing, a population more likely to be diagnosed at later stages.[3–5] Similarly, pooled analyses from clinical trials of metastatic colorectal cancer

Department of Surgery, Division of Surgical Oncology, Duke University Medical Center, Box 3966, 10 Bryan Searle Drive, 466G Seeley G. Mudd Building, Durham, NC 27710, USA
* Corresponding author.
E-mail address: Michael.Lidsky@duke.edu
Twitter: @BerkAykutMD (B.A.); @michael_lidsky (M.E.L.)

Surg Oncol Clin N Am 32 (2023) 119–141
https://doi.org/10.1016/j.soc.2022.07.009
1055-3207/23/© 2022 Elsevier Inc. All rights reserved.

(mCRC) patients show that younger patients have worse progression-free (PFS) and overall survival (OS).[6] Emerging data also suggest that the different embryologic origins of midgut and hindgut colon segments result in distinct molecular profiles of right-sided and left-sided colon cancers, respectively.[7,8] Right-sided tumors tend to be poorly differentiated and more frequently harbor *KRAS* mutations, and patients with liver metastases from right-sided cancers have a worse OS rate because they often present at later stages and are older at diagnosis.[9,10] Contrarily, left-sided colon cancers tend to have higher rates of distant metastases but are more commonly well-differentiated and *KRAS* wild-type, which is associated with improved response to cytotoxic and targeted therapy and a better prognosis.[11,12] Although 20% of CRC patients present with synchronous liver metastases, half of all patients with initially non-metastatic disease progress and develop liver and lung metastases.[13,14] Notably, the liver is recognized as the most common site of CRC metastasis due to the portal venous drainage, and metastases to the liver remain the most common cause of disease-specific mortality. Left untreated, 5-year OS approaches 0% for patients with colorectal liver metastases (CRLM).[15] Hence, the management of CRLM has evolved into a complex field. Today, patients with mCRC are evaluated by multidisciplinary teams, inclusive of surgeons, medical oncologists, and radiation oncologists. Optimal management of CRLM consists of an individualized treatment strategy based on patient and tumor factors, including age, comorbidities, sidedness, the location and extent of disease, as well as molecular profile. Although hepatic resection is the backbone of curative-intent treatment, management of CRLM has become increasingly multimodal during the last decade and includes the use of downstaging chemotherapy, ablation techniques, and locoregional therapy, each of which are reviewed herein.

Imaging of Colorectal Liver Metastases

During the past 2 decades, hepatic metastasectomy has emerged as a safe and promising therapy to improve outcomes in patients with CRLM.[16] The current guidelines for resection of CRLM recommend removal of all macroscopic disease with negative margins while leaving sufficient functioning liver.[17] Therefore, preoperative imaging plays a vital role in adequately identifying and characterizing the extent of disease within the liver, defining relevant anatomy, estimating the remnant liver volume, and importantly identifying extrahepatic disease that may often preclude hepatectomy. Historically, ultrasonography was the method of choice to identify CRLM; however, technological advances in computed tomography (CT), MRI, and PET have led to improved detection of occult lesions and better delineation of hepatic anatomy. Although multiphase (triphasic) CT has emerged as the modality of choice for detecting liver metastases for CRC, it is limited in detecting CRLM in obese patients, CRLM less than 10 mm, or CRLM in patients with significant chemotherapy-associated steatosis.[18,19] While liver metastases typically seem as hypoattenuating lesions, the addition of arterial and portal venous phase imaging can be helpful to define liver vascular anatomy. Compared with CT, MRI with diffusion-weighted imaging and hepatocyte-specific contrast agents facilitates improved detection of subcentimeter lesions with a sensitivity of up to 95% despite generating typically lower resolution images.[20] With no randomized data comparing CT and MRI, the choice of imaging modality is often institution-dependent, although comparative analyses are underway to determine if MRI adds value to clinical decision-making beyond CT alone.[21] Besides CT and MRI, selective use of PET imaging using the glucose analog ^{18}F-fluorodeoxyglucose may be of value in detecting occult extrahepatic disease.

Resectable Colorectal Liver Metastases

Surgical management of resectable colorectal liver metastases

Surgical resection remains the backbone of CRLM therapy and is the only potentially curative treatment. In a recent study including 1211 patients undergoing resection for CRLM, Creasy and colleagues reported a median disease-specific survival of 4.9 years and an observed cure rate of 20%.[22] As technical advancements in liver surgery have propelled the evolution of hepatic resection for CRLM, many attempts have been made to stratify patients with liver disease to determine their prognosis after surgery. Risk scores such as the Fong score (Clinical Risk Score) have been proposed to define oncologic resectability.[23] In their seminal study, which incorporated data from 1001 patients, Fong and colleagues proposed a clinical risk score that proved to be highly predictive of the outcome. This score is calculated from 5 prognostic criteria, including (1) nodal status of the primary lesion, (2) disease-free interval from diagnosis of the primary lesion to the discovery of liver metastases less than 12 months, (3) greater than 1 hepatic metastases, (4) size of largest metastasis greater than 5 cm, and (5) preoperative carcinoembryonic antigen (CEA) level greater than 200 ng/mL. Based on these criteria, patients can be stratified as either low or high risk. Patients with a low clinical risk score of 0 to 2 have a more favorable outcome with a 5-year survival rate of 52.3%. In contrast, patients with a high clinical risk score of 3 to 5 have a much more guarded prognosis with a 5-year survival rate of 20.2%.[24] Other scores that are commonly calculated for patients with CLRM are the Nagashima, Nordlinger, and Konopke scores.[16,25,26] Although most studies investigating the value of stratification schema are limited by small sample size and institutional variation in practice and referral patterns, such clinical risk scores are valuable tools to predict long-term survival of patients with CRLM and reinforce the importance of oncologic and biologic considerations in the management of this disease.

Technical resectability is also debated, and while definitions may vary, a commonly used description of unresectable disease includes that in which margin negative resection would require the removal of all 3 hepatic veins, both portal veins, or the retrohepatic vena cava, and/or leave fewer than 2 adequately perfused and drained segments of the liver.[24] Today, the combination of parenchymal preserving resection and ablation techniques, neoadjuvant therapy to downsize tumors, and strategies to increase hepatic reserve have expanded the criteria of resectability to include any patient in whom all disease can be removed with a negative margin and sufficient future liver remnant (FLR). As such, the determination of resectability is a highly nuanced and individualized approach and is optimally assessed by an experienced hepatic surgeon. A lack of input from a liver surgeon may have devastating impact on patient outcomes, as demonstrated by Vega and colleagues, who reported that more than 44% of patients destined for palliative chemotherapy by a multidisciplinary tumor board without a liver surgeon present were considered potentially resectable after retrospective review by independent liver surgeons.[27]

With the shift of focus away from the diseased liver to the FLR, several tools have been developed to predict postoperative liver function and avoid posthepatectomy liver failure (PHLF). One such tool is indocyanine green (ICG) clearance testing, although its ability to accurately predict mortality is still under debate. ICG is a water-soluble dye that binds to albumin and is exclusively cleared from the bloodstream by the liver. As such, it allows for a real-time assessment of postoperative residual liver function in addition to preoperative volumetric analyses, which remains the most widely used tool.[28] In addition to patient-specific factors, surgical factors influence the risk of PHLF. These include intraoperative blood loss greater than

1200 mL, need for vascular resection, skeletonization of the hepatoduodenal ligament, resection of greater than 50% liver volume, and major hepatectomy.[29]

In contrast to fixed factors that are predictive of prognosis, resection margin status has been investigated as a predictor of outcome. Although historically an R0 margin width of 1 cm has been considered optimal in the resection of CRLM, Pawlik and colleagues reported a similar outcome in patients with negative resection margins, regardless of margin width.[30,31] Rather, it is thought that tumor biology (eg, molecular profile) is a more important predictor than margin width for local recurrence and long-term survival. Accordingly, anatomic resection (AR) has been observed to increase disease-free survival (DFS) to 33.8 months compared with 10.5 months in the non-AR group for *KRAS* mutant CRLM.[32] These findings provide further evidence that individual tumor biology dictates local recurrence in CRLM.

To achieve the goal of metastasectomy with a successful R0 resection, many patients undergo an AR, defined by the resection of one or more anatomic liver segments. However, there is no difference in the proportion of R0 resections in patients undergoing parenchymal-sparing hepatectomy (PSH) versus AR.[33] Moreover, PSH has recently been shown to have oncological outcomes comparable with AR.[34] Although some studies report similar perioperative morbidity and mortality rates for AR and PSH, others have shown improved morbidity and mortality in patients undergoing PSH due to the reduced magnitude of resection and what is typically an increased FLR.[35–37] Additionally, the reduced volume of resected liver with PSH can expand the number of patients with CRLM eligible for repeat hepatic resection at the time of recurrence, which occurs in 70% to 80% of patients.[38] As such, AR was identified as an independent factor associated with the inability to undergo repeat resection for recurrent CRLM.[39]

In concert with continued efforts to pursue parenchymal-sparing resections, there has been a steady decline in major hepatic resections during the past 20 years. One factor that has facilitated parenchymal preservation for advanced disease is the use of ablative therapies. The trend in decreased major hepatectomies accompanied by an increase in ablation is associated with a decrease in overall complications from 53.2% to 19.9% and an improvement in perioperative mortality from 5.2% to 1.6%.[35] Ablative therapies include radiofrequency ablation (RFA), which can improve OS rates compared with chemotherapy alone for lesions that are otherwise not amenable to resection.[40,41] RFA is safe and effective, although it has only limited effectiveness adjacent to vascular structures due to the heat sink phenomenon. Similarly, microwave ablation (MWA) has been shown to be equally effective as hepatic resection in a small randomized controlled trial (RCT) consisting of 30 patients.[42] Compared with RFA, MWA can produce much faster heating and larger volume ablation zones that are less susceptible to near heat sink. Although MWA has limited use in the treatment of subcapsular or high-risk location (adjacent to central biliary tree) metastases, it is becoming more popular due to its effectiveness in metastases measuring more than 3 cm. Other percutaneous ablative techniques that have gained acceptance as treatment modalities for CRLM include cryoablation and irreversible electroporation. Today, local ablative techniques are commonly used to complement hepatic resection when complete resection of all metastases is not possible, as well as to facilitate parenchymal preservation.

Efforts to reduce surgical stress are paralleled by a trend toward increased use of minimally invasive techniques in liver surgery. Laparoscopic liver surgery for CRLM is associated with reduced blood loss (median difference 147 mL), shorter hospital stays (median difference 2.4 days), and reduced morbidity (odds ratio [OR] 0.64, 95% CI 0.55–0.75; $P < .00001$) compared with open resection techniques.[43]

Importantly, the OSLO COMET trial and other studies report similar rates of resection free margins for both laparoscopic and open surgery without differences in disease recurrence, 3-year or 5-year survival, suggesting noninferiority for these oncologic endpoints.[44,45]

Chemotherapy for Resectable Colorectal Liver Metastases

Theoretic benefits of chemotherapy for resectable CRLM include treating micrometastatic disease in the liver and systemically to decrease the risk of recurrence, downstaging disease to lessen the extent of liver resection required, as well as to test biology and improve selection of patients most likely to benefit from hepatectomy. Adjuvant chemotherapy for resected CRLM, however, has not been shown to improve OS for this patient population. A 2006 RCT suggested adjuvant fluorouracil may improve DFS; however, no improvement was observed in OS.[46] Similar findings were observed by Mitry and colleagues, where 2 European RCTs were combined to improve statistical power to detect a difference in survival.[47] Despite this analysis, adjuvant fluorouracil, although associated with a potential improvement of PFS (hazard ratio [HR] 1.32; 95% CI 1.00–1.76; $P = .058$), did not result in an improvement in OS (HR 1.32; 95% CI 0.95 - 1.82; $P = .095$). To address critiques of early studies that included the use of antiquated single-agent regimens, Ychou and colleagues conducted an RCT comparing adjuvant 5-fluorouracil/leucovorin and irinotecan (FOLFIRI) versus fluorouracil but neither PFS or OS were improved with this modern regimen.[48] Most recently, the Japan Clinical Oncology Group reported JCOG0603, which randomized patients with resected CRLM to adjuvant modified 5-fluorouracil/leucovorin and oxaliplatin (mFOLFOX6) versus surveillance. In this study, which included treatment-naïve patients, adjuvant mFOLFOX6 did improve DFS (HR 0.67; 95% CI, 0.50–0.92; $P = .006$) but not OS.[49] In fact, OS was worse in patients receiving mFOLFOX6 (71.2% for hepatectomy followed by chemotherapy vs 83.1% for hepatectomy alone), which was theorized to be due to chemotherapy-induced liver damage, imbalanced posttrial therapies, poor adherence to adjuvant chemotherapy, and/or induction of chemoresistance following elimination of chemosensitive tumor cells.

Despite lack of data supporting adjuvant chemotherapy for patients with resectable CRLM, some advocate for neoadjuvant chemotherapy. The rationale for neoadjuvant chemotherapy in this population includes optimizing the chances of an R0 resection, downstaging disease to facilitate parenchymal preserving hepatectomy, and improving patient selection for liver resection. In the landmark European Organization For Research And Treatment Of Cancer (EORTC) 40983 trial, 364 patients with 4 or fewer resectable CRLM across 78 hospitals in Europe were randomized to perioperative FOLFOX4 or surgery alone.[50] Notably, perioperative chemotherapy led to an 8.1% increase in PFS at 3 years (from 28.1%, 95.66% CI 21.2–36.6 to 36.2%, 95.66% CI 28.7–43.8; HR 0.77, 0.60–1.00; $P = .041$; **Fig. 1A**). Subgroup analysis of patients undergoing resection revealed an even more pronounced benefit of 9.2% (from 33.2%, 25.3–41.2 to 42.4%, 34.0–50.5; HR 0.73, 0.55–0.97; $P = .025$). However, with long-term follow-up, EORTC 40983 did not reveal an improvement in median OS (61.3 months for the perioperative cohort vs 54.3 months for the surgery alone cohort; $P = .34$; **Fig. 1B**).[51] Not only did perioperative chemotherapy fail to improve OS for this patient population, additional findings in EORTC 40983 include increased postoperative morbidity in the perioperative chemotherapy arm (25% vs 16%; $P = .04$). The excess morbidity was primarily related to biliary fistula (8% vs 4%), prolonged hepatic failure (6% vs 3%), and intra-abdominal infection (7% vs 2%). Of note, only 7% of patients progressed during the course of preoperative chemotherapy, with the number of patients resected in each arm being identical. These data indicate that short-course

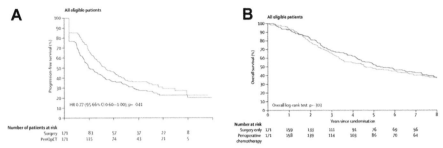

Fig. 1. Perioperative chemotherapy for resectable CRLM improves Progression-free survival but not Overall Survival. (*A*) Perioperative chemotherapy led to an 8.1% increase in PFS at 3 years in all eligible patients. (*B*) 5-year overall survival was 51.2% in the perioperative chemotherapy group versus 47.8% in the surgery-only group. PeriOpCT, perioperative chemotherapy consisting of 5-FU, leucovorin and oxaliplatin. (Reprinted with permission from Elsevier. The Lancet Oncol, Vol 14, Issue 12, 2021, p.1208-15, Nordlinger et al., Perioperative FOLFOX4 chemotherapy and surgery versus surgery alone for resectable liver metastases from colorectal cancer (EORTC 40983): long-term results of a randomised, controlled, phase 3 trial, https://doi.org/10.1016/S1470-2045(13)70447-9.)

FOLFOX in patients with oligometastatic disease is an inadequate strategy to identify patients who would least likely benefit from exploration or resection. As such, the role of neoadjuvant chemotherapy for resectable CRLM remains controversial because it may delay surgery and cause hepatotoxicity. Ongoing trials such as the CHARISMA trial may answer whether subgroups of patients with primary resectable CRLM characterized as high-risk by the Fong Clinical Risk Score could benefit from neoadjuvant chemotherapy.[52]

Targeted therapies have also been studied in the neoadjuvant setting. The New EPOC study was a randomized controlled trial aimed to assess the benefit of cetuximab added to perioperative chemotherapy (FOLFOX, XELOX, or FOLFIRI) in patients with resectable *KRAS* wild-type CRLM. With an overall median follow-up of 20.7 months, PFS was noted to be significantly shorter in the chemotherapy plus cetuximab group compared with the chemotherapy alone group (14.1 months, 95% CI 11.8–15.9 vs 20.5 months, 95% CI 16.8–26.7; HR 1.48, 95% CI 1.04–2.12; $P = .030$).[53] Moreover, OS was shorter in the cetuximab group on long-term follow-up (55.4 vs 81.0 months, HR 1.45, 95% CI 1.02–2.05; $P = .036$), suggesting that cetuximab in combination with chemotherapy cannot be recommended for patients with resectable CRLM.[54]

Hepatic Artery Infusion Therapy for Resectable Colorectal Liver Metastases

Although standard systemic regimens have not been shown to improve survival for resectable CRLM, adjuvant hepatic artery infusion (HAI) was reported to improve outcomes in this population. Although normal liver parenchyma receives dual blood supply from the portal venous and arterial circulation, hepatic metastases derive their blood supply from the hepatic artery.[55] Based on this finding, Clarkson and colleagues first introduced hepatic arterial chemotherapy in 1961.[56] Their method entailed catheterization of the common hepatic artery via the brachial artery, allowing for continuous antimetabolite infusion. To further minimize systemic chemotoxic effects, Sullivan and colleagues from the Lahey Hospital described a modified technique that included ligation of all nonhepatic branches of the hepatic artery.[57] With the advent of intraoperative dye studies that ensure exclusively hepatic perfusion before initiating therapy, HAI has gained increased enthusiasm during the past decades, although it still remains a therapy that is restricted to few select centers. Despite limitations in availability of this therapy, Kemeny and colleagues demonstrated that liver-directed therapy with HAI may improve outcomes when combined with systemic therapy in the adjuvant setting after complete resection of CRLM.[58] In the 1999 RCT, adjuvant HAI not only resulted in an improvement in hepatic-recurrence free survival from 60% to 90% at 2 years but also yielded an improvement in 2-year OS from 72% to 86% (P = .03). Recent studies suggest that hepatic resection followed by adjuvant HAI combined with systemic chemotherapy can achieve 5-year and 10-year survival rates as high as 78% and 61%, respectively.[59] Similarly, Koerkamp and colleagues recently reported that perioperative HAI was associated with increased OS (67 months with HAI vs 44 months without HAI, P < .001).[60] The largest association between HAI and improved outcomes was also found for patients with a low clinical risk score and no extrahepatic disease. Regarding somatic mutations in patients with resected CRLM, adjuvant HAI is also associated with improved OS (HR 0.53, P < .002) independent of *KRAS* mutational status in a retrospective analysis of 674 patients.[61] Based on these data, adjuvant HAI is the only therapy that has been shown to improve OS in a randomized trial, and contemporary retrospective analyses continue to suggest encouraging outcomes in the adjuvant setting.

Potentially Resectable and Unresectable Colorectal Liver Metastases

Chemotherapy for potentially resectable and unresectable colorectal liver metastases
Upfront surgery is feasible in only 15% to 25% of patients with CRLM.[62] As such, studies have investigated the role of chemotherapeutic strategies for potentially resectable and unresectable CRLM with the goal of downstaging to resectable status (**Table 1**). In their landmark study, Adam and colleagues reported that chemotherapy with FOLFOX, FOLFIRI, or FOLFIRINOX, allowed 12.5% of patients with initially unresectable CRLM to undergo hepatic resection.[63] In a smaller series consisting of 40 patients, the addition of irinotecan to 5-FU and folinic acid increased the resection rate in patients with initially unresectable liver metastases to 32.5%.[64] Importantly, cumulative 3-year and 5-year survival rates are comparable among patients undergoing curative-intent hepatectomy after conversion to resectable status compared with patients with resectable CRLM at diagnosis.[65] More recently, the randomized phase II METHEP trial investigated whether intensified chemotherapy can further increase resection rates and improve outcomes in patients with CRLM.[66] A total of 125 patients were randomly assigned to standard FOLFOX or FOLFIRI, or intensified chemotherapy with high-dose irinotecan (FOLFIRI-HD), high-dose oxaliplatin (FOLFOX7) or triplet therapy with FOLFIRINOX. Although the rate of toxicity was higher in patients receiving intensified chemotherapy, patients in the FOLFIRINOX arm had the best conversion to resection rate, with 67% of patients ultimately undergoing liver resection, compared with only 40% to 59% in the remaining arms.

Identification of biomarkers and development of monoclonal antibodies targeting epidermal growth factor receptor (EGFR) and vascular endothelial growth factors (VEGF) have further expanded the therapeutic arsenal for the treatment of CRC and CRLM. In the phase II CELIM trial, 114 patients with unresectable CRLM were randomly assigned to receive anti-EGFR therapy (cetuximab) with either FOLFOX or FOLFIRI.[67,68] The primary endpoint was defined as tumor response assessed by the response evaluation criteria in solid tumors criteria. Notably, although there was no significant difference in the response rate, retrospective analysis of the *KRAS* mutation status revealed a response rate of 70% (95% CI 58–81) in patients with wild-type *KRAS* compared with only 41% (95% CI 22–61) in patients with *KRAS*-mutated

Table 1
Key clinical trials of perioperative chemotherapy for potentially resectable and unresectable colorectal liver metastases

Study Name	Author	Year	Number of patients	KRAS status	Treatment	Control	DFS or PFS	OS	Resection Rate (including all R status)	R0 Resection Rate
	Adam et al.[63]	2004	1439	Not reported	FOLFOX/FOLFIRI/FOLFIRINOX and secondary resection	Primary resection	22% and 17% at 5 and 10 y (secondary resection) Not reported (primary resection)	33% and 23% at 5 and 10 y (secondary resection) 48% and 30% at 5 and 10 y (primary resection)	12.5% after neoadjuvant chemotherapy	Not reported
	Pozzo et al.[64]	2004	40	Not reported	FOLFIRI	n/a	14.3 mo	Not reached	40% after neoadjuvant chemotherapy	32.5% after neoadjuvant chemotherapy
CRYSTAL	Van Cutsem et al.[69]	2009	599	wt/mut	Cetuximab-FOLFIRI	FOLFIRI	9.9 mo (Cetuximab-FOLFIRI; wt-KRAS) 8.7 mo (FOLFIRI; wt-KRAS) 7.6 mo (Cetuximab-FOLFIRI; mut-KRAS) 8.1 mo (FOLFIRI; mut-KRAS)	24.9 mo (Cetuximab-FOLFIRI; wt-KRAS) 21.0 mo (FOLFIRI; wt-KRAS) 17.5 mo (Cetuximab-FOLFIRI; mut-KRAS) 17.7 mo (FOLFIRI; mut-KRAS)	7% (Cetuximab-FOLFIRI) 3.7% (FOLFIRI)	4.8% (Cetuximab-FOLFIRI) 1.7% (FOLFIRI)
OPUS	Bokemeyer et al.[70,71]	2009	337	wt/mut	Cetuximab-FOLFOX-4	FOLFOX-4	7.7 mo (Cetuximab-FOLFOX-4; wt-KRAS) 7.2 mo (FOLFOX-4; wt-KRAS) 5.5 mo (Cetuximab-FOLFOX-4; mut-KRAS) 8.6 mo (FOLFOX-4; mut-KRAS)	22.8 mo (Cetuximab-FOLFOX-4; wt-KRAS) 18.5 mo (FOLFOX-4; wt-KRAS) 13.4 mo (Cetuximab-FOLFOX-4; mut-KRAS) 17.5 mo (FOLFOX-4; mut-KRAS)	Not reported	9.8% (Cetuximab-FOLFOX-4; wt-KRAS) 4.1% (FOLFOX-4; wt-KRAS) 1.9% (Cetuximab-FOLFOX-4; mut-KRAS) 2.1% (FOLFOX-4; mut-KRAS)

CELIM	Folprecht et al.[67,68]	2010	114	wt/mut	Cetuximab-FOLFOX-6	Cetuximab-FOLFIRI	11.2 mo (Cetuximab-FOLFOX-6) 10.5 mo (Cetuximab-FOLFIRI)	35.8 mo (Cetuximab-FOLFOX-6) 29 mo (Cetuximab-FOLFIRI)	42% (Cetuximab-FOLFOX-6) 44% (Cetuximab-FOLFIRI)	38% (Cetuximab-FOLFOX-6) 30% (Cetuximab-FOLFIRI)
METHEP	Ychou et al.[66]	2013	125	wt/mut	FOLFIRI-HD/ FOLFOX7/ FOLFIRINOX	FOLFIRI/ FOLFOX4	12.1 mo (FOLFIRI-HD) 8.5 mo (FOLFOX-7) 14.1 mo (FOLFIRINOX) 9.2 mo (Controls)	29.4 mo (FOLFIRI-HD) 26.9 mo (FOLFOX-7) 48.8 mo (FOLFIRINOX) 17.7 mo (Controls)	59.4% (FOLFIRI-HD) 43.3% (FOLFOX-7) 66.7% (FOLFIRINOX) 40% (Controls)	25% (FOLFIRI-HD) 23.3% (FOLFOX-7) 30% (FOLFIRINOX) 23.3% (Controls)
FIRE-3	Heinemann et al.[74]	2014	592	Wt	Cetuximab-FOLFIRI	Bevacizumab-FOLFIRI	10 mo (Cetuximab-FOLFIRI) 10.3 mo (Bevacizumab-FOLFIRI)	28.7 mo (Cetuximab-FOLFIRI) 25 mo (Bevacizumab-FOLFIRI)	12% (Cetuximab-FOLFIRI) 14% (Bevacizumab-FOLFIRI)	Not reported
OLIVIA	Gruenberger et al.[72]	2015	80	Wt	Bevacizumab-FOLFOXIRI	Bevacizumab-mFOLFOX-6	18.6 mo (Bevacizumab-FOLFOXIRI) 12.5 mo (Bevacizumab-mFOLFOX-6)	Not reached (Bevacizumab-FOLFOXIRI) 32.2 mo (Bevacizumab-mFOLFOX-6)	61% (Bevacizumab-FOLFOXIRI) 49% (Bevacizumab-mFOLFOX-6)	49% (Bevacizumab-FOLFOXIRI) 23% (Bevacizumab-mFOLFOX-6)
ATOM	Oki et al.[76]	2019	122	Wt	Bevacizumab-mFOLFOX-6	Cetuximab-mFOLFOX-6	11.5 mo (Bevacizumab-mFOLFOX-6) 14.8 mo (Cetuximab-mFOLFOX-6)	Not reported	56.1% (Bevacizumab-mFOLFOX-6) 49.2% (Cetuximab-mFOLFOX-6)	43.9% (Bevacizumab-mFOLFOX-6) 37.3% (Cetuximab-mFOLFOX-6)
BECOME	Tang et al.[73]	2020	241	Mut	Bevacizumab-mFOLFOX-6	mFOLFOX-6	9.5 mo (Bevacizumab-mFOLFOX-6) 5.6 mo (mFOLFOX-6)	25.7 mo (Bevacizumab-mFOLFOX-6) 20.5 mo (mFOLFOX-6)	Not reported	22.3 (Bevacizumab-mFOLFOX-6) 5.8% (mFOLFOX-6)

tumors (P = .008). Moreover, in a retrospective but blinded evaluation of resectability, 41 (60%) of 68 patients were judged to be resectable after neoadjuvant chemotherapy, compared with 22 (32%) of 68 patients at baseline. Despite this difference of 19 (28%) patients perceived to have converted to resectable status (P < .0001), only 34% of patients actually underwent R0 resection. The CRYSTAL trial also evaluated the impact of cetuximab, which showed a HR of 0.85 (95% CI 0.72–0.99; P = .048) for PFS with FOLFIRI-cetuximab as compared with the FOLFIRI alone.[69] Similarly, the OPUS study showed that the addition of cetuximab to FOLFOX-4 significantly improved PFS (HR 0.567; P = .0064) and response (OR 2.551; P = .0027) in patients with *KRAS* wild-type mCRC.[70,71]

In the phase II OLIVIA trial, patients with initially unresectable CRLM were randomized to anti-VEGF therapy (bevacizumab) plus modified FOLFOX or FOLFOXIRI.[72] In patients assigned to bevacizumab-FOLFOXIRI, the resection rate was 61% (95% CI 45–76) compared with 49% (95% CI 32–65) in the bevacizumab-mFOLFOX group; however, R0 resection rates were 49% and 23%, respectively. The observed increase in resection rate with bevacizumab-FOLFOXIRI also translated into prolonged PFS (18.6 months vs 11.5 months). Importantly, these multiagent regimens came at the cost of morbidity: 38 bevacizumab–FOLFOXIRI patients (95%) and 31 bevacizumab–mFOLFOX-6 patients (84%) experienced a grade 3 or greater toxicity event such as neutropenia, diarrhea, or febrile neutropenia. More recently, the BECOME trial tested whether adding bevacizumab to chemotherapy can improve resection rates in initially unresectable *RAS* mutant CRLM.[73] Although it is unclear which subsets of patients were converted, the R0 resection rate was 22.3% in the mFOLFOX plus bevacizumab group compared with 5.8% in the mFOLFOX group, suggesting bevacizumab can increase resection rates in *RAS*-mutant CRLM (P < .01).

To compare the effectiveness of cetuximab and bevacizumab, the multicenter FIRE-3 trial randomized patients with *KRAS* wild-type CRLM to either FOLFIRI plus cetuximab or bevacizumab as first-line treatment.[74] Interestingly, although no differences were observed in median PFS, patients in the cetuximab arm had a longer median OS than patients in the bevacizumab arm (28.7 vs 25.0 months, HR 0.77, 95% CI 0.62–0.96; P = .017). In a follow-up study of FIRE-3, the advantage of cetuximab over bevacizumab could only be observed in patients with CRLM and left-sided primary tumors.[75] As such, patients with *KRAS* wild-type CRLM from left-sided primary tumors may be considered for cytotoxic therapy in combination with anti-EGFR therapy, whereas those with right-sided primary tumors should be considered for bevacizumab, if addition of a biologic agent is deemed important. These results are congruent with the more recent ATOM trial from Japan, which demonstrated a median tumor shrinkage rate of 38% at 8 weeks in the cetuximab arm versus 25% in the bevacizumab arm. However, no differences were identified in the resection rate or PFS in that study.[76] As such, the choice of a neoadjuvant chemotherapy regimen for unresectable CRLM remains a complex and highly individualized decision.

Future Liver Remnant Augmentation Strategies: Two-Stage Hepatectomy with Portal Vein Embolization and Associating Liver Partition and Portal Vein Ligation for Staged hepatectomy

Although an FLR of approximately 25% to 30% is generally considered to be sufficient to maintain liver function in patients without liver disease, a larger future remnant liver is recommended for patients with chemotherapy-associated steatohepatitis and hepatic dysfunction to avoid PHLF.[77] To this end, several methods have been proposed to induce compensatory hypertrophy of the FLR and increase resectability in patients with extensive bilobar liver metastases. The concept of a two-stage hepatectomy

(TSH) was first introduced by Adam and colleagues as an approach involving an initial limited resection of the less affected side of the liver, followed by contralateral liver resection after a period of liver hypertrophy.[78] However, a high postoperative death rate of 15% after the second-stage procedure in this series prompted the development of an alternate 2-stage strategy involving portal vein embolization (PVE) to accelerate the liver hypertrophy process.[79] The hypertrophic potential of the liver was first demonstrated in a rabbit model by Rous and Larimore in the 1920s and is based on previous observations by James Cantlie from 1897.[80,81] However, it was not until 1975 that Honjo and colleagues introduced portal vein ligation (PVL) as part of a 2-stage extended hepatectomy approach, marking the first clinical implementation of compensatory liver hypertrophy triggered by portal vein occlusion.[82–84] Soon after, Kinoshita and Makuuchi described the strategy to induce liver hypertrophy by injection of embolizing agents in one of the portal branches in 1990. Although PVE results in ipsilateral atrophy with compensatory hypertrophy of the FLR, the absolute FLR volume seems to be less important than the kinetic growth rate (KGR). In a study by Shindoh and colleagues from MD Anderson Cancer Center, a KGR, defined as the volume of liver hypertrophy per week, exceeding 2%, was associated with decreased rates of PHLF.[85] Further, when the KGR exceeded 2% and the standardized FLR volume surpassed 30%, liver-related mortality was not observed. In a similar analysis from Memorial Sloan Kettering Cancer Center, Leung and colleagues reported a growth rate greater than 2.66% per week was necessary to mitigate the risk of PHLF.[86] As such, common practice today includes determination of the FLR volume, the degree of hypertrophy (final FLR volume − initial FLR volume), and KGR, all of which are considered before hepatectomy is performed. With these considerations now known, a contemporary series evaluated the safety and success rate of TSH with PVE. This series demonstrated a 5-year survival rate of 51% in the TSH group compared with 15% in nonsurgically treated patients ($P = .005$).[87] Importantly, the median number and size of CRLM did not differ between both groups, indicating that complete TSH is associated with excellent oncologic outcomes: 90-day mortality rate was 6% with a 49% morbidity rate after the second stage of hepatectomy, consistent with previously reported mortality and morbidity rates after TSR. In patients who do not respond to PVE, hepatic vein embolization (HVE) has been proposed as an additional strategy to increase FLR volume and achieve resectability.[88]

Beyond PVE and total venous deprivation strategies (PVE + HVE) with TSH, the associating liver partition with PVL for staged hepatectomy (ALPPS) technique, described by Schnitzbauer and colleagues, triggers a spectacularly rapid regeneration of the FLR and reduces the interval between the stage 1 and 2 hepatectomies from 4 to 6 weeks to only 7 to 14 days.[89] Despite an up to 80% reduction in the time needed to allow for sufficient FLR hypertrophy compared with PVE or PVL alone, ALPPS has gained fervent criticism due to concerns over mortality rates of up to 25%.[90] The multicenter randomized LIGRO trial was designed to assess these concerns and systematically compare ALPPS to TSH with PVL or PVE.[91] Although 87% of the patients in the ALPPS arm reached an FLR of more than 30% within just 7 days, only 30% of patients in the TSH group reached this milestone. Even after 4 weeks, only 47% of patients in the TSH group reached a 30% FLR, highlighting the extent of regeneration that can be achieved with ALPPS. Notably, the LIGRO study demonstrated a significant increase in the primary outcome of resection rate from 57% (95% CI 43–72) in the TSH arm to 92% (95% CI 84–100) in the ALPPS arm. Similarly, the estimated median survival in the ALPPS group was 46 months compared with 26 months in the TSH group in a follow-up study (95% CI 34–59 and 16–36, respectively; $P = .028$; **Fig. 2**).[92] Importantly, the LIGRO trial reported morbidity to be similar with 43% of the patients in

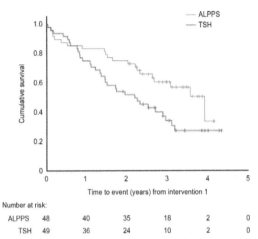

Fig. 2. ALPPS improves Overall Survival in patients with CRLM and an insufficient FLR compared with TSH. Overall survival curves for all included patients are shown. Estimated median survival in the ALPPS group was 46 months compared with 26 months in the TSH group. (*From* Hasselgren et al. ALPPS Improves Survival Compared With TSH in Patients Affected of CRLM: Survival Analysis From the Randomized Controlled Trial LIGRO. Ann Surg 2021 Mar 1;273(3):442-448.)

the ALPPS group and TSH group experiencing a grade IIIa or greater complication by Clavien–Dindo classification. Similarly, the 90-day mortality from the final intervention was 8.3% in the ALPPS group and 6.1% in the TSH group (*P* = .68), indicating similar rates of severe complications and mortality in this trial. In light of the LIGRO trial being conducted at high-volume ALPPS centers with tremendous experience, a meta-analysis inclusive of 90 studies and 4352 patients suggested ALPPS may be associated with higher morbidity and mortality rates.[93] Compared with TSH, ALPPS was associated with a trend toward increased morbidity (73% vs 59%; *P* = .16) and mortality (14% vs 7%; *P* = .19) after completion of second stage of either approach. As such, ALPPS remains controversial among hepatobiliary surgeons.

Hepatic Artery Infusion for Unresectable Colorectal Liver Metastases

Notably, although only 50% to 70% of patients with CRLM respond to first-line systemic chemotherapy, patients who fail to convert to resection ultimately reach dose-limiting toxicity and transition to second-line chemotherapy or maintenance chemotherapy. Unfortunately, response to second-line chemotherapy is typically only 5% to 20%.[94] In an RCT comparing second-line FOLFIRI with and without bevacizumab, the response rate in the combined arm was only 5% and median OS was only 11 months from the time of initiation of this regimen.[95] For patients whose therapy is de-escalated to maintenance capecitabine, PFS is improved by 2 months (3.9 vs 1.9 months, HR 0.44, 95% CI 0.33–0.57; *P* < .0001) but there is no difference in OS (15.2 vs 14.8 months; *P* = .98) compared with active monitoring (surveillance).[96] Given the limitations of systemic therapy in this population, HAI has been shown to improve survival and convert patients to resection in prospective studies. In the most recent randomized trial, the CALGB 9481 study compared HAI with FUDR alone to systemic 5-fluorouracil alone. Although these treatment arms are now both considered to be outdated regimens, Kemeny and colleagues reported an improvement in median survival (24.4 vs 20 months; *P* = .0034), longer time to hepatic progression

(9.8 vs 7.3 months; $P = .034$), and improved quality of life for patients with unresectable CRLM receiving HAI versus systemic therapy.[97] In a more recent phase II single-arm study, D'Angelica and colleagues evaluated the role of HAI combined with modern chemotherapy as a conversion strategy for patients with unresectable CRLM.[98] In this study of heavily pretreated patients (67% had already received 2–3 lines of chemotherapy) with a high disease burden (median 13 tumors), the response rate for the cohort was 73%.[98,99] Chemotherapy-naïve patients had a response rate of 86%, whereas the response rate was 67% even in previously treated patients.[98,99] Moreover, HAI combined with modern chemotherapy yielded a median OS and PFS of 38 months and 13 months, respectively. Notably, there was a significant difference in OS between chemotherapy-naive patients and those who had previously received chemotherapy (76.6 vs 29.7 months $P = .022$; **Fig. 3**A). Importantly, 52% of patients with extensive CRLM converted to resection. In the long-term follow-up landmark analysis of patients who converted to resection within 12 months of initiating HAI, 5-year survival was 63%, similar to survival endpoints in patients who are resectable at diagnosis (**Fig. 3**B).[98,99]

Although results with HAI for unresectable CRLM are encouraging, there remains ongoing skepticism regarding the safety, feasibility, and efficacy of this therapy outside of Memorial Sloan Kettering Cancer Center where this therapy has been pioneered and optimized since the 1980s. Beyond the approximately 20% of patients who experience a pump-specific complication related to the pocket, device, catheter, or artery, the major safety consideration is biliary sclerosis (defined as requiring an invasive biliary procedure); however, in the modern era, this serious complication from FUDR toxicity occurs in 2% to 8% of patients, with the risk being highest in the adjuvant setting.[59,98–100] In part due to awareness of these outcomes as well as

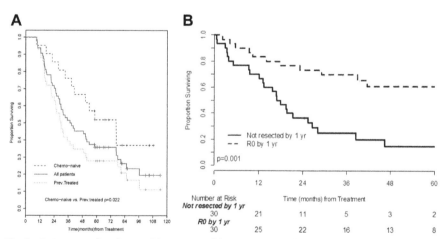

Fig. 3. Outcomes of patients with unresectable CRLM treated with HAI and systemic therapy in a nonrandomized, single-arm phase II study. (*A*) Landmark analysis demonstrated a median 3-year OS of 80% in patients who converted to and underwent resection within 12 months of initiating HAI versus 26% for those who did not convert. Time 0 to 12 months from start of treatment. (*B*) Overall survival stratified by prior chemotherapy exposure. Median survival was 38 months for all patients, 76.6 months for chemo-naïve patients and 29.7 months for previously treated patients. (*From* Pak et al. Prospective phase II trial of combination hepatic artery infusion and systemic chemotherapy for unresectable colorectal liver metastases: Long term results and curative potential. J Surg Oncol 2018 Mar;117(4):634-643. https://doi.org/10.1002/jso.24898.)

unacceptable outcomes with available systemic chemotherapy, there is renewed enthusiasm for HAI with rapid expansion of new HAI programs nationwide and world-wide.[101-104] Although it is anticipated that HAI will continue to expand, thereby improving access to many more patients, modern-day multicenter randomized trials are desperately needed to determine the exact role of HAI in standardized algorithms for patients.

Transplantation for Unresectable Colorectal Liver Metastases

Although liver transplantation is considered the standard of care for eligible patients with hepatocellular carcinoma, there are only limited data on the role of liver transplantation for CRLM. In their prospective SECA-II study, Dueland and colleagues reported OS at 1, 3, and 5 years of 100%, 83%, and 83%, respectively.[105] The median DFS was 13.7 months, with 1, 2, and 3 years DFS rates of 53%, 44%, and 35%, respectively. More recently, the group from Oslo, Norway published their results comparing highly selected patients who underwent hepatectomy after PVE versus liver transplant. The results of this study indicate that liver transplantation was associated with a 5-year OS of 33.4% compared with 6.7% for patients treated with PVE and liver resection.[106] In a subgroup analysis, 5-year OS was 45.3% for patients with liver transplantation for primary left-sided tumors compared with 0% for patients with an ascending colon primary tumor (P<.01). Patients receiving PVE only had a median OS of only 10.9 months, and 8 patients receiving liver resection after PVE had a median OS of 29.8 months. Consistent with these outcomes, a multicenter analysis for living-donor liver transplant from North America and the Netherlands reported acceptable donor morbidity with estimated 1.5-year recipient PFS and OS rates of 62% and 100%, respectively.[107] Because it becomes clear that transplant likely has a role in the management of patients with unresectable CRLM, recurrence seems inevitable, suggesting the importance of ongoing investigation to optimize patient selection for transplantation.

Immunotherapy

Immunotherapy has opened a new era in the management of numerous cancer types that are presumed to be immunogenic and characterized by a high tumor mutation burden. Although most CRLM do not represent disease entities with a high tumor neo-antigen density, multiple strategies have been explored to enhance their immunogenicity. The REGONIVO trial evaluated the role of regorafenib and nivolumab in microsatellite stable or mismatch repair-proficient mCRC. Surprisingly, patients with liver metastases had a significantly lower response rate (8.3%) than those with lung metastases without any liver involvement (63.6%).[108] Recently, Mettu and colleagues reported that patients with refractory microsatellite/mismatch repair stable mCRC benefitted from cotargeting VEGF and programmed cell death 1 or programmed cell death ligand 1 (HR for PFS was 0.66; 95% CI 0.44–0.99).[109] Similar to the findings of the REGONIVO trial, the response rate was higher among patients without liver metastases (23.1%) compared with patients with liver metastasis (5.8%). One possible explanation for this finding comes from a recent study by Yu and colleagues investigating antitumor immunity in patients with liver metastases.[110] In a syngeneic murine model of CRC, tumor-antigen restricted cytotoxic T lymphocytes were found to undergo apoptosis on interaction with macrophages within liver metastases. As such, liver metastases might corrupt antitumor immunity and mediate resistance to immunotherapy.

DISCUSSION

During the course of their illness, nearly half of all patients diagnosed with CRC will develop metastatic disease in the liver. With CRC being one of the most common cancer diagnoses in men and women, CRLM represents the final stage of a complex multistep biological process and is a significant cause of morbidity and mortality worldwide. Although studies on the natural history of CRLM show few or no patients surviving beyond 3 years, the last few decades have seen enormous strides in the surgical and medical management of CRLM. Currently, resection of CRLM with the goal to achieve an R0 margin remains the only opportunity for cure. The extent of hepatic resection needed to achieve this goal is mainly dictated by the size, location, and the number of liver metastases. Resectability is best determined by an experienced liver surgeon who can then deploy parenchymal preserving approaches to eradicate all hepatic disease while minimizing morbidity. The decisions to use chemotherapy for resectable CRLM, and in what sequence with resection if at all, remain complex, and without clear evidence for a survival advantage with these therapies, such decisions should be tailored to each individual patient and their disease. Management strategies for patients who are not clearly resectable at diagnosis or are technically unresectable seem to be more straightforward at the outset; however, with modern systemic therapy regimens combined with aggressive surgical approaches including TSH with PVE, ALPPS, and/or liver-directed therapy with HAI, efforts may be focused on maximizing response to downstage CRLM and convert the patient to a resectable situation.

For patients with CRLM, it remains important to establish goals of therapy early on, such that treatment decisions can be formulated accordingly. As is evident from the literature included herein, evaluation of resectability, sequencing of surgery with chemotherapy, selection of the optimal chemotherapy regimen, and/or consideration of other modalities of treatment including liver-directed therapy with HAI, remains nuanced and best determined by a multidisciplinary team.

CLINICS CARE POINTS

- Higher-level evidence is needed for assessment of safety and patient outcomes in regard to the role of neoadjuvant chemotherapy for resectable CRLM.
- Determination of the optimal modality of treatment for each patient requires a multidisciplinary team.

DISCLOSURE

The authors have nothing to disclose.

REFERENCES

1. Siegel RL, Miller KD, Goding Sauer A, et al. Colorectal cancer statistics, 2020. CA Cancer J Clin 2020;70(3):145–64. https://doi.org/10.3322/caac.21601.
2. Dekker E, Tanis PJ, Vleugels JLA, et al. Colorectal cancer. Lancet 2019; 394(10207):1467–80. https://doi.org/10.1016/S0140-6736(19)32319-0.
3. Kneuertz PJ, Chang GJ, Hu CY, et al. Overtreatment of young adults with colon cancer: more intense treatments with unmatched survival gains. JAMA Surg 2015;150(5):402–9. https://doi.org/10.1001/jamasurg.2014.3572.

4. Liang JT, Huang KC, Cheng AL, et al. Clinicopathological and molecular biological features of colorectal cancer in patients less than 40 years of age. Br J Surg 2003;90(2):205–14. https://doi.org/10.1002/bjs.4015.

5. Siegel RL, Torre LA, Soerjomataram I, et al. Global patterns and trends in colorectal cancer incidence in young adults. Gut 2019;68(12):2179–85. https://doi.org/10.1136/gutjnl-2019-319511.

6. Lieu CH, Renfro LA, de Gramont A, et al. Association of age with survival in patients with metastatic colorectal cancer: analysis from the ARCAD Clinical Trials Program. J Clin Oncol 2014;32(27):2975–84. https://doi.org/10.1200/JCO.2013.54.9329.

7. Nitsche U, Stogbauer F, Spath C, et al. Right Sided Colon Cancer as a Distinct Histopathological Subtype with Reduced Prognosis. Dig Surg 2016;33(2):157–63. https://doi.org/10.1159/000443644.

8. Gervaz P, Bucher P, Morel P. Two colons-two cancers: paradigm shift and clinical implications. J Surg Oncol 2004;88(4):261–6. https://doi.org/10.1002/jso.20156.

9. Yahagi M, Okabayashi K, Hasegawa H, et al. The Worse Prognosis of Right-Sided Compared with Left-Sided Colon Cancers: a Systematic Review and Meta-analysis. J Gastrointest Surg 2016;20(3):648–55. https://doi.org/10.1007/s11605-015-3026-6.

10. Brule SY, Jonker DJ, Karapetis CS, et al. Location of colon cancer (right-sided versus left-sided) as a prognostic factor and a predictor of benefit from cetuximab in NCIC CO.17. Eur J Cancer 2015;51(11):1405–14. https://doi.org/10.1016/j.ejca.2015.03.015.

11. Engstrand J, Nilsson H, Stromberg C, et al. Colorectal cancer liver metastases - a population-based study on incidence, management and survival. BMC Cancer 2018;18(1):78. https://doi.org/10.1186/s12885-017-3925-x.

12. Petrelli F, Tomasello G, Borgonovo K, et al. Prognostic Survival Associated With Left-Sided vs Right-Sided Colon Cancer: A Systematic Review and Meta-analysis. JAMA Oncol 2017;3(2):211–9. https://doi.org/10.1001/jamaoncol.2016.4227.

13. Vayrynen V, Wirta EV, Seppala T, et al. Incidence and management of patients with colorectal cancer and synchronous and metachronous colorectal metastases: a population-based study. BJS Open 2020;4(4):685–92. https://doi.org/10.1002/bjs5.50299.

14. Andres A, Mentha G, Adam R, et al. Surgical management of patients with colorectal cancer and simultaneous liver and lung metastases. Br J Surg 2015;102(6):691–9. https://doi.org/10.1002/bjs.9783.

15. Wagner JS, Adson MA, Van Heerden JA, et al. The natural history of hepatic metastases from colorectal cancer. A comparison with resective treatment. Ann Surg 1984;199(5):502–8. https://doi.org/10.1097/00000658-198405000-00002.

16. Nordlinger B, Guiguet M, Vaillant JC, et al. Surgical resection of colorectal carcinoma metastases to the liver. A prognostic scoring system to improve case selection, based on 1568 patients. Assoc Francaise de Chirurgie. Cancer 1996;77(7):1254–62.

17. Garden OJ, Rees M, Poston GJ, et al. Guidelines for resection of colorectal cancer liver metastases. Gut 2006;55(Suppl 3:iii):1–8. https://doi.org/10.1136/gut.2006.098053.

18. Hekimoglu K, Ustundag Y, Dusak A, et al. Small colorectal liver metastases: detection with SPIO-enhanced MRI in comparison with gadobenate

dimeglumine-enhanced MRI and CT imaging. Eur J Radiol 2011;77(3):468–72. https://doi.org/10.1016/j.ejrad.2009.09.002.

19. Sahani DV, Bajwa MA, Andrabi Y, et al. Current status of imaging and emerging techniques to evaluate liver metastases from colorectal carcinoma. Ann Surg 2014;259(5):861–72. https://doi.org/10.1097/SLA.0000000000000525.

20. Muhi A, Ichikawa T, Motosugi U, et al. Diagnosis of colorectal hepatic metasta-ses: comparison of contrast-enhanced CT, contrast-enhanced US, superpara-magnetic iron oxide-enhanced MRI, and gadoxetic acid-enhanced MRI. J Magn Reson Imaging 2011;34(2):326–35. https://doi.org/10.1002/jmri.22613.

21. Gorgec B, Hansen I, Kemmerich G, et al. Clinical added value of MRI to CT in patients scheduled for local therapy of colorectal liver metastases (CAMINO): study protocol for an international multicentre prospective diagnostic accuracy study. BMC Cancer 2021;21(1):1116. https://doi.org/10.1186/s12885-021-08833-1.

22. Creasy JM, Sadot E, Koerkamp BG, et al. Actual 10-year survival after hepatic resection of colorectal liver metastases: what factors preclude cure? Surgery 2018;163(6):1238–44. https://doi.org/10.1016/j.surg.2018.01.004.

23. Fong Y, Fortner J, Sun RL, et al. Clinical score for predicting recurrence after he-patic resection for metastatic colorectal cancer: analysis of 1001 consecutive cases. Ann Surg 1999;230(3):309–18. https://doi.org/10.1097/00000658-199909000-00004 ; discussion 318-21.

24. Mann CD, Metcalfe MS, Leopardi LN, et al. The clinical risk score: emerging as a reliable preoperative prognostic index in hepatectomy for colorectal metasta-ses. Arch Surg 2004;139(11):1168–72. https://doi.org/10.1001/archsurg.139.11.1168.

25. Nagashima I, Takada T, Adachi M, et al. Proposal of criteria to select candidates with colorectal liver metastases for hepatic resection: comparison of our scoring system to the positive number of risk factors. World J Gastroenterol 2006;12(39):6305–9. https://doi.org/10.3748/wjg.v12.i39.6305.

26. Konopke R, Kersting S, Distler M, et al. Prognostic factors and evaluation of a clinical score for predicting survival after resection of colorectal liver metasta-ses. Liver Int 2009;29(1):89–102. https://doi.org/10.1111/j.1478-3231.2008.01845.x.

27. Vega EA, Salehi O, Nicolaescu D, et al. Correction to: Failure to Cure Patients with Colorectal Liver Metastases: The Impact of the Liver Surgeon. Ann Surg Oncol 2021;28(Suppl 3):879. https://doi.org/10.1245/s10434-021-10185-w.

28. Akita H, Sasaki Y, Yamada T, et al. Real-time intraoperative assessment of resid-ual liver functional reserve using pulse dye densitometry. World J Surg 2008;32(12):2668–74. https://doi.org/10.1007/s00268-008-9752-0.

29. Kauffmann R, Fong Y. Post-hepatectomy liver failure. Hepatobiliary Surg Nutr 2014;3(5):238–46. https://doi.org/10.3978/j.issn.2304-3881.2014.09.01.

30. Margonis GA, Sergentanis TN, Ntanasis-Stathopoulos I, et al. Impact of Surgical Margin Width on Recurrence and Overall Survival Following R0 Hepatic Resec-tion of Colorectal Metastases: A Systematic Review and Meta-analysis. Ann Surg 2018;267(6):1047–55. https://doi.org/10.1097/SLA.0000000000002552.

31. Pawlik TM, Scoggins CR, Zorzi D, et al. Effect of surgical margin status on sur-vival and site of recurrence after hepatic resection for colorectal metastases. Ann Surg 2005;241(5):715–22. https://doi.org/10.1097/01.sla.0000160703.75808.7d, discussion 722-4.

32. Margonis GA, Buettner S, Andreatos N, et al. Anatomical Resections Improve Disease-free Survival in Patients With KRAS-mutated Colorectal Liver

Metastases. Ann Surg 2017;266(4):641–9. https://doi.org/10.1097/SLA. 0000000000002367.

33. Muratore A, Ribero D, Zimmitti G, et al. Resection margin and recurrence-free survival after liver resection of colorectal metastases. Ann Surg Oncol 2010; 17(5):1324–9. https://doi.org/10.1245/s10434-009-0770-4.

34. Matsumura M, Mise Y, Saiura A, et al. Parenchymal-Sparing Hepatectomy Does Not Increase Intrahepatic Recurrence in Patients with Advanced Colorectal Liver Metastases. Ann Surg Oncol 2016;23(11):3718–26. https://doi.org/10. 1245/s10434-016-5278-0.

35. Kingham TP, Correa-Gallego C, D'Angelica MI, et al. Hepatic parenchymal preservation surgery: decreasing morbidity and mortality rates in 4,152 resections for malignancy. J Am Coll Surg 2015;220(4):471–9. https://doi.org/10.1016/j. jamcollsurg.2014.12.026.

36. Deng G, Li H, Jia GQ, et al. Parenchymal-sparing versus extended hepatectomy for colorectal liver metastases: A systematic review and meta-analysis. Cancer Med 2019;8(14):6165–75. https://doi.org/10.1002/cam4.2515.

37. Moris D, Ronnekleiv-Kelly S, Rahnemai-Azar AA, et al. Parenchymal-Sparing Versus Anatomic Liver Resection for Colorectal Liver Metastases: a Systematic Review. J Gastrointest Surg 2017;21(6):1076–85. https://doi.org/10.1007/ s11605-017-3397-y.

38. Matsuki R, Mise Y, Saiura A, et al. Parenchymal-sparing hepatectomy for deep-placed colorectal liver metastases. Surgery 2016;160(5):1256–63. https://doi. org/10.1016/j.surg.2016.06.041.

39. Mise Y, Aloia TA, Brudvik KW, et al. Parenchymal-sparing Hepatectomy in Colorectal Liver Metastasis Improves Salvageability and Survival. Ann Surg 2016; 263(1):146–52. https://doi.org/10.1097/SLA.0000000000001194.

40. Ruers T, Punt C, Van Coevorden F, et al. Radiofrequency ablation combined with systemic treatment versus systemic treatment alone in patients with non-resectable colorectal liver metastases: a randomized EORTC Intergroup phase II study (EORTC 40004). Ann Oncol 2012;23(10):2619–26. https://doi.org/10. 1093/annonc/mds053.

41. Siperstein AE, Berber E, Ballem N, et al. Survival after radiofrequency ablation of colorectal liver metastases: 10-year experience. Ann Surg 2007;246(4):559–65. https://doi.org/10.1097/SLA.0b013e318155a7b6 ; discussion 565-7.

42. Shibata T, Niinobu T, Ogata N, et al. Microwave coagulation therapy for multiple hepatic metastases from colorectal carcinoma. Cancer 2000;89(2):276–84.

43. Cheng Y, Zhang L, Li H, et al. Laparoscopic versus open liver resection for colorectal liver metastases: a systematic review. J Surg Res 2017;220:234–46. https://doi.org/10.1016/j.jss.2017.05.110.

44. Syn NL, Kabir T, Koh YX, et al. Survival Advantage of Laparoscopic Versus Open Resection For Colorectal Liver Metastases: A Meta-analysis of Individual Patient Data From Randomized Trials and Propensity-score Matched Studies. Ann Surg 2020;272(2):253–65. https://doi.org/10.1097/SLA.0000000000003672.

45. Fretland AA, Dagenborg VJ, Bjornelv GMW, et al. Laparoscopic Versus Open Resection for Colorectal Liver Metastases: The OSLO-COMET Randomized Controlled Trial. Ann Surg 2018;267(2):199–207. https://doi.org/10.1097/SLA. 0000000000002353.

46. Portier G, Elias D, Bouche O, et al. Multicenter randomized trial of adjuvant fluorouracil and folinic acid compared with surgery alone after resection of colorectal liver metastases: FFCD ACHBTH AURC 9002 trial. J Clin Oncol 2006; 24(31):4976–82. https://doi.org/10.1200/JCO.2006.06.8353.

47. Mitry E, Fields AL, Bleiberg H, et al. Adjuvant chemotherapy after potentially curative resection of metastases from colorectal cancer: a pooled analysis of two randomized trials. J Clin Oncol 2008;26(30):4906–11. https://doi.org/10.1200/JCO.2008.17.3781.

48. Ychou M, Raoul JL, Douillard JY, et al. A phase III randomised trial of LV5FU2 + irinotecan versus LV5FU2 alone in adjuvant high-risk colon cancer (FNCLCC Accord02/FFCD9802). Ann Oncol 2009;20(4):674–80. https://doi.org/10.1093/annonc/mdn680.

49. Kanemitsu Y, Shimizu Y, Mizusawa J, et al. Hepatectomy Followed by mFOL-FOX6 Versus Hepatectomy Alone for Liver-Only Metastatic Colorectal Cancer (JCOG0603): A Phase II or III Randomized Controlled Trial. J Clin Oncol 2021; 39(34):3789–99. https://doi.org/10.1200/JCO.21.01032.

50. Nordlinger B, Sorbye H, Glimelius B, et al. Perioperative chemotherapy with FOLFOX4 and surgery versus surgery alone for resectable liver metastases from colorectal cancer (EORTC Intergroup trial 40983): a randomised controlled trial. Lancet 2008;371(9617):1007–16. https://doi.org/10.1016/S0140-6736(08)60455-9.

51. Nordlinger B, Sorbye H, Glimelius B, et al. Perioperative FOLFOX4 chemotherapy and surgery versus surgery alone for resectable liver metastases from colorectal cancer (EORTC 40983): long-term results of a randomised, controlled, phase 3 trial. Lancet Oncol 2013;14(12):1208–15. https://doi.org/10.1016/S1470-2045(13)70447-9.

52. Ayez N, van der Stok EP, de Wilt H, et al. Neo-adjuvant chemotherapy followed by surgery versus surgery alone in high-risk patients with resectable colorectal liver metastases: the CHARISMA randomized multicenter clinical trial. BMC Cancer 2015;15:180. https://doi.org/10.1186/s12885-015-1199-8.

53. Primrose J, Falk S, Finch-Jones M, et al. Systemic chemotherapy with or without cetuximab in patients with resectable colorectal liver metastasis: the New EPOC randomised controlled trial. Lancet Oncol 2014;15(6):601–11. https://doi.org/10.1016/S1470-2045(14)70105-6.

54. Bridgewater JA, Pugh SA, Maishman T, et al. Systemic chemotherapy with or without cetuximab in patients with resectable colorectal liver metastasis (New EPOC): long-term results of a multicentre, randomised, controlled, phase 3 trial. Lancet Oncol 2020;21(3):398–411. https://doi.org/10.1016/S1470-2045(19)30798-3.

55. Breedis C, Young G. The blood supply of neoplasms in the liver. Am J Pathol 1954;30(5):969–77.

56. Clarkson B, Young C, Dierick W, et al. Effects of continuous hepatic artery infusion of antimetabolites on primary and metastatic cancer of the liver. Cancer 1962;15:472–88.

57. Sullivan RD, Norcross JW, Watkins E Jr. Chemotherapy of Metastatic Liver Cancer by Prolonged Hepatic-Artery Infusion. N Engl J Med 1964;270:321–7. https://doi.org/10.1056/NEJM196402132700701.

58. Kemeny N, Huang Y, Cohen AM, et al. Hepatic arterial infusion of chemotherapy after resection of hepatic metastases from colorectal cancer. N Engl J Med 1999;341(27):2039–48. https://doi.org/10.1056/NEJM199912303412702.

59. Kemeny NE, Chou JF, Boucher TM, et al. Updated long-term survival for patients with metastatic colorectal cancer treated with liver resection followed by hepatic arterial infusion and systemic chemotherapy. J Surg Oncol 2016;113(5):477–84. https://doi.org/10.1002/jso.24189.

60. Groot Koerkamp B, Sadot E, Kemeny NE, et al. Perioperative Hepatic Arterial Infusion Pump Chemotherapy Is Associated With Longer Survival After Resection of Colorectal Liver Metastases: A Propensity Score Analysis. J Clin Oncol 2017;35(17):1938–44. https://doi.org/10.1200/JCO.2016.71.8346.

61. Gholami S, Kemeny NE, Boucher TM, et al. Adjuvant Hepatic Artery Infusion Chemotherapy is Associated With Improved Survival Regardless of KRAS Mutation Status in Patients With Resected Colorectal Liver Metastases: A Retrospective Analysis of 674 Patients. Ann Surg 2020;272(2):352–6. https://doi.org/10.1097/SLA.0000000000003248.

62. Altendorf-Hofmann A, Scheele J. A critical review of the major indicators of prognosis after resection of hepatic metastases from colorectal carcinoma. Surg Oncol Clin N Am 2003;12(1):165–92. https://doi.org/10.1016/s1055-3207(02)00091-1, xi.

63. Adam R, Delvart V, Pascal G, et al. Rescue surgery for unresectable colorectal liver metastases downstaged by chemotherapy: a model to predict long-term survival. Ann Surg 2004;240(4):644–57. https://doi.org/10.1097/01.sla.0000141198.92114.f6 [discussion: 657-8].

64. Pozzo C, Basso M, Cassano A, et al. Neoadjuvant treatment of unresectable liver disease with irinotecan and 5-fluorouracil plus folinic acid in colorectal cancer patients. Ann Oncol 2004;15(6):933–9. https://doi.org/10.1093/annonc/mdh217.

65. Bismuth H, Adam R, Levi F, et al. Resection of nonresectable liver metastases from colorectal cancer after neoadjuvant chemotherapy. Ann Surg 1996;224(4):509–20. https://doi.org/10.1097/00000658-199610000-00009 [discussion 520-2].

66. Ychou M, Rivoire M, Thezenas S, et al. A randomized phase II trial of three intensified chemotherapy regimens in first-line treatment of colorectal cancer patients with initially unresectable or not optimally resectable liver metastases. The METHEP trial. Ann Surg Oncol 2013;20(13):4289–97. https://doi.org/10.1245/s10434-013-3217-x.

67. Folprecht G, Gruenberger T, Bechstein WO, et al. Tumour response and secondary resectability of colorectal liver metastases following neoadjuvant chemotherapy with cetuximab: the CELIM randomised phase 2 trial. Lancet Oncol 2010;11(1):38–47. https://doi.org/10.1016/S1470-2045(09)70330-4.

68. Folprecht G, Gruenberger T, Bechstein W, et al. Survival of patients with initially unresectable colorectal liver metastases treated with FOLFOX/cetuximab or FOLFIRI/cetuximab in a multidisciplinary concept (CELIM study). Ann Oncol 2014;25(5):1018–25. https://doi.org/10.1093/annonc/mdu088.

69. Van Cutsem E, Kohne CH, Hitre E, et al. Cetuximab and chemotherapy as initial treatment for metastatic colorectal cancer. N Engl J Med 2009;360(14):1408–17. https://doi.org/10.1056/NEJMoa0805019.

70. Bokemeyer C, Bondarenko I, Hartmann JT, et al. Efficacy according to biomarker status of cetuximab plus FOLFOX-4 as first-line treatment for metastatic colorectal cancer: the OPUS study. Ann Oncol 2011;22(7):1535–46. https://doi.org/10.1093/annonc/mdq632.

71. Bokemeyer C, Bondarenko I, Makhson A, et al. Fluorouracil, leucovorin, and oxaliplatin with and without cetuximab in the first-line treatment of metastatic colorectal cancer. J Clin Oncol 2009;27(5):663–71. https://doi.org/10.1200/JCO.2008.20.8397.

72. Gruenberger T, Bridgewater J, Chau I, et al. Bevacizumab plus mFOLFOX-6 or FOLFOXIRI in patients with initially unresectable liver metastases from colorectal

cancer: the OLIVIA multinational randomised phase II trial. Ann Oncol 2015; 26(4):702–8. https://doi.org/10.1093/annonc/mdu580.

73. Tang W, Ren L, Liu T, et al. Bevacizumab Plus mFOLFOX6 Versus mFOLFOX6 Alone as First-Line Treatment for RAS Mutant Unresectable Colorectal Liver-Limited Metastases: The BECOME Randomized Controlled Trial. J Clin Oncol 2020;38(27):3175–84. https://doi.org/10.1200/JCO.20.00174.

74. Heinemann V, von Weikersthal LF, Decker T, et al. FOLFIRI plus cetuximab versus FOLFIRI plus bevacizumab as first-line treatment for patients with metastatic colorectal cancer (FIRE-3): a randomised, open-label, phase 3 trial. Lancet Oncol 2014;15(10):1065–75. https://doi.org/10.1016/S1470-2045(14) 70330-4.

75. Heinemann V, von Weikersthal LF, Decker T, et al. FOLFIRI plus cetuximab or bevacizumab for advanced colorectal cancer: final survival and per-protocol analysis of FIRE-3, a randomised clinical trial. Br J Cancer 2021;124(3): 587–94. https://doi.org/10.1038/s41416-020-01140-9.

76. Oki E, Emi Y, Yamanaka T, et al. Randomised phase II trial of mFOLFOX6 plus bevacizumab versus mFOLFOX6 plus cetuximab as first-line treatment for colorectal liver metastasis (ATOM trial). Br J Cancer 2019;121(3):222–9. https://doi. org/10.1038/s41416-019-0518-2.

77. Tucker ON, Heaton N. The 'small for size' liver syndrome. Curr Opin Crit Care 2005;11(2):150–5. https://doi.org/10.1097/01.ccx.0000157080.11117.45.

78. Adam R, Laurent A, Azoulay D, et al. Two-stage hepatectomy: A planned strategy to treat irresectable liver tumors. Ann Surg 2000;232(6):777–85. https://doi. org/10.1097/00000658-200012000-00006.

79. Jaeck D, Oussoultzoglou E, Rosso E, et al. A two-stage hepatectomy procedure combined with portal vein embolization to achieve curative resection for initially unresectable multiple and bilobar colorectal liver metastases. Ann Surg 2004; 240(6):1037–49. https://doi.org/10.1097/01.sla.0000145965.86383.89 [discussion: 1049-51].

80. Rous P, Larimore LD. Relation of the Portal Blood to Liver Maintenance : A Demonstration of Liver Atrophy Conditional on Compensation. J Exp Med 1920;31(5):609–32. https://doi.org/10.1084/jem.31.5.609.

81. van Gulik TM, van den Esschert JW. James Cantlie's early messages for hepatic surgeons: how the concept of pre-operative portal vein occlusion was defined. HPB (Oxford) 2010;12(2):81–3.

82. Kinoshita H, Sakai K, Hirohashi K, et al. Preoperative portal vein embolization for hepatocellular carcinoma. World J Surg 1986;10(5):803–8. https://doi.org/10. 1007/BF01655244.

83. Makuuchi M, Thai BL, Takayasu K, et al. Preoperative portal embolization to increase safety of major hepatectomy for hilar bile duct carcinoma: a preliminary report. Surgery 1990;107(5):521–7.

84. Honjo I, Suzuki T, Ozawa K, et al. Ligation of a branch of the portal vein for carcinoma of the liver. Am J Surg 1975;130(3):296–302. https://doi.org/10.1016/ 0002-9610(75)90389-x.

85. Shindoh J, Truty MJ, Aloia TA, et al. Kinetic growth rate after portal vein embolization predicts posthepatectomy outcomes: toward zero liver-related mortality in patients with colorectal liver metastases and small future liver remnant. J Am Coll Surg 2013;216(2):201–9. https://doi.org/10.1016/j.jamcollsurg.2012.10.018.

86. Leung U, Simpson AL, Araujo RL, et al. Remnant growth rate after portal vein embolization is a good early predictor of post-hepatectomy liver failure. J Am

Coll Surg 2014;219(4):620–30. https://doi.org/10.1016/j.jamcollsurg.2014. 04.022.

87. Brouquet A, Abdalla EK, Kopetz S, et al. High survival rate after two-stage resection of advanced colorectal liver metastases: response-based selection and complete resection define outcome. J Clin Oncol 2011;29(8):1083–90. https://doi.org/10.1200/JCO.2010.32.6132.

88. Hwang S, Lee SG, Ko GY, et al. Sequential preoperative ipsilateral hepatic vein embolization after portal vein embolization to induce further liver regeneration in patients with hepatobiliary malignancy. Ann Surg 2009;249(4):608–16. https:// doi.org/10.1097/SLA.0b013e31819ecc5c.

89. Schnitzbauer AA, Lang SA, Goessmann H, et al. Right portal vein ligation combined with in situ splitting induces rapid left lateral liver lobe hypertrophy enabling 2-staged extended right hepatic resection in small-for-size settings. Ann Surg 2012;255(3):405–14. https://doi.org/10.1097/SLA.0b013e31824856f5.

90. Kang D, Schadde E. Hypertrophy and Liver Function in ALPPS: Correlation with Morbidity and Mortality. Visc Med 2017;33(6):426–33. https://doi.org/10.1159/ 000479477.

91. Sandstrom P, Rosok BI, Sparrelid E, et al. ALPPS Improves Resectability Compared With Conventional Two-stage Hepatectomy in Patients With Advanced Colorectal Liver Metastasis: Results From a Scandinavian Multicenter Randomized Controlled Trial (LIGRO Trial). Ann Surg 2018;267(5):833–40. https://doi.org/10.1097/SLA.0000000000002511.

92. Hasselgren K, Rosok BI, Larsen PN, et al. ALPPS Improves Survival Compared With TSH in Patients Affected of CRLM: Survival Analysis From the Randomized Controlled Trial LIGRO. Ann Surg 2021;273(3):442–8. https://doi.org/10.1097/ SLA.0000000000003701.

93. Eshmuminov D, Raptis DA, Linecker M, et al. Meta-analysis of associating liver partition with portal vein ligation and portal vein occlusion for two-stage hepatectomy. Br J Surg 2016;103(13):1768–82. https://doi.org/10.1002/bjs.10290.

94. Tournigand C, Andre T, Achille E, et al. FOLFIRI followed by FOLFOX6 or the reverse sequence in advanced colorectal cancer: a randomized GERCOR study. J Clin Oncol 2004;22(2):229–37. https://doi.org/10.1200/JCO.2004. 05.113.

95. Bennouna J, Sastre J, Arnold D, et al. Continuation of bevacizumab after first progression in metastatic colorectal cancer (ML18147): a randomised phase 3 trial. Lancet Oncol 2013;14(1):29–37. https://doi.org/10.1016/S1470-2045(12)70477-1.

96. Adams RA, Fisher DJ, Graham J, et al. Capecitabine Versus Active Monitoring in Stable or Responding Metastatic Colorectal Cancer After 16 Weeks of First-Line Therapy: Results of the Randomized FOCUS4-N Trial. J Clin Oncol 2021;39(33): 3693–704. https://doi.org/10.1200/JCO.21.01436.

97. Kemeny NE, Niedzwiecki D, Hollis DR, et al. Hepatic arterial infusion versus systemic therapy for hepatic metastases from colorectal cancer: a randomized trial of efficacy, quality of life, and molecular markers (CALGB 9481). J Clin Oncol 2006;24(9):1395–403. https://doi.org/10.1200/JCO.2005.03.8166.

98. D'Angelica MI, Correa-Gallego C, Paty PB, et al. Phase II trial of hepatic artery infusional and systemic chemotherapy for patients with unresectable hepatic metastases from colorectal cancer: conversion to resection and long-term outcomes. Ann Surg 2015;261(2):353–60. https://doi.org/10.1097/SLA. 0000000000000614.

99. Pak LM, Kemeny NE, Capanu M, et al. Prospective phase II trial of combination hepatic artery infusion and systemic chemotherapy for unresectable colorectal liver metastases: Long term results and curative potential. J Surg Oncol 2018; 117(4):634–43. https://doi.org/10.1002/jso.24898.

100. Allen PJ, Nissan A, Picon AI, et al. Technical complications and durability of hepatic artery infusion pumps for unresectable colorectal liver metastases: an institutional experience of 544 consecutive cases. J Am Coll Surg 2005; 201(1):57–65. https://doi.org/10.1016/j.jamcollsurg.2005.03.019.

101. Chakedis J, Beal EW, Sun S, et al. Implementation and early outcomes for a surgeon-directed hepatic arterial infusion pump program for colorectal liver metastases. J Surg Oncol 2018;118(7):1065–73. https://doi.org/10.1002/jso.25249.

102. Creasy JM, Napier KJ, Reed SA, et al. Implementation of a Hepatic Artery Infusion Program: Initial Patient Selection and Perioperative Outcomes of Concurrent Hepatic Artery Infusion and Systemic Chemotherapy for Colorectal Liver Metastases. Ann Surg Oncol 2020. https://doi.org/10.1245/s10434-020-08972-y.

103. Dhir M, Jones HL, Shuai Y, et al. Hepatic Arterial Infusion in Combination with Modern Systemic Chemotherapy is Associated with Improved Survival Compared with Modern Systemic Chemotherapy Alone in Patients with Isolated Unresectable Colorectal Liver Metastases: A Case-Control Study. Ann Surg Oncol 2017;24(1):150–8. https://doi.org/10.1245/s10434-016-5418-6.

104. Muaddi H, D'Angelica M, Wiseman JT, et al. Safety and feasibility of initiating a hepatic artery infusion pump chemotherapy program for unresectable colorectal liver metastases: A multicenter, retrospective cohort study. J Surg Oncol 2021;123(1):252–60. https://doi.org/10.1002/jso.26270.

105. Dueland S, Syversveen T, Solheim JM, et al. Survival Following Liver Transplantation for Patients With Nonresectable Liver-only Colorectal Metastases. Ann Surg 2020;271(2):212–8. https://doi.org/10.1097/SLA.0000000000003404.

106. Dueland S, Yaqub S, Syversveen T, et al. Survival Outcomes After Portal Vein Embolization and Liver Resection Compared With Liver Transplant for Patients With Extensive Colorectal Cancer Liver Metastases. JAMA Surg 2021;156(6): 550–7. https://doi.org/10.1001/jamasurg.2021.0267.

107. Hernandez-Alejandro R, Ruffolo LI, Sasaki K, et al. Recipient and Donor Outcomes After Living-Donor Liver Transplant for Unresectable Colorectal Liver Metastases. JAMA Surg 2022. https://doi.org/10.1001/jamasurg.2022.0300.

108. Fukuoka S, Hara H, Takahashi N, et al. Regorafenib Plus Nivolumab in Patients With Advanced Gastric or Colorectal Cancer: An Open-Label, Dose-Escalation, and Dose-Expansion Phase Ib Trial (REGONIVO, EPOC1603). J Clin Oncol 2020;38(18):2053–61. https://doi.org/10.1200/JCO.19.03296.

109. Mettu NB, Ou FS, Zemla TJ, et al. Assessment of Capecitabine and Bevacizumab With or Without Atezolizumab for the Treatment of Refractory Metastatic Colorectal Cancer: A Randomized Clinical Trial. JAMA Netw Open 2022;5(2): e2149040. https://doi.org/10.1001/jamanetworkopen.2021.49040.

110. Yu J, Green MD, Li S, et al. Liver metastasis restrains immunotherapy efficacy via macrophage-mediated T cell elimination. Nat Med 2021;27(1):152–64. https://doi.org/10.1038/s41591-020-1131-x.

Surgeon-Led Clinical Trials in Pancreatic Cancer

Akhil Chawla, MD[a,b], Cristina R. Ferrone, MD[c],*

KEYWORDS

- Pancreatic cancer • Clinical trials • Chemotherapy • Radiation

KEY POINTS

- Pancreatic cancer
- Clinical trials
- Neoadjuvant therapy
- Chemotherapy
- Radiation

BACKGROUND

With an increase in systemic options available for metastatic pancreatic cancer, there has recently been a rise in key clinical trials focused on localized pancreatic cancer. Many of these reports have been practice-defining and have altered the design of subsequent clinical trials. The results have raised key questions for clinical trial investigators to clarify the future standard of care. The utilization of multi-agent chemotherapy regimens in the localized disease setting has sparked cooperative group and international collaborations in an effort to better understand the optimal regimen in the neoadjuvant and adjuvant disease settings. In addition, sophisticated techniques in radiation oncology, including the increasing familiarity with hypofractionated radiation, have boosted its use in the perioperative setting. Key to many of these trials has been the utilization of imaging criteria to define eligibility criteria, which aim to increase the level of quality control and standardization. However, we have learned that therein lies a significant amount of subjectivity in interpretation between each classification, requiring an increased sophistication in terms of trial design. This review highlights key clinical trials in localized pancreatic cancer over the past decade, with an emphasis on surgeon-led efforts to highlight the significant investigations that have ultimately paved the way for future prospective studies in pancreatic cancer.

---

[a] Division of Surgical Oncology, Department of Surgery, Northwestern Medicine Regional Medical Group, Northwestern University Feinberg School of Medicine, 676 N. St. Clair St., Suite 650Chicago, IL 60611, USA; [b] Robert H. Lurie Comprehensive Cancer Center, Chicago, IL, USA; [c] Department of Surgery, Massachusetts General Hospital, Boston, MA, USA
* Corresponding author. Wang 460, 15 Parkman Street, Boston, MA 02114.
E-mail address: CFERRONE@mgh.harvard.edu

Surg Oncol Clin N Am 32 (2023) 143–151
https://doi.org/10.1016/j.soc.2022.08.001
1055-3207/23/© 2022 Elsevier Inc. All rights reserved.
surgonc.theclinics.com

ADJUVANT TRIALS IN PANCREATIC CANCER

The establishment of standard combination chemotherapy regimens such as fluoro-uracil, leucovorin, irinotecan, and oxaliplatin (FOLFIRINOX) and gemcitabine with albumin-bound paclitaxel (nab-paclitaxel) in the localized disease space have stemmed from key multi-institutional randomized clinical trials performed in the met-astatic disease setting.[1,2] These trials ultimately led to a broad acceptance of well-defined multi-agent combination chemotherapy regimens in metastatic pancreatic cancer due to increased efficacy when compared with single-agent therapy. The increased experience managing the multi-agent chemotherapy-induced toxicity has subsequently also improved. The significant improvement in the survival of patients with metastatic pancreatic ductal adenocarcinomas (PDAC) prompted the switch from single-agent therapy[3–5] to multi-agent therapy.[6–10]

European Study Group for Pancreatic Cancer (ESPAC)-4 Trial

The landmark ESPAC-4 randomized phase III trial established the first standard multidrug adjuvant therapy regimen for pancreatic cancer.[6] In this multi-center trial led by the Eu-ropean Study Group for Pancreatic Cancer, 732 patients were randomized from six coun-tries to either gemcitabine with capecitabine or gemcitabine treatment alone within 12 weeks of surgery. The primary endpoint of this trial was overall survival (OS) with the intent to treat the population of patients who received at least one cycle of adjuvant ther-apy. Patients randomized to gemcitabine with capecitabine were found to have a median OS of 28.0 months compared with 25.5 months in the gemcitabine alone arm (hazard ratio [HR] 0.82; 95% confidence interval [CI] 0.68–0.98; $P = 0.032$). Importantly, patients who received combination therapy had overall good tolerability of the dual-agent regimen, with an acceptable level of toxicity using a dose reduction protocol.[6]

Adjuvant Therapy for Patients With Resected Pancreatic Cancer (APACT) Trial

The APACT trial evaluated gemcitabine and nab-paclitaxel in the adjuvant setting. The phase III multicenter trial randomized 866 patients to receive the combined adjuvant regimen or to receive adjuvant gemcitabine alone. After a median follow-up of 38.5 months, gemcitabine and nab-paclitaxel did not improve disease-free survival (DFS) compared with the gemcitabine group (19.4 vs 18.8 months, HR 0.88; 95%CI: 0.73–1.06; $P = .1824$), which was the primary endpoint of the study. Importantly, DFS in this study was *independently assessed*, as opposed to *investigator assessed*, with hopes to decrease investigator bias due to lack of imaging reliability for recurrent dis-ease. These results had initially only been presented in abstract form.[11] Recently, the updated 5-year analysis was reported for this study. The OS, a secondary endpoint in the trial, which did not reach statistical significance in the original report, was confirmed to be improved with the combination regimen when compared with gemcitabine alone. The median OS in the gemcitabine and nab-paclitaxel arm was 41.8 months, compared with 37.7 months (HR 0.80; 95% CI: 0.678–0.947; $P = .0091$). Although the results of this study are slowly gaining traction in clinical practice, this study served to establish gem-citabine and nab-paclitaxel as an adjuvant regimen option in pancreatic cancer.[12]

Unicancer Partenariat de Recherche en Oncologie Digestive (PRODIGE) 24/Canadian Cancer Trials Group (CCTG) PA.6 Trial

The Unicancer PRODIGE 24/CCTG PA.6 trial led by the Partenariat de Recherche en Oncologie Digestive intergroup and the Canadian Cancer Trials Group established modified FOLFIRINOX (mFOLFIRINOX) as the standard adjuvant chemotherapy regimen for pancreatic cancer patients with good performance status.[13] In this multi-institutional phase III European Trial, eligible patients restricted to a postoperative CA 19-9 serum level of less than 180 U/m were randomized to receive 6 months of adjuvant mFOLFIRINOX or adjuvant gemcitabine within 3 to 12 weeks of surgical resection.[13] The primary endpoint for the trial was DFS. After a median follow-up of 69.7 months, patients treated in the mFOLFIRINOX arm showed a 5-year DFS rate of 26.1% versus 19.0% in the gemcitabine arm (HR 0.66; 95% CI 0.54–0.82; P = .0001). Medial OS in the mFOLFIRINOX arm was 53.5 months in comparison to 35.5 months in patients who received adjuvant gemcitabine (HR 0.68; 95% CI 0.54–0.85; P = .0009).[14] Favorable survival outcomes were seen in both arms of this trial when compared with prior adjuvant gemcitabine trials likely because of the eligibility restriction of good performance status and low CA 19 to 9 levels. In addition, patients in the gemcitabine arm who recurred are likely to have benefited from contemporary treatment regimens at the time of disease progression.

These landmark adjuvant therapy trials highlight the value of combination chemotherapy in the adjuvant disease setting for patients with the surgically resected disease if their performance status allows them to tolerate their associated toxicities.

NEOADJUVANT CHEMOTHERAPY TRIALS

Experience in terms of efficacy and toxicity of mFOLFIRINOX and gemcitabine-based combination regimens has allowed investigators to evaluate combination regimens in the neoadjuvant setting. The utilization of combination systemic therapy in the adjuvant setting has been shown to improve DFS and OS in the above-described landmark trials.[6,12,13] However, approximately half of the patients who undergo pancreatic resection are unable to complete intended adjuvant chemotherapy.[15,16] Treatment with preoperative chemotherapy may lead to enhanced rates of tolerability for patients, particularly when compared with patients receiving multi-agent regimens after recovering from pancreatic surgery.[17] Therefore, there has been an increased emphasis on the utilization of neoadjuvant and perioperative combination therapies in localized pancreatic cancer.

Study Group of Preoperative Therapy for Pancreatic Cancer (PREP)-02/Japanese Study Group of Adjuvant Therapyfor Pancreatic Cancer (JSAP)05 Trial

The Japanese PREP-02/JSAP05 trial, which began in 2013, was the first multi-institutional randomized trial to report results on the use of perioperative chemotherapy. In total, 362 patients were enrolled at 57 centers over a 3-year period.[18] Patients with localized pancreatic cancer without any evidence of arterial involvement were enrolled after histologic confirmation and central randomization to either a perioperative therapy arm or an adjuvant therapy arm. Venous vascular involvement to any extent was allowed. Patients (n = 182) in the perioperative arm received two cycles of neoadjuvant gemcitabine and S-1, an oral 5-fluorouracil derivative[19] not available in the United States, followed by an operation and adjuvant S-1 for 6 months. Patients randomized to the adjuvant therapy arm (n = 180) received 6 months of adjuvant S-1. Preoperative therapy improved OS to 36.7 months compared with 28.8 months in the adjuvant therapy arm (HR 0.72; P = .015).[20] These results were among the first prospective randomized data to show that preoperative chemotherapy leads to nodal downstaging; patients in the perioperative arm were found to have nodal metastases in 59.6% of patients compared with 81.5% of patients in the adjuvant therapy arm. In addition, neoadjuvant chemotherapy therapy did not lead to any difference in surgical outcomes including morbidity, operative time, intraoperative bleeding, rate of reoperation, or operative mortality. Although this study was the first randomized multi-institutional trial to show the benefit of perioperative therapy, by design, patients in the perioperative arm received two extra months of systemic therapy, when compared with the adjuvant arm. Therefore, this trial did not definitively address the optimal sequencing of therapy in resectable pancreatic cancer.

Southwestern Oncology Group (SWOG) S1505 Trial

The Southwest Oncology Group's 1505 trial evaluated two standard multi-agent perioperative chemotherapy regimens. Patients with resectable pancreatic cancer by National Comprehensive Cancer Network (NCCN)/Intergroup criteria,[21,22] and confirmed via a post hoc central radiologic eligibility review were eligible. In total, 147 patients were randomized to perioperative mFOLFIRINOX therapy or therapy with perioperative gemcitabine and nab-paclitaxel. Patients received 12 weeks of neoadjuvant therapy, followed by an operation, and 12 weeks of adjuvant therapy.

After central radiologic review, 43 patients were ultimately excluded leaving 103 eligible patients for analysis.[23] Statistical analysis for the primary endpoint included OS with a "pick the winner" design, stratified by performance status. The trial failed to meet the pre-specified threshold and there was no difference in median OS between the two multi-agent regimens.[16] The median OS of patients treated with mFOLFIRINOX was 22.4 months and 23.6 months for those treated with gemcitabine and nab-paclitaxel.[16] Of 103 eligible patients who underwent neoadjuvant therapy, 26 dropped out due to progression of disease and treatment toxicity.[23] Of the 77 patients who went to the operating room, 73 underwent a curative-intent resection. A margin-negative resection was achieved in 85% of these cases. However, only 60% were able to begin their adjuvant therapy after recovering from the operation, with less than half of the patients in each arm completing all protocol-defined therapy.[16,23]

Taken together, the results of the SWOG S1505 trial did not yield a clear direction regarding a superior multi-agent neoadjuvant regimen. However, there were key lessons that were recognized from the trial results. Confirming what has been shown in previously reported single-arm phase II studies,[7,8,24] the SWOG S1505 results corroborate high rates of therapy completion using multi-agent chemotherapy, with 84% to 85% of patients completing all preoperative chemotherapy. However, with 36% of all patients not undergoing an operation due to disease progression during neoadjuvant chemotherapy,[23] increased equipoise has been raised regarding the efficacy of the neoadjuvant strategy for all patients with technically resectable disease. Another key takeaway from this trial involved the need for a prospective radiologic review. Nearly a third of patients enrolled in the SWOG S1505 were determined to be ineligible after post hoc central radiology review, underscoring the importance of integrating a prospective central radiologic eligibility review into trial design.

Alliance A021806 Trial

The ALLIANCE A021806 trial randomizes patients with resectable pancreatic cancer to perioperative or adjuvant chemotherapy. This phase III randomized controlled trial seeks to elucidate the role of neoadjuvant chemotherapy in patients with resectable pancreatic cancer. Patients with resectable pancreatic cancer based on the NCCN/Intergroup definition are eligible for the study. The protocol includes a preregistration phase which involves a prospective central radiologic eligibility review for confirmation of resectable disease status. Patients are then randomized to a Perioperative Arm or an Adjuvant Arm. The Perioperative Arm includes treatment with eight cycles of neoadjuvant mFOLFIRINOX treatment, followed by surgical resection, and four cycles of adjuvant mFOLFIRINOX. The Adjuvant Arm includes upfront surgery followed by 12 cycles of adjuvant mFOLFIRINOX. Restaging scans are performed every 2 months in both arms of the study.

The primary endpoint for this trial is 2-year OS. Secondary endpoints include DFS, margin-negative resection rate, locoregional recurrence rate, and distant recurrence rate. Importantly, this trial will directly assess the tolerability of mFOLFIRINOX therapy in the perioperative versus the adjuvant setting with the dose-intensity of chemotherapy delivered as well as adverse events in each arm evaluated as a secondary endpoint. Built-in is the key quality of life correlatives that will serve to better elucidate how patients may tolerate each strategy. Currently, there is no level one phase III evidence to guide the clear use of neoadjuvant mFOLFIRINOX treatment of resectable pancreatic cancer. Although institutional bias exists, there is significant variability in national practice patterns. Therefore, the ALLIANCE A021806 trial aims to establish a new standard of care for patients with resectable disease.

RADIATION TRIALS

Radiation therapy continues to be controversial in the management of pancreatic adenocarcinoma. Furthermore, the total dose and dosing schedule to achieve the optimal outcome continue to be under investigation.

PREOPANC-1 Trial

The most recent phase III trial involving radiation therapy for patients with resectable and borderline PDAC is the PREOPANC-1 study from the Netherlands.[25] This study involved 16 centers and randomized 246 patients with either resectable or borderline pancreatic cancer to receive preoperative chemoradiotherapy, which consisted of three cycles of gemcitabine, with the second cycle combined with radiotherapy, followed by an operation and four cycles of adjuvant gemcitabine or to an immediate operation and six cycles of adjuvant gemcitabine. Median OS by intention to treat was 16.0 months in patients treated with preoperative chemoradiotherapy and 14.3 months in patients treated with immediate surgery (hazard ratio, 0.78; 95% CI, 0.58–1.05; $P = .096$). The R0 resection rate was 71% (51 of 72) in patients who received preoperative chemoradiotherapy and 40% (37 of 92) in patients assigned to an immediate operation ($P < .001$). Preoperative chemoradiotherapy was associated with a significantly better DFS, locoregional failure-free interval, rate of pathologic lymph nodes, perineural invasion, and venous invasion. Survival analysis of patients who underwent tumor resection and started adjuvant chemotherapy showed improved survival with preoperative chemoradiotherapy (35.2 v 19.8 months; $P = .029$). The proportion of patients who suffered serious adverse events was 52% versus 41% ($P = .096$). After a median follow-up of 27 months the intent to treat analysis did not show an OS difference and the predefined subgroup of patients with suspected resectable PDAC showed no significant difference in OS or DFS. However, after a median follow-up of 59 months, neoadjuvant gemcitabine-based chemoradiotherapy followed by surgery and adjuvant gemcitabine improved OS compared with upfront surgery and adjuvant gemcitabine in patients with borderline resectable pancreatic cancer (5-year OS 20.5% vs 6.5%).[25]

Alliance A021501

The Alliance for Clinical Oncology Trial A021501, a recently completed randomized phase II trial, enrolling 134 patients with biopsy-confirmed pancreatic ductal adenocarcinoma that meets centrally reviewed anatomic criteria on imaging for the borderline resectable disease were randomized to receive either eight cycles of mFOLFIRINOX or seven cycles of mFOLFIRINOX followed by stereotactic body radiation therapy (33–40 Gy in five fractions). Patients without evidence of disease progression following preoperative therapy underwent pancreatectomy and, if able, received four additional cycles of postoperative modified fluorouracil, leucovorin, irinotecan, and oxaliplatin (mFOLFOX). The primary endpoint is an 18-month OS rate of patients enrolled in each of the two treatment arms. This has not yet been published. An interim analysis of the margin-negative resection rate within each arm was performed which mandated the closure of the radiation arm. Although the radiation arm did not show an improvement in the margin negative resection rates, the trial was not powered to evaluate the benefit of radiation in the overall treatment of pancreatic adenocarcinoma. Therefore, definitive conclusions cannot be made regarding the utility of radiation treatment in this disease.

Despite improvement in local control rates,[25] there continues to be institutional, regional, and international biases evaluating the role of radiation in the care of patients with borderline and locally advanced pancreatic adenocarcinoma. Two Phase II clinical trials conducted at the Massachusetts General Hospital for borderline and locally advanced pancreatic cancer patients support the use of radiation in these patient populations.[7,8] Both trials enrolled 50 patients each, of whom 32 and 34 patients went on to surgical resection in the borderline and locally advanced populations, respectively. Most of the patients in both trials received eight cycles of neoadjuvant FOLFIRINOX followed by 50.4 Gy of radiation with 5-fluorouracil. The margin-negative resection rate was 97% in borderline resectable patients[7] and 88% in locally advanced patients.[8] Both trials showed impressive disease-free and OS rates of 48.6 months and 64.5 months, respectively, in borderline resectable patients[7] and 21.3 months and 33.0 months, respectively, in locally advanced patients.[8]

Locally Advanced Trials

The treatment of locally advanced diseases has improved significantly because of more effective systemic therapies, better radiation treatments, and more aggressive surgical approaches. Over the last decade, a larger number of patients who present with locally advanced diseases are being considered for surgical resection. However, the optimal preoperative treatment for locally advanced pancreatic cancer continues to be explored.

Massachusetts General Hospital (MGH) 13-051

The MGH single institution Phase II clinical trial for locally advanced PDAC enrolled 50 patients, of whom 34 (69%) went on to surgical resection.[8] Of these patients 80% completed all 8 cycles of FOLFIRINOX, but 51% (25/49) had a grade 3 or greater toxicity from chemotherapy. Of the 34 patients who underwent resection, 30 (88%) had a margin-negative resection, which was the primary endpoint of the study. For resected patients, median progression-free survival was 21.3 months and median OS was 33.0 months.[8]

Neoadjuvant Chemotherapy in Locally Advanced Pancreatic Cancer (NEOLAP)

The NEOLAP Phase II trial compared the efficacy and safety of nab-paclitaxel plus gemcitabine with nab-paclitaxel plus gemcitabine followed by FOLFIRINOX as multidrug induction chemotherapy regimens in locally advanced pancreatic cancer.[26] Twenty-eight centers in Germany randomized 130 patients to either the nab-paclitaxel plus gemcitabine group (64 patients) or the sequential FOLFIRINOX group (66 patients). Surgical exploration after completed induction chemotherapy was done in 63% (40/64) of patients and 36% were resected in the nab-paclitaxel plus gemcitabine group, whereas 64% (42/66) patients were explored and 44% resected in the sequential FOLFIRINOX group. After a median follow-up of 24.9 months, the median OS was 18.5 months in the nab-paclitaxel plus gemcitabine group and 20.7 months in the sequential FOLFIRINOX group (HR 0.86; 95%CI 0.55–1.36; P = .53). Of all the secondary endpoints evaluated, only histopathological downstaging was improved in the sequential FOLFIRINOX group (ypT1/2 stage: 20/29 (69%) versus 4/23 (17%), P = .0003; ypN0 stage: 15/29 (52%) versus 4/23 (17%), P = .02). Although both regimens resulted in similar resection rates and OS, the encouraging changes in the histopathologic profiles with treatment sequencing need to be further explored.

SUMMARY

Advances in multimodality therapy have allowed pancreatic cancer patients to continue to have improved progression-free and OS rates. Clinical trials are confirming improved margin-negative resection rates and decreased rates of nodal involvement resulting in encouraging OS rates. However, despite these improvements most of the patients will continue to present distantly as their first site of recurrence.[27] Internationally there is consensus that patients with borderline and locally advanced pancreatic cancer should receive neoadjuvant systemic chemotherapy. The role of radiation therapy in pancreatic cancer continues to be discussed. For resectable pancreatic cancer, the standard of care is upfront resection, and the role of neoadjuvant therapy will hopefully be answered with the Alliance A021806 clinical trial. Improving our understanding of the biology of pancreatic cancer will result in improved individualized systemic treatments to further raise the survival of pancreatic cancer patients.

CLINICS CARE POINTS

- Multimodality therapy is essential to optimize the treatment of patients with pancreatic cancer.
- Neoadjuvant therapy in patients with borderline and locally advanced pancreatic ductal adenocarcinomas has improved margin-negative resection rates and overall survival.
- The role of neoadjuvant therapy in resectable pancreatic cancer has not been clarified and the standard of care continues to be upfront resection.

DISCLOSURE

Ferrone: Consultant for Intraop

REFERENCES

1. Von Hoff DD, Ervin T, Arena FP, et al. Increased survival in pancreatic cancer with nab-paclitaxel plus gemcitabine. N Engl J Med 2013;369(18):1691–703. https://doi.org/10.1056/NEJMoa1304369.
2. Conroy T, Paillot B, François E, et al. Irinotecan plus oxaliplatin and leucovorin-modulated fluorouracil in advanced pancreatic cancer–a Groupe Tumeurs Digestives of the Federation Nationale des Centres de Lutte Contre le Cancer study. J Clin Oncol 2005;23(6):1228–36. https://doi.org/10.1200/JCO.2005.06.050.
3. Oettle H, Neuhaus P, Hochhaus A, et al. Adjuvant chemotherapy with gemcitabine and long-term outcomes among patients with resected pancreatic cancer: the CONKO-001 randomized trial. JAMA 2013;310(14):1473–81. https://doi.org/10.1001/jama.2013.279201.

4. Neoptolemos JP, Stocken DD, Friess H, et al. A randomized trial of chemoradio-therapy and chemotherapy after resection of pancreatic cancer. N Engl J Med 2004;350(12):1200–10. https://doi.org/10.1056/NEJMoa032295.

5. Maeda A, Boku N, Fukutomi A, et al. Randomized Phase III Trial of Adjuvant Chemotherapy with Gemcitabine versus S-1 in Patients with Resected Pancreatic Cancer: Japan Adjuvant Study Group of Pancreatic Cancer (JASPAC-01). Jpn J Clin Oncol 2008;38(3):227–9. https://doi.org/10.1093/jjco/hym178.

6. Neoptolemos JP, Palmer DH, Ghaneh P, et al. Comparison of adjuvant gemcita-bine and capecitabine with gemcitabine monotherapy in patients with resected pancreatic cancer (ESPAC-4): a multicentre, open-label, randomised, phase 3 trial. Lancet 2017;389(10073):1011–24. https://doi.org/10.1016/s0140-6736(16)32409-6.

7. Murphy JE, Wo JY, Ryan DP, et al. Total Neoadjuvant Therapy With FOLFIRINOX Followed by Individualized Chemoradiotherapy for Borderline Resectable Pancreatic Adenocarcinoma: A Phase 2 Clinical Trial. JAMA Oncol 2018. https://doi.org/10.1001/jamaoncol.2018.0329.

8. Murphy JE, Wo JY, Ryan DP, et al. Total Neoadjuvant Therapy With FOLFIRINOX in Combination With Losartan Followed by Chemoradiotherapy for Locally Advanced Pancreatic Cancer: A Phase 2 Clinical Trial. JAMA Oncol 2019. https://doi.org/10.1001/jamaoncol.2019.0892.

9. Katz MH, Shi Q, Ahmad SA, et al. Preoperative Modified FOLFIRINOX Treatment Followed by Capecitabine-Based Chemoradiation for Borderline Resectable Pancreatic Cancer: Alliance for Clinical Trials in Oncology Trial A021101. JAMA Surg 2016;151(8):e161137. https://doi.org/10.1001/jamasurg.2016.1137.

10. Jang JY, Han Y, Lee H, et al. Oncological Benefits of Neoadjuvant Chemoradia-tion With Gemcitabine Versus Upfront Surgery in Patients With Borderline Resect-able Pancreatic Cancer: A Prospective, Randomized, Open-label, Multicenter Phase 2/3 Trial. Ann Surg 2018;268(2):215–22. https://doi.org/10.1097/sla.0000000000002705.

11. Tempero MA, Reni M, Riess H, et al. APACT: phase III, multicenter, international, open-label, randomized trial of adjuvant nab-paclitaxel plus gemcitabine (nab-P/G) vs gemcitabine (G) for surgically resected pancreatic adenocarcinoma. J Clin Oncol 2019;37(15_suppl):4000. https://doi.org/10.1200/JCO.2019.37.15_suppl.4000.

12. Tempero M, O'Reilly E, Van Cutsem E, et al. LBA-1 Phase 3 APACT trial of adju-vant nab-paclitaxel plus gemcitabine (nab-P + Gem) vs gemcitabine (Gem) alone in patients with resected pancreatic cancer (PC): Updated 5-year overall survival. Ann Oncol 2021;32:S226. https://doi.org/10.1016/j.annonc.2021.06.009.

13. Conroy T, Hammel P, Hebbar M, et al. FOLFIRINOX or Gemcitabine as Adjuvant Therapy for Pancreatic Cancer. N Engl J Med 2018;379(25):2395–406. https://doi.org/10.1056/NEJMoa1809775.

14. Conroy T, Hammel P, Turpin A, et al. LBA57 Unicancer PRODIGE 24/CCTG PA6 trial: Updated results of a multicenter international randomized phase III trial of adjuvant mFOLFIRINOX (mFFX) versus gemcitabine (gem) in patients (pts) with resected pancreatic ductal adenocarcinomas (PDAC). Ann Oncol 2021;32:S1334. https://doi.org/10.1016/j.annonc.2021.08.2137.

15. Hsu CC, Herman JM, Corsini MM, et al. Adjuvant chemoradiation for pancreatic adenocarcinoma: the Johns Hopkins Hospital-Mayo Clinic collaborative study. Ann Surg Oncol 2010;17(4):981–90. https://doi.org/10.1245/s10434-009-0743-7.

16. Sohal D, Duong MT, Ahmad SA, et al. SWOG S1505: Results of perioperative chemotherapy (peri-op CTx) with mfolfirinox versus gemcitabine/nab-paclitaxel

(Gem/nabP) for resectable pancreatic ductal adenocarcinoma (PDA). J Clin Oncol 2020;38(15_suppl):4504. https://doi.org/10.1200/JCO.2020.38.15_suppl. 4504.

17. Chawla A, Ferrone CR. Neoadjuvant Therapy for Resectable Pancreatic Cancer: An Evolving Paradigm Shift. Front Oncol 2019;9:1085. https://doi.org/10.3389/fonc.2019.01085.

18. Unno M, Motoi F, Matsuyama Y, et al. Randomized phase II/III trial of neoadjuvant chemotherapy with gemcitabine and S-1 versus upfront surgery for resectable pancreatic cancer (Prep-02/JSAP-05). J Clin Oncol 2019;37(4_suppl):189. https://doi.org/10.1200/JCO.2019.37.4_suppl.189.

19. de Bono JS, Twelves CJ. The oral fluorinated pyrimidines. Invest New Drugs 2001;19(1):41–59. https://doi.org/10.1023/a:1006404701008.

20. Satoi S, Unno M, Motoi F, et al. The effect of neoadjuvant chemotherapy with gemcitabine and S-1 for resectable pancreatic cancer (randomized phase II/III trial; Prep-02/JSAP-05). J Clin Oncol 2019;37(15_suppl):4126. https://doi.org/10.1200/JCO.2019.37.15_suppl.4126.

21. Katz MH, Marsh R, Herman JM, et al. Borderline resectable pancreatic cancer: need for standardization and methods for optimal clinical trial design. Ann Surg Oncol 2013;20(8):2787–95. https://doi.org/10.1245/s10434-013-2886-9.

22. NCCN. National Comprehensive Cancer Network (NCCN) Clinical Practice Guidelines in Oncology, Pancreatic Adenocarcinoma Version 1.2022. National Comprehensive Cancer Network. Available at: https://www.nccn.org/professionals/physician_gls/pdf/pancreatic.pdf. Accessed 05/01/2022.

23. Ahmad SA, Duong M, Sohal DPS, et al. Surgical Outcome Results From SWOG S1505: A Randomized Clinical Trial of mFOLFIRINOX Versus Gemcitabine/Nab-paclitaxel for Perioperative Treatment of Resectable Pancreatic Ductal Adenocarcinoma. Ann Surg 2020. https://doi.org/10.1097/SLA.0000000000004155.

24. de W Marsh R, Talamonti MS, Baker MS, et al. Primary systemic therapy in resectable pancreatic ductal adenocarcinoma using mFOLFIRINOX: A pilot study. J Surg Oncol 2018;117(3):354–62. https://doi.org/10.1002/jso.24872.

25. Versteijne E, Suker M, Groothuis K, et al. Preoperative Chemoradiotherapy Versus Immediate Surgery for Resectable and Borderline Resectable Pancreatic Cancer: Results of the Dutch Randomized Phase III PREOPANC Trial. J Clin Oncol 2020;38(16):1763–73. https://doi.org/10.1200/jco.19.02274.

26. Kunzmann V, Siveke JT, Algül H, et al. Nab-paclitaxel plus gemcitabine versus nab-paclitaxel plus gemcitabine followed by FOLFIRINOX induction chemotherapy in locally advanced pancreatic cancer (NEOLAP-AIO-PAK-0113): a multicentre, randomised, phase 2 trial. Lancet Gastroenterol Hepatol 2021;6(2):128–38. https://doi.org/10.1016/S2468-1253(20)30330-7.

27. Chawla A, Qadan M, Castillo CF, et al. Prospective Phase II Trials Validate the Effect of Neoadjuvant Chemotherapy on Pattern of Recurrence in Pancreatic Adenocarcinoma. Ann Surg 2020. https://doi.org/10.1097/SLA.0000000000004585.

Primary Colorectal Cancer

Alexander Dowli, MD[a], Alessandro Fichera, MD[a,*],
James Fleshman, MD[a]

KEYWORDS

- Minimally invasive surgery • Colectomy • Proctectomy • Colon cancer
- Rectal cancer

KEY POINTS

- Laparoscopy for colon cancer is safe and has equivalent oncologic outcomes when compared to open surgery. Further evidence is needed for rectal cancer.
- Apart from cost, no differences have been noted between laparoscopic and robotic colorectal surgery.
- In patients with rectal cancer, total neoadjuvant therapy is associated with higher complete response rates. Further evidence is needed to assess long-term oncologic outcomes.
- In select patients with rectal cancer, watch and wait therapy may be considered as a safe alternative to definitive surgery.

INTRODUCTION/SYNOPSIS

Over the last few decades, the colorectal surgery world has seen a paradigm shift in the care of patients. The introduction of minimally invasive techniques led to the development of procedures resulting in reduced patient morbidity and hospital stay. The vetting process of minimally invasive colorectal surgery involved rigorous studies to ensure that oncologic outcomes were not being compromised. In this article, we discuss the most relevant randomized controlled trials that support the practice of minimally invasive colorectal surgery.

The multimodal treatment of rectal cancer has developed rapidly, resulting in improved survival and decreased morbidity and mortality. In this review, we also present the latest evidence behind the multidisciplinary approach to rectal cancer.

Funding: None.
Disclosure: The authors have nothing to disclose.
[a] Division of Colorectal Surgery, Department of Surgery, Baylor University Medical Center, Dallas, TX, USA
* Corresponding author. 3409 Worth StreetWorth Tower, Suite 600Dallas, TX 75246.
E-mail address: alessandro.fichera@bswhealth.org

SURGICAL TECHNIQUE–COLON CANCER

Minimally invasive techniques were first considered in colorectal surgery in the early 1990s.[1] With that it was important to know if these techniques were offering the same oncologic outcome as open techniques.

The laparoscopy-assisted colectomy versus open colectomy for treatment of non-metastatic colon cancer trial, also known as the BARCELONA trial, was the first trial comparing open and laparoscopic colectomy for nonmetastatic colon cancer.[2] The authors enrolled 219 patients over a 5-year period; 111 in the laparoscopic colectomy group and 108 in the open colectomy group. Patients were followed up for a median of 43 months. Patients in the laparoscopic arm had a shorter hospital stay and decreased morbidity. Perioperative mortality was similar in both groups. The authors found that when compared to open colectomy, laparoscopic colectomy was associated with a reduced risk of tumor relapse and a reduced risk of death from cancer, with these differences being seen only in stage III patients (freedom from recurrence, $P = 0 \cdot 04$; overall survival, $P = 0 \cdot 02$; cancer-related survival, $P = 0 \cdot 006$).[2] Of note, the trial involved a small number of surgeons. The findings of this study when it comes to stage III colon cancer have not been duplicated (**Fig. 1**).

The COlon cancer Laparoscopic or Open Resection (COLOR) trial randomized 1076 patients with colon cancer, in Europe and the United States, to open or laparoscopic colectomy.[3] These patients were followed up for a median of 53 months. There was no difference in number of lymph nodes harvested, resection margin positivity, perioperative morbidity, or mortality. For all stages, the 3-year disease-free survival was 76.2% in the open colectomy group and 74.2% in the laparoscopic colectomy ($P = 0.7$). Similarly, no difference was found in overall survival, 84.2% in the open colectomy group versus 81.8% in the laparoscopic colectomy ($P = 0.45$).[3]

A trial from the Clinical Outcomes of Surgical Therapy Study (COST trial) group investigated the noninferiority of laparoscopic colectomy for stage I-III colon cancer.[4] This study involved 48 institutions with trained and credentialed surgeons. The study randomized 872 patients with colon cancer to open or laparoscopic colectomy. The average follow-up duration was 4.4 years. As expected, the laparoscopic group had a shorter hospital stay and lower intravenous narcotics use ($P < 0.001$). Intraoperative and postoperative complications at discharge and 60 days, 30-day postoperative mortality, readmission, and reoperation were comparable between groups. Resection margins were less than 5 cm in 5% of the laparoscopic group and 6% of the open colectomy group ($P = 0.52$). Cancer recurrence rates were similar in both groups, 16% laparoscopic surgery versus 18% open surgery ($P = 0.32$). Surgical wound recurrence was less than 1% in either group ($P = 0.50$). Overall survival at 3 years was comparable between both groups, 85% in the open group and 86% laparoscopic group ($P = 0.51$). No difference was found in any stage of colon cancer. The feared increase in peritoneal carcinomatosis and wound implantation due to a laparoscopic approach did not occur.[4]

The 5-year follow-up of the COST trial was reported in the *Annals of Surgery*.[5] The median follow-up duration was 7 years. Laparoscopic colectomy was found to be noninferior to open colectomy after 5-year follow-up. Disease-free 5-year survival (laparoscopic 69.2%, open 68.4%, $P = 0.94$) and overall 5-year survival (laparoscopic 76.4%, open 74.6%, $P = 0.93$) were similar for both groups. Recurrence rates and sites of first recurrence were similar between both groups (**Fig. 2**).

The COST trial was a noninferiority trial requiring a smaller number of subjects. Of note, this was the first surgical trial to use unedited videos to credential surgeons to take part in the study. Survival and recurrence rates were better than those in the

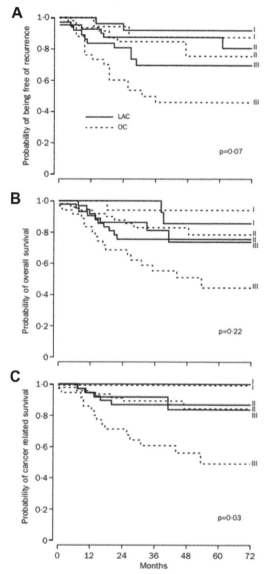

Fig. 1. (A) Freedom from recurrence, (B) overall survival, and (C) cancer-related survival in stages I, II, and III colon cancer after laparoscopic versus open colectomy.[2]

Surveillance, Epidemiology, and End Results Program database (SEER) in the same timeframe suggesting that surgeon training and skills improve outcomes.[5]

SURGICAL TECHNIQUE–RECTAL CANCER

Even though laparoscopic resection of colon cancer was shown to be noninferior to open resection, there was speculation that laparoscopic proctectomy may not achieve adequate oncologic resection due to the difficulty of dissection within the

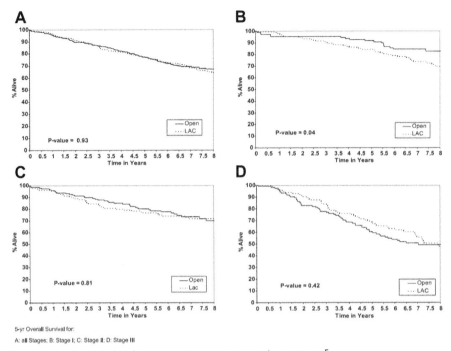

Fig. 2. Overall survival in laparoscopic versus open colon surgery.[5]

confines of the pelvis and assessing resection margins laparoscopically without a hand to feel for hard tumor.[6] Therefore, several trials were performed to answer this question.

The short-term endpoints of conventional versus laparoscopic-assisted surgery in patients with colorectal cancer (MRC-CLASICC trial) from the United Kingdom addressed the differences in laparoscopic and open surgery outcomes in patients with colon and rectal cancer.[7] The smaller group of rectal cancer patients had a higher incidence of positive circumferential resection margins (CRM) and longitudinal margins. No difference was found in proportion of Dukes C2 tumors or in-hospital mortality. The increase in positive resection margins occurred in those patients undergoing anterior resection in the laparoscopic surgery group, 12% versus 6%. This difference was not statistically significant, $P = 0.19.$[7]

The laparoscopic versus open surgery for rectal cancer (COLOR II) trial was a randomized controlled trial from 30 centers in Europe that randomized 1044 patients to laparoscopic and open proctectomy.[8] Blood loss was less in laparoscopic surgery (median 200 mL vs 400 mL, $P < 0.0001$). Return of bowel function was faster, and hospital stay was shorter, by 1 day in the laparoscopic group. R0 resection was comparable between both groups (laparoscopic 88% vs open 92%; $P = 0.250$). A rather high positive CRM was noted in 10% of both groups ($P = 0.850$). There was no difference in the distance to distal resection margin (average 3 cm in both groups, $P = 0.676$). Morbidity and mortality at 4 weeks after surgery were similar in both groups. Operative times for laparoscopic procedures were significantly longer (240 min vs 188 min, $P < 0.0001$). The patient population included patients with stage I-III rectal cancers at all levels of the rectum (0–15 cm) who did not receive neoadjuvant therapy in all indicated cases.[8]

The American College of Surgeons Oncology Group/Alliance for Clinical Trials Z6051 randomized controlled trial objective was to compare disease-free survival and recurrence after open versus laparoscopic surgery for patients who had received neoadjuvant therapy for stage II/III rectal cancer within 12 cm from the anal verge.[9] The primary outcome was to compare a composite score that consisted of circumferential radial margin greater than 1 mm, distal margin without tumor, and completeness of total mesorectal excision (TME). Simply put, the composite score defined successful oncologic resection (**Table 1**).

There were 222 patients that underwent open TME and 240 patients that underwent laparoscopic TME. Patients underwent abdominoperineal resection (23.3%) or low anterior resection (76.7%). Successful resection, as defined by the composite score, occurred in 86.9% of open resection cases and 81.7% of laparoscopic resection cases, $P = 0.41$. In 93.5% of the cases, the quality of the TME specimen was complete (77.1%) and nearly complete (16.5%). Negative circumferential radial margin was observed in 92.3% of open resections versus 87.9% of laparoscopic resections, $P = 0.11$. The distal margin was negative in more than 98% of patients and was equivalent between groups, $P = 0.91$. Operative time was significantly longer for laparoscopic resection on average (266.2 vs 220.6 minutes; $P < 0.001$). Overall length of stay, severe complications, or readmission within 30 days did not differ significantly between groups.[9]

The second report of the American College of Surgeon Oncology Group (ACOSOG) Z6051 trial presented the long-term results on disease-free survival and recurrence after open versus laparoscopic surgery for stage II/III rectal cancer.[10] A total of 462 patients were randomized; 240 for laparoscopic and 222 for open surgery (this open group included hybrid hand assist technique where the TME was done with open instruments). Median follow-up duration was 47.9 months. The trial found no significant difference in 2-year disease-free survival (79.5% vs 83.2%), locoregional recurrence (4.6% vs 4.5%), or distant recurrence (14.6% vs 16.7%) for laparoscopic versus open surgery, respectively. Disease-free survival was impacted by unsuccessful resection ($P = 0.006$) showing the importance of an adequate total mesolectal excision technique (**Fig. 3**).[10]

The ALaCaRT trial (Effect of Laparoscopic-Assisted Resection vs Open Resection on Pathological Outcomes in Rectal Cancer) from Australia and New Zealand was a randomized clinical trial that also aimed to show noninferiority of laparoscopic versus open proctectomy, based on the ACOSOG Z6051 protocol.[11] The authors randomized 486 patients to each treatment modality. However, noninferiority was not established as both complete TME and CRM were superior in the open surgery group ($P = .06$). There was no difference in obtaining a distal clear margin ($P = 0.67$).[11]

Table 1			
Surgical success outcomes[9]			
	Laparoscopic Resection	**Open Resection**	**P Value**
CRM > 1 mm or distance = NA	87.9 (83.8 to 92.0)	92.3 (88.8 to 95.8)	.11
Distal margin negative	98.3 (96.7 to 99.95)	98.2 (96.5 to 99.95)	.91
Complete or nearly complete TME	92.1 (88.7 to 95.5)	95.1 (92.2 to 97.9)	.20
Successful resection			
Modified intent to treat	81.7 (76.8 to 86.6)	86.9 (82.5 to 91.4)	.41
Pre protocol	81.7 (76.5 to 86.9)	86.9 (82.5 to 91.4)	.41

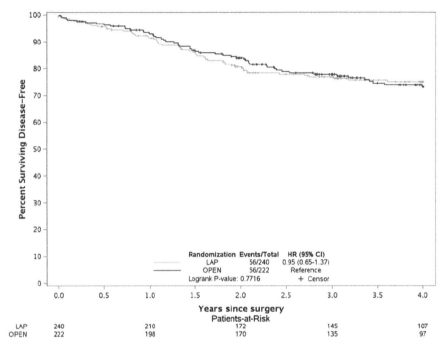

Fig. 3. Disease-free survival of open versus laparoscopic resection of stage II to III rectal cancer.[10]

From South Korea came the COREAN trial, open versus laparoscopic surgery for mid-rectal or low rectal cancer after neoadjuvant chemoradiotherapy.[12] It used the same protocol as ACOSOG Z6051 and ALACART trials to compare laparoscopic and open surgery in patients with mid-rectal or low rectal cancer, after neoadjuvant chemoradiotherapy. The trial randomized 340 patients to open or laparoscopic arms. Patients were stratified according to preoperative chemotherapy regimen and sex. Operating time was longer in laparoscopic cases (mean 244.9 minutes vs 197.0 minutes, $P < 0.0001$). Patients treated laparoscopically showed faster recovery of bowel function (38.5 hours vs 60 hours, $P < 0.001$). No oncologic difference was found between the groups studied. Specifically, macroscopic quality of the TME ($P = 0.414$), involvement of the CRM ($P = 0.770$), and the number of harvested lymph nodes ($P = 0.085$) were not different between laparoscopic and open TME.[12] Of note, this study did not use the composite score, while the previous 2 studies did.

The majority of the evidence shown above reflects oncologic noninferiority of laparoscopic colorectal surgery as compared to open surgery. The robotic technique for rectal cancer resection needs to be examined as well. One of the first randomized controlled trials to address robotic proctectomy was the ROLARR trial (Effect of Robotic-Assisted vs Conventional Laparoscopic Surgery on Risk of Conversion to Open Laparotomy Among Patients Undergoing Resection for Rectal Cancer).[13] This was a multicenter, international trial comparing robot-assisted versus laparoscopic surgery for the treatment of rectal cancer. This included 471 patients. The primary end point was conversion to open surgery. The conversion rate was 12.2% for laparoscopic surgery versus 8.1% for robotic surgery, with no statistical significance ($P = 0.16$). Other endpoints studied included CRM positivity, intact TME, intraoperative complications, postoperative complication within 30 days and 180 days, and 30-day mortality. No statistically significant differences were found for those variables.[13]

The only difference between the 2 operative methods was cost. The cost of robotic surgery averaged $13,668, whereas the cost of laparoscopic surgery averaged $12,556 ($P = 0.02$).[13]

A randomized controlled trial from Korea looking at robotic versus laparoscopic proctectomy found no difference in the quality of TME, rate of positive resection margins, number of harvested lymph nodes, morbidity, and bowel function recovery.[14] On quality-of-life questionnaire, the robot-assisted group had better sexual function at 1 year ($P = 0.03$).[14]

Preoperative Therapy Trials for Rectal Cancer

In this section, we discuss the current evidence supporting the use of neoadjuvant therapy for rectal cancer, focusing on TME trials as the standard of care in terms of proper oncologic surgical technique.[10]

The Dutch trial, "Preoperative radiotherapy combined with total mesorectal excision for resectable rectal cancer", looked at preoperative short-course radiotherapy in combination with TME.[15] A total of 1861 patients, with no evidence of metastatic disease, were randomly assigned to TME preceded by 5×5 Gy radiotherapy or TME alone. The overall survival rate at 2 years was similar in both groups; 81.8% in the surgery-alone group versus 82% in the preoperative radiation and surgery group ($P = 0.84$). At 2 years, the local recurrence rate of the preoperative radiation and surgery group was lower than that of the surgery-alone group, 2.4% versus 8.2%, respectively, ($P < 0.001$).[15]

Long-term outcomes of this trial were also reported.[16] The median follow-up duration was 12 years. Local recurrence, the primary endpoint, was 5% in the group that received radiation versus 11% in the surgery-alone group ($P < 0.0001$). In patients with stage III rectal cancer and a negative circumferential resection margin, 10-year survival was at 50% in the group receiving neoadjuvant radiotherapy versus 40% in the surgery-alone group ($P = 0.032$).

The preoperative versus postoperative chemoradiotherapy for rectal cancer trial, also known as the GERMAN trial, investigated the differences between preoperative versus postoperative chemoradiation.[17] A total of 823 patients with stage II or III rectal cancer were studied. The overall 5-year survival between both groups was similar; 76% for the preoperative group and 74% for the postoperative group ($P = 0.80$). Acute toxicity was found to be higher in the postoperative treatment group, 40% versus 27% ($P = 0.001$). At 5 years, the local recurrence rate was found to be higher in the postoperative treatment group, 13% versus 6% ($P = 0.006$). When looking at patients who were initially thought to need an abdominoperineal resection, there was a higher sphincter preservation rate in the preoperative chemoradiation group.[17]

The study also reported its long-term outcomes.[18] At 10 years, there was no difference in overall survival, 59.6% versus 59.9% ($P = 0.85$). However, preoperative chemoradiation group had a lower local recurrence rate (7.1% vs 10.1%, $P = 0.048$).[18]

The Trans-Tasman Radiation Oncology Group trial, a randomized trial of short-course radiotherapy versus long-course chemoradiation comparing rates of local recurrence in patients with T3 rectal cancer, studied the differences between short-course and long-course neoadjuvant therapies.[19] Short-course radiation was defined as radiotherapy at 5×5 Gy in 1 week, early surgery, and 6 courses of adjuvant chemotherapy. Long-course radiation was defined as 50.4 Gy, 1.8 Gy/fraction, delivered in 5.5 weeks, with a continuous infusion of fluorouracil 225 mg/m^2 per day. Surgery followed in 4 to 6 weeks, followed by 4 courses of chemotherapy. A total of 326 patients were randomized to each modality. The median follow-up duration was 5.9 years. At 3 years, local recurrence was 7.5% for the short-course group versus 4.4% for the long-course group and was found not to be statistically significant (*P* = 0.24). Similarly, there was no difference in overall survival; 74% versus 70% for the short-course versus long-course group (*P* = 0.62).[19]

Another trial that looked at short-course radiation was the Stockholm III trial, tumor regression after radiotherapy for rectal cancer.[20] This trial randomized patients to 3 groups: short-course radiation with surgery within 1 week, short-course radiation with surgery after 4-8 weeks, and long-course radiation with surgery after 4-8 weeks. Short-course radiation with a delay in surgery was found to have the highest rate of pathologic complete response, 10.4% versus 0.3% in the short-course radiotherapy with immediate surgery group and 2.2% in the long-course radiotherapy group. Pathologic complete response was also found to correlate with improved overall survival (**Fig. 4**).[20]

Among the patient groups studied in the Stockholm III trial, analysis was performed to look at the optimal timing for surgery.[21] Overall, oncological outcomes were similar among the 3 groups.[21]

It was noted however, that short-course radiation therapy with surgery 1 week later had a higher rate of postoperative complications (53% vs 41% with delay, *P* = 0.001) (**Fig. 5**).[21]

To understand which therapy had the most effect on disease recurrence, the RAPIDO trial was designed, "Short-course radiotherapy followed by chemotherapy before TME versus preoperative chemoradiotherapy, TME, and optional adjuvant chemotherapy in locally advanced rectal cancer."[22] This trial specifically addressed patients with locally advanced rectal adenocarcinoma with high-risk features on MRI.

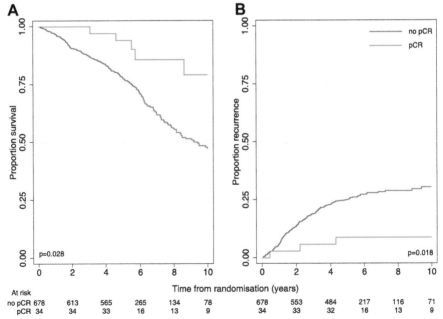

Fig. 4. Kaplan-Meier's estimates by pathologic response. (*A*) Overall survival. (*B*) Time to recurrence.[20]

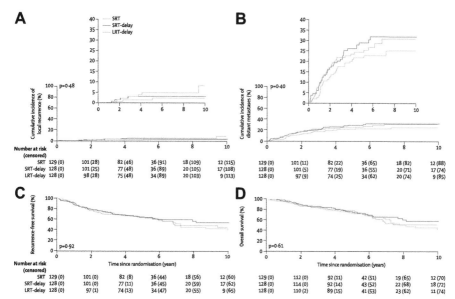

Fig. 5. Local recurrence (*A*), distant metastases (*B*), recurrence-free survival (*C*), and overall survival (*D*) in 3-arm randomization. SRT, short-course radiotherapy (5 × 5 Gy with surgery within 1 week); SRT-delay, short-course radiotherapy (5 × 5 Gy with surgery after 4–8 weeks); LRT-delay, long-course radiotherapy (25 × 2 Gy with surgery after 4–8 weeks).[21]

The trial studied 2 treatment strategies. The standard of care treatment group received long-course radiation therapy, with simultaneous twice-daily oral capecitabine followed by TME. In addition, adjuvant chemotherapy was optional, given only if required by hospital policy, in the form of 8 cycles of capecitabine and oxaliplatin (CAPOX) or 12 cycles of folinic acid, fluorouracil, and oxaliplatin (FOLFOX4). The experimental group received short-course radiotherapy, followed by 6 cycles of CAPOX chemotherapy or 9 cycles of FOLFOX4 followed by TME. The primary endpoint of the trial was any disease-related treatment failure at 3 years, such as locoregional failure, distant metastasis, or a treatment-related death. A total of 912 patients were randomized (450 in the standard of care group, 462 in the experimental group). The average follow-up duration was 4.6 years. Disease-related treatment failure was 30.4% in the standard of care group versus 23.7% in the experimental group (*P* = 0.019). In the experimental group, the rate of pathological complete response was 28% compared to 14% in the standard of care group (*P* < 0.0001). The difference could be indicative of the increased efficacy of preoperative full-course chemotherapy as opposed to adjuvant chemotherapy the patients received in the standard of care group. Mortality was equivalent in both groups with 4 patients in each treatment arm.[22]

Further investigation into the optimal timing to deliver nonsurgical therapies for locally advanced rectal cancer was performed in a trial called "Effect of adding mFOLFOX6 after neoadjuvant chemoradiation in locally advanced rectal cancer", from the Timing of Rectal Cancer Response to Chemoradiation Consortium, also known as the TIMING study.[23] The primary endpoint was complete pathological response. All patients received chemoradiation. Following this, patients were randomized into 4 groups. Group 1 patients had surgery, TME, 6–8 weeks after chemoradiation (continuous infusion of fluorouracil and radiotherapy). Group 2-4 patients received 2, 4, or 6 cycles of mFOLFOX6 (leucovorin calcium, also known as folinic acid, fluorouracil, and oxaliplatin), respectively, between chemoradiation and TME (**Fig. 6**).

Pathological complete response was 18% for group 1, 25% for group 2, 30% for group 3, and 38% for group 4 with statistical significance, $P = 0.036$. This study introduced the concept of total neoadjuvant therapy for the treatment of locally advanced rectal cancer.[23]

A study from France found that induction chemotherapy with folinic acid, fluorouracil irinotecan, and oxaliplatin (FOLFIRINOX) prior to preoperative chemoradiotherapy improved outcomes when compared to preoperative chemoradiotherapy followed by adjuvant chemotherapy. This trial is known as the PRODIGE 23 trial—Neoadjuvant chemotherapy with FOLFIRINOX and preoperative chemoradiotherapy for patients with locally advanced rectal cancer (UNICANCER-PRODIGE 23).[24] Patients were randomized to standard of care or total neoadjuvant chemotherapy. The standard of care group received chemoradiotherapy, TME, followed by chemotherapy. The total neoadjuvant chemotherapy group received neoadjuvant chemotherapy with FOLFIRINOX, chemoradiotherapy, TME, followed by adjuvant chemotherapy. The primary endpoint was disease-free survival at 3 years, 69% in the standard of care group versus 76% in the total neoadjuvant chemotherapy group ($P = 0.034$). These data further highlighted the value of neoadjuvant chemotherapy.[24]

WATCH AND WAIT FOR RECTAL CANCER

Given the high pathologic complete response rates obtained with modern neoadjuvant regimens including total neoadjuvant therapy (TNT), the concept of nonoperative management (NOM) of rectal cancer or watch and wait (W&W) in selected patients was introduced. The first article describing a W&W strategy came from Brazil.[25] Habr-Gama and colleagues reviewed 265 patients with resectable distal rectal adenocarcinoma that were treated initially by long-course neoadjuvant chemoradiation

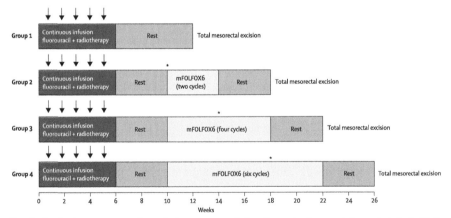

Fig. 6. Radiotherapy was given 5 days per week for 5 weeks (*arrows*) for a total of 45 Gy with a minimum boost of 5·4 Gy. Fluorouracil was given as a 225-mg/m² per day continuous infusion for 7 days per week during radiation therapy for 5–6 weeks. FOLFOX6 was given in 2-week cycles of leucovorin 200 mg/m² or 400 mg/m² and oxaliplatin 85 mg/m² in a 2-hour infusion, bolus fluorouracil 400 mg/m² on day 1, and a 46-hour infusion of fluorouracil 2400 mg/m². Interim assessments were done by proctoscopic examination. TME was done if the patient had stable or progressive disease.[23]

consisting of 5-FU, leucovorin, and 5040 cGy.[25] Those with an incomplete clinical response were offered surgery. Following this, a comparison was made between patients who underwent surgery and achieved a complete pathologic response and patients who had a complete clinical response that did not undergo surgery. After neoadjuvant therapy, 71 patients exhibited a complete clinical response and did not undergo surgery. Twenty-two patients had an incomplete clinical response followed by a complete pathological response. In the surgery group, there were 9 permanent colostomies and 7 temporary diverting ileostomies. Systemic recurrences were present in 3 patients of each group. There were 2 locoregional recurrences in the observation group. Five-year disease-free survival was 83% in the surgery group versus 92% in the observation group. Five-year overall survival was 88% in the surgery group versus 100% in the observation group. This was the first study that showed that in patients with complete clinical response after neoadjuvant therapy, there may be a role for NOM. Of note, less than 27% of patients in either group were node-positive prior to receiving treatment.[25]

The same group then looked at patients with node-positive, nonmetastatic disease.[26] The comparison was between patients with baseline node-positive disease and those with node-negative disease. Patients that achieved a complete clinical response after neoadjuvant therapy were then managed nonoperatively. Overall, 135 with node-negative disease and 62 with node-positive disease had a complete clinical response and were subsequently managed nonoperatively ($P = 0.13$). There were no significant differences in 5-year overall cancer-specific survival, distant metastasis-free survival, or organ preservation (**Fig. 7**).

With this information, there was an interest in seeing the effects of local excision on rectal cancer patients after neoadjuvant chemotherapy. The Organ preservation with chemoradiotherapy plus local excision for rectal cancer: 5-year results of the GRECCAR 2 randomized trial, also known as the GRECCAR 5 study, was a randomized multicenter prospective trial.[27] Patient selection included pretreatment clinical stage T2 or T3 lower rectal adenocarcinoma, maximum size of 4 cm, and good clinical response to neoadjuvant chemoradiotherapy (residual tumor ≤ 2 cm). Patients were randomized to TME (71 patients) or local excision (74 patients). Of note, for the local excision group, a TME was offered if the pathological tumor stage returned as T2 or T3. Patients were followed up for 5 years. In the local excision group, 26 out of 74 patients ultimately required TME. When analyzing the data in an intent to treat fashion, there was no difference between the local excision and TME groups with regard to metastatic disease (18% vs 19%; $P = 0.73$) or overall survival (84% vs 82% $P = 0.85$). This suggested that, in select patients with an excellent clinical response, local excision may be an option as an alternative to TME.[27]

The largest data set of rectal cancer patients treated with the W&W strategy is the International Watch & Wait Database.[28] In its latest published analysis at the time of this publication, the database had 1009 registered patients. A total of 880 patients achieved a complete clinical response after neoadjuvant therapy. Pretreatment clinical nodal stage of patients was N0 in 35%, N1 in 31%, N2 in 19%, and unknown in 15%. At 2 years, 25.2% of patients experienced local regrowth. Ninety-seven percent of local recurrence was intraluminal. This highlights the importance of close luminal follow-up. Of note, 88% of local recurrence occurred in the first 2 years. Eight percent of patients had distant metastasis. At 5 years, the overall survival was 85%.[28]

The latest prospective trial at the time of this publication looking at W&W strategy for rectal cancer is the "organ preservation of rectal adenocarcinoma" (OPRA) trial.[29] Patients with rectal adenocarcinoma that were of MRI stage II and III were randomized to 2 different groups. The first group, the induction group which included 152 patients,

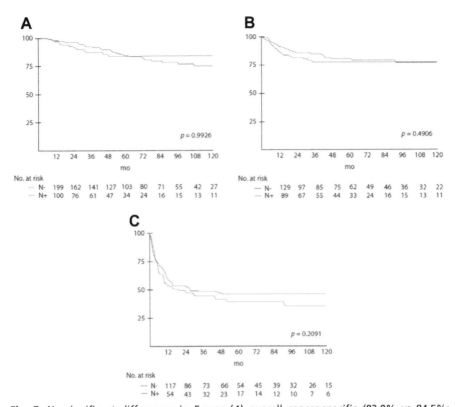

Fig. 7. No significant differences in 5-year (*A*) overall cancer-specific (83.9% vs 84.5%; *P* = 0.99), (*B*) distant metastases-free (77.5% vs 80.5%; *P* = 0.49), or (*C*) surgery-free (organ-preservation) survival (39.7% vs 46.8%; *P* = 0.20) between cN+ and cN0 patients.[26]

received 4 months of FOLFOX (leucovorin calcium [folinic acid], fluorouracil, and oxaliplatin) or CAPEOX (capecitabine plus oxaliplatin) before fluorouracil- or capecitabine-based chemoradiotherapy. The second group, the consolidation group which included 155 patients, received 4 months of FOLFOX or CAPEOX after fluorouracil- or capecitabine-based chemoradiotherapy. Patients underwent restaging at 8-12 weeks after completing TNT with digital rectal examination, MRI, and flexible sigmoidoscopy. Patients with an incomplete response were offered TME. Patients with near-complete or complete clinical response were offered W&W. After a median follow-up of 2 years, disease-free survival and distant metastasis-free survival were similar between both groups. However, the rate of organ preservation was higher in the consolidation group (58% vs 43%, *P* = 0.01). The authors concluded that, in patients with locally advanced rectal cancer that achieve a complete clinical response to TNT, W&W is possible and may result in organ preservation in about half the patients without affecting survival. Consolidation chemotherapy resulted in a higher rate of organ preservation than induction chemotherapy.[29]

TRANS-ANAL TOTAL MESORECTAL EXCISION

Trans-anal surgery for rectal cancer has gained popularity in some centers, especially for distal rectal cancers that are more easily approached with this method versus the transabdominal technique. The endoscope or robot has been added to this approach as well, and this was found to be feasible in case series.[30–32] These techniques are sometimes being referred to as NOTES–TME (natural orifice translumenal endoscopic surgery TME).

Rasulov and colleagues[33] reported an RCT involving 45 patients. The aim was to investigate the difference between laparoscopic TME and trans-anal total mesorectal excision (TaTME). There were 23 patients in the laparoscopic group and 22 in the TaTME group. Inclusion criteria were primary operable rectal cancer or rectal cancer with good response to neoadjuvant chemoradiotherapy. Both groups were comparable in terms of body mass index, age, and stage of disease. The median distance from the anal verge was 6.5 cm for the TaTME group and 7 cm for the laparoscopic group. The average operative time was comparable between both arms—320 minutes for TaTME and 305 minutes in the laparoscopic group. The average estimated blood loss was less than 100 mL for both groups. The median distal margin of resection was similar, 21 mm for the TaTME group and 23 mm for the laparoscopic group.

Transanal extraction of the specimen was more common in the TaTME group—86% vs 48% ($P = 0.021$). Complications were equivalent between both groups, 27% versus 26%. Quality of the TME did not differ between groups ($P = 0.859$), with unsatisfactory TME occurring around 18% of the time. The authors concluded that overall, the 2 methods were comparable.[33]

A randomized controlled trial from China aimed to study the pathological results between laparoscopic TME and TaTME.[34] There were 133 patients in the laparoscopic group and 128 patients in the TaTME group. Tumor characteristics and demographics were similar between the groups. The TME was nearly complete or complete in all patients. The TaTME group did not have any patients with a positive distal resection margin, while the laparoscopic group had 2 such patients (1.5%, $P = 0.498$). The distance between the tumor and distal resection margin only differed by 1 mm between the 2 groups ($P = 0.745$). A positive circumferential resection margin occurred in 2 patients in each arm ($P = 0.674$). The number of lymph nodes resected was also similar, 16 in the laparoscopic group and 15 in the TaTME group. The authors concluded that the pathological outcomes between TaTME and laparoscopic transabdominal TME were comparable.[34]

Other trials are currently in progress comparing TaTME to other methods. The CO-LOR III trial, a multicenter randomized clinical trial comparing transanal TME versus laparoscopic TME for mid-rectal and low rectal cancers, is currently underway.[35] The primary endpoint of the study is involvement of the circumferential radial margin. There are a few secondary endpoints including completeness of the TME, morbidity and mortality, local recurrence, disease-free and overall survival, proportion of sphincter-saving procedures, and quality of life.[35] Another study protocol from Spain aims to study TaTME versus laparoscopic low anterior resection.[36]

SUMMARY

Laparoscopic surgery for colon cancer is safe and has equivalent oncologic outcomes when compared to open surgery. Further evidence is needed for laparoscopic surgery in rectal cancer. Regardless of the modality, a complete TME is crucial for locoregional control. Apart from cost, no differences have been noted between laparoscopic and robotic colorectal surgeries. In patients with rectal cancer, total neoadjuvant therapy followed by TME offers the best chance for cure. W&W for rectal cancer is a developing field, with the latest data suggesting that consolidation chemotherapy after chemoradiation may offer patients the best chance for organ preservation. Further research is needed to guide patient selection in this treatment strategy.

REFERENCES

1. Phillips EH, Franklin M, Carroll BJ, et al. Laparoscopic colectomy. Ann Surg 1992; 216(6):703–7.
2. Lacy AM, García-Valdecasas JC, Delgado S, et al. Laparoscopy-assisted colectomy versus open colectomy for treatment of non-metastatic colon cancer: a randomised trial. Lancet 2002;359(9325):2224–9.
3. Buunen M, Veldkamp R, Hop WC, et al. Survival after laparoscopic surgery versus open surgery for colon cancer: long-term outcome of a randomised clinical trial. Lancet Oncol 2009;10(1):44–52.
4. Nelson H, Sargent DJ, Wieand HS, et al. A comparison of laparoscopically assisted and open colectomy for colon cancer. N Engl J Med 2004;350(20):2050–9.
5. Fleshman J, Sargent DJ, Green E, et al. Laparoscopic colectomy for cancer is not inferior to open surgery based on 5-year data from the COST Study Group trial. Ann Surg 2007;246(4):655–62 [discussion: 662-4].
6. Krane MK, Fichera A. Laparoscopic rectal cancer surgery: where do we stand? World J Gastroenterol 2012;18(46):6747–55.
7. Guillou PJ, Quirke P, Thorpe H, et al. Short-term endpoints of conventional versus laparoscopic-assisted surgery in patients with colorectal cancer (MRC CLASICC trial): multicentre, randomised controlled trial. Lancet 2005;365(9472):1718–26.
8. van der Pas MH, Haglind E, Cuesta MA, et al. Laparoscopic versus open surgery for rectal cancer (COLOR II): short-term outcomes of a randomised, phase 3 trial. Lancet Oncol 2013;14(3):210–8.
9. Fleshman J, Branda M, Sargent DJ, et al. Effect of laparoscopic-assisted resection vs open resection of stage ii or iii rectal cancer on pathologic outcomes: the ACOSOG Z6051 randomized clinical trial. JAMA 2015;314(13):1346–55.
10. Fleshman J, Branda ME, Sargent DJ, et al. Disease-free survival and local recurrence for laparoscopic resection compared with open resection of stage II to III rectal cancer: follow-up results of the ACOSOG Z6051 randomized controlled trial. Ann Surg 2019;269(4):589–95.
11. Stevenson AR, Solomon MJ, Lumley JW, et al. Effect of laparoscopic-assisted resection vs open resection on pathological outcomes in rectal cancer: the ALaCaRT randomized clinical trial. JAMA 2015;314(13):1356–63.
12. Kang SB, Park JW, Jeong SY, et al. Open versus laparoscopic surgery for mid or low rectal cancer after neoadjuvant chemoradiotherapy (COREAN trial): short-term outcomes of an open-label randomised controlled trial. Lancet Oncol 2010;11(7):637–45.
13. Jayne D, Pigazzi A, Marshall H, et al. Effect of robotic-assisted vs conventional laparoscopic surgery on risk of conversion to open laparotomy among patients undergoing resection for rectal cancer: the ROLARR randomized clinical Trial. JAMA 2017;318(16):1569–80.
14. Kim MJ, Park SC, Park JW, et al. Robot-assisted versus laparoscopic surgery for rectal cancer: a phase II open label prospective randomized controlled trial. Ann Surg 2018;267(2):243–51.
15. Kapiteijn E, Marijnen CA, Nagtegaal ID, et al. Preoperative radiotherapy combined with total mesorectal excision for resectable rectal cancer. N Engl J Med 2001;345(9):638–46.

16. van Gijn W, Marijnen CA, Nagtegaal ID, et al. Preoperative radiotherapy combined with total mesorectal excision for resectable rectal cancer: 12-year follow-up of the multicentre, randomised controlled TME trial. Lancet Oncol 2011;12(6):575–82.

17. Sauer R, Becker H, Hohenberger W, et al. Preoperative versus postoperative chemoradiotherapy for rectal cancer. N Engl J Med 2004;351(17):1731–40.

18. Sauer R, Liersch T, Merkel S, et al. Preoperative versus postoperative chemoradiotherapy for locally advanced rectal cancer: results of the German CAO/ARO/AIO-94 randomized phase III trial after a median follow-up of 11 years. J Clin Oncol 2012;30(16):1926–33.

19. Ngan SY, Burmeister B, Fisher RJ, et al. Randomized trial of short-course radiotherapy versus long-course chemoradiation comparing rates of local recurrence in patients with T3 rectal cancer: Trans-Tasman Radiation Oncology Group trial 01.04. J Clin Oncol 2012;30(31):3827–33.

20. Erlandsson J, Lörinc E, Ahlberg M, et al. Tumour regression after radiotherapy for rectal cancer - Results from the randomised Stockholm III trial. Radiother Oncol 2019;135:178–86.

21. Erlandsson J, Holm T, Pettersson D, et al. Optimal fractionation of preoperative radiotherapy and timing to surgery for rectal cancer (Stockholm III): a multicentre, randomised, non-blinded, phase 3, non-inferiority trial. Lancet Oncol 2017;18(3):336–46.

22. Bahadoer RR, Dijkstra EA, van Etten B, et al. Short-course radiotherapy followed by chemotherapy before total mesorectal excision (TME) versus preoperative chemoradiotherapy, TME, and optional adjuvant chemotherapy in locally advanced rectal cancer (RAPIDO): a randomised, open-label, phase 3 trial. Lancet Oncol 2021;22(1):29–42.

23. Garcia-Aguilar J, Chow OS, Smith DD, et al. Effect of adding mFOLFOX6 after neoadjuvant chemoradiation in locally advanced rectal cancer: a multicentre, phase 2 trial. Lancet Oncol 2015;16(8):957–66.

24. Conroy T, Bosset JF, Etienne PL, et al. Neoadjuvant chemotherapy with FOLFIRINOX and preoperative chemoradiotherapy for patients with locally advanced rectal cancer (UNICANCER-PRODIGE 23): a multicentre, randomised, open-label, phase 3 trial. Lancet Oncol 2021;22(5):702–15.

25. Habr-Gama A, Perez RO, Nadalin W, et al. Operative versus nonoperative treatment for stage 0 distal rectal cancer following chemoradiation therapy: long-term results. Ann Surg 2004;240(4):711–7 [discussion: 717-8].

26. Habr-Gama A, São Julião GP, Vailati BB, et al. Organ preservation among patients with clinically node-positive rectal cancer: is it really more dangerous? Dis Colon Rectum 2019;62(6):675–83.

27. Rullier E, Vendrely V, Asselineau J, et al. Organ preservation with chemoradiotherapy plus local excision for rectal cancer: 5-year results of the GRECCAR 2 randomised trial. Lancet Gastroenterol Hepatol 2020;5(5):465–74.

28. van der Valk MJM, Hilling DE, Bastiaannet E, et al. Long-term outcomes of clinical complete responders after neoadjuvant treatment for rectal cancer in the International Watch & Wait Database (IWWD): an international multicentre registry study. Lancet 2018;391(10139):2537–45.

29. Garcia-Aguilar J, Patil S, Gollub MJ, et al. Organ Preservation in Patients With Rectal Adenocarcinoma Treated With Total Neoadjuvant Therapy. J Clin Oncol 2022;40(23):2546–56.

30. Jeong WJ, Choi BJ, Lee SC. Pure natural orifice transluminal endoscopic surgery for rectal cancer: Ta-TME and CME without abdominal assistance. Asian J Surg 2019;42(2):450–7.

31. Marks JH, Salem JF, Adams P, et al. initial clinical experience with single-port robotic transanal total mesorectal excision (SP rTaTME). Tech Coloproctol 2021; 25(6):721–6.

32. Zorron R, Phillips HN, Wynn G, et al. "Down-to-Up" transanal NOTES Total mesorectal excision for rectal cancer: Preliminary series of 9 patients. J Minim Access Surg 2014;10(3):144–50.

33. Rasulov AO, Mamedli ZZ, Dzhumabaev KE, et al. [Total mesorectal excision in rectal cancer management: laparoscopic or transanal?]. Khirurgiia (Mosk) 2016;(5):37–44.

34. Zeng Z, Luo S, Chen J, et al. Comparison of pathological outcomes after transanal versus laparoscopic total mesorectal excision: a prospective study using data from randomized control trial. Surg Endosc 2020;34(9):3956–62.

35. Deijen CL, Velthuis S, Tsai A, et al. COLOR III: a multicentre randomised clinical trial comparing transanal TME versus laparoscopic TME for mid and low rectal cancer. Surg Endosc 2016;30(8):3210–5.

36. Serra-Aracil X, Zárate A, Mora L, et al. Study protocol for a multicenter prospective controlled and randomized trial of transanal total mesorectal excision versus laparoscopic low anterior resection in rectal cancer. Int J Colorectal Dis 2018; 33(5):649–55.

Evidence for the Current Management of Soft-tissue Sarcoma and Gastrointestinal Stromal Tumors and Emerging Directions

Fahima Dossa, MD, PhD[a], Rebecca A. Gladdy, MD, PhD[a,b,c],*

KEYWORDS

- Soft-tissue sarcoma • Extremity sarcoma • Retroperitoneal sarcoma
- Gastrointestinal stromal tumor • Radiotherapy • Chemotherapy

KEY POINTS

- Soft-tissue sarcomas (STS) are a family of biologically diverse tumors with differing clinical courses and response to treatment.
- Radiotherapy (RT) improves local control for extremity STS; level 1 evidence questions the efficacy of RT for retroperitoneal sarcoma (RPS), where the response may vary by histology.
- Evidence for routine neoadjuvant/adjuvant chemotherapy in STS is lacking. The role of neoadjuvant chemotherapy for high-risk RPS is yet to be defined.
- Use of targeted therapy has fundamentally changed the treatment of gastrointestinal stromal tumors.
- Global collaborations have contributed significantly to our understanding of sarcoma and will continue to be critical for tailoring multimodal treatment.

INTRODUCTION

Sarcomas are rare mesenchymal tumors that comprise less than 1% of adult malignancies and 15% of pediatric malignancies. More than 70 types of sarcoma exist, with heterogeneity in biology, treatment response, and prognosis.[1,2] Although surgery

Conflicts of Interest: none.
^a Department of Surgery, University of Toronto, Stewart Building, 149 College Street, Toronto, Ontario M5T 1P5, Canada; ^b Division of Surgical Oncology, Department of Surgery, Mount Sinai Hospital and Princess Margaret Cancer Centre, University of Toronto, Toronto, Canada; ^c Sinai Health System, 600 University Avenue, Suite 1225, Toronto, Ontario M5G 1X5, Canada
* Corresponding author. Sinai Health System, 600 University Avenue, Suite 1225, Toronto, Ontario M5G 1X5, Canada.
E-mail address: Rebecca.Gladdy@sinaihealth.ca

Surg Oncol Clin N Am 32 (2023) 169–184
https://doi.org/10.1016/j.soc.2022.07.010

remains the primary curative therapy for most sarcoma types, the rarity of the disease, coupled with the variable biologic and clinical behavior, necessitates highly coordinated multimodal management, best offered at expert centers.[3–6]

In this review, we will provide a brief overview of historical studies that inform our current management of soft-tissue sarcoma (STS) and provide an update on current clinical trials and future research directions in STS. We will pay particular attention to gastrointestinal stromal tumors (GISTs), the most common gastrointestinal sarcoma. We also highlight the challenges in studying rare cancers and the importance of global collaborations in advancing our understanding of these tumors.

SOFT-TISSUE SARCOMA
Surgery

Extremity soft-tissue sarcoma—limb-sparing surgery is achieved in >90% of patients

Historically, the standard treatment for extremity sarcoma was radical excision with amputation. Seminal work by Rosenberg and colleagues,[7] established the role of a more limited limb-sparing approach. In a randomized study of patients with localized extremity STS, limb-sparing resection with adjuvant radiotherapy (RT) was associated with higher local recurrence than amputation but no statistically significant difference in 5-year overall survival (OS)—88% versus 83% for amputation and limb-sparing surgery, respectively. Limb-sparing resections are now the standard treatment of extremity STS and are achieved in >90% of patients with advances in limb reconstruction.[8–10]

Retroperitoneal soft-tissue sarcoma (retroperitoneal sarcoma)—extent of surgical resection continues to be debated

Analogous to the approaches of amputation and limb-sparing surgery in extremity STS, options for retroperitoneal sarcoma (RPS) include systematic compartmental resection of the tumor along with adjacent organs, irrespective of involvement, to incorporate a "margin" of uninvolved tissue, versus more limited organ-sparing surgery. Several issues, including retrospective study designs and inherent selection biases, limit conclusions that can be drawn from existing studies.[11] To date, there are no prospective trials evaluating whether a more aggressive surgical approach is associated with lower rates of local recurrence.

Radiation

Extremity soft-tissue sarcoma

The purpose of radiotherapy is to improve local control. Early experiences in the treatment of extremity STS revealed high local recurrence rates, reaching over 60% in some series.[12] RT was therefore adopted in an attempt to improve local control. The first prospective evidence of the efficacy of RT was demonstrated by Pisters and colleagues,[13] who randomized 164 patients with primary or recurrent resected extremity and superficial trunk STS to adjuvant brachytherapy (BT) versus no further therapy. BT patients demonstrated improved 5-year local control rates (82% vs 69%, $p = 0.04$) but no difference in 5-year disease-specific survival (84% vs 81%, $p = 0.65$) when compared with no further treatment (median follow-up 76 months). In subgroup analysis, the BT benefit was limited to high-grade disease only (5-year local control 89% vs 66% for BT and no further treatment groups, respectively, $p = 0.0025$), establishing a role for adjuvant RT in patients at highest risk for local recurrence.

Subsequent studies explored the use of external beam radiotherapy (EBRT). In a prospective study of patients with extremity STS who were randomized to adjuvant EBRT (45 Gy with 18 Gy boost to the tumor bed) versus no RT, adjuvant treatment was associated with lower local recurrence rates among patients with both high-

and low-grade disease, with durable effects at long-term follow-up.[14] Similar to Pisters and colleagues, there were no differences in OS between randomized groups, confirming the role of RT in local disease control only.

Preoperative radiotherapy is associated with acute wound complications but less long-term toxicity. In the National Cancer Institute of Canada Sarcoma 2 (NCIC-SR2) study,[15] patients with extremity STS were randomized to preoperative (50 Gy over 25 fractions) versus postoperative RT (66 Gy over 33 fractions). The primary endpoint was major wound complications within 120 days of surgery (reoperation, complex wound care, and readmission). The trial was closed early as a significant difference in the primary outcome was found—patients treated with preoperative RT had a higher frequency of wound complications than patients treated with postoperative RT (35% vs 17%, respectively; $p = 0.01$), with complications occurring almost exclusively in patients with lower extremity tumors.[15] Long-term follow-up, however, found greater rates of subcutaneous tissue fibrosis, edema, and joint stiffness at 2 years with postoperative RT, including lower functional scores.[16] Beyond lower rates of late radiation-associated toxicity, preoperative treatment offers the potential benefit of downsizing tumors and sterilizing margins, and lower costs and greater convenience with fewer fractions administered than postoperative treatment.[17]

A subsequent phase II trial by O'Sullivan and colleagues[18] evaluated whether image-guided intensity-modulated radiotherapy (IG-IMRT), which provides more accurate delivery of radiation, was associated with fewer complications. Seventy patients with lower-extremity STS enrolled between 2005 and 2009 were treated with preoperative IG-IMRT of 50 Gy over 25 fractions. Among the 59 evaluable patients, 30.5% developed acute wound complications within 120 days—lower than the 42.9% rate of the historical preop RT cohort from the NCIC-SR2 trial—however, statistical significance was not reached.

The potential for image-guided radiotherapy (IGRT) to reduce late toxicities has also been explored in the Radiation Therapy Oncology Group (RTOG)-0630 trial, a prospective phase II study.[17] In this study, patients with upper and lower extremity STS underwent preoperative IGRT (total dose 50 Gy over 25 fractions) with surgery performed 4 to 8 weeks later. Among the 57 patients assessed for late toxicities at 2 years, 10.5% had developed at least one grade ≥ 2 toxicity (as compared with 37% in NCIC-SR2,[15] $p < 0.001$). Acute wound complications developed among 36.6% of patients but cannot be directly compared with the results of O'Sullivan and colleagues[18] because of differences in study design and outcome ascertainment (eg, inclusion of both upper and lower extremity STS, time point of assessment, differences in RT technique). Taken together, however, these trials suggest IGRT can significantly reduce late radiation-associated toxicities.

Despite these studies, controversy still exists regarding the modality and sequencing of RT for the treatment of extremity STS. With the adoption of more accurate IG-IMRT, clinicians are exploring whether postoperative RT can be administered at doses and fractionation similar to preoperative treatment, potentially reducing toxicity while still providing adequate local control. An ongoing Canadian phase III study planning to enroll 206 patients with extremity and truncal STS will compare acute wound complications among patients treated with preoperative versus postoperative IMRT, both administered at 50 Gy over 25 fractions (NCT02565498, 50/50 Trial). Postoperative patients with positive surgical margins will additionally receive 16 Gy boost in eight fractions. Secondary outcomes include acute and late radiation toxicity, patient function, local recurrence-free survival, metastasis free-survival, and OS. Study completion is estimated for December 2022.

Future directions: histotype-specific studies. Whereas previous studies of patients with extremity STS have enrolled patients of diverse histotypes, ongoing studies recognizing the heterogeneity in biologic behavior and treatment response restrict enrollment to specific histotypes based on known patterns of response. One recent example is the Dose Reduction of Preoperative Radiotherapy in Myxoid Liposarcoma (DoReMY) study, a prospective phase II trial conducted at 9 sarcoma centers in the United States and Europe.[19] Myxoid liposarcoma (MLPS) has been shown to have robust pathological responses to preoperative RT and occurs in younger patients who are at risk of functional consequences of late radiation-associated toxicity. This study, therefore, evaluated whether patients with MLPS of the extremity or trunk could undergo radiation dose de-escalation while still maintaining excellent treatment responses. A total of 79 enrolled patients underwent preoperative RT with 36 Gy administered over 18 fractions. The primary endpoint was extensive pathologic treatment response (treatment effects in $\geq$50% tumor volume), where success was defined as $\geq$70% of resection specimens showing an extensive response. Extensive response was observed in 91% of patients; with a median follow-up of 25 months, local control was 100%. Six percent of patients had major wound complications and 14% experienced grade $\geq$2 late toxic effects. The results of this trial, therefore, suggest that dose reduction can safely and effectively be used in MLPS. Finally, this study serves as a paradigm for future investigation of histotype-directed treatment.

Retroperitoneal soft-tissue sarcoma (retroperitoneal sarcoma)
The role of radiotherapy in the treatment of retroperitoneal sarcoma continues to evolve. Retroperitoneal tumors account for 15% of STS.[20–22] Although surgery remains the cornerstone of treatment, anatomic constraints limit the ability to achieve an R0 resection. Multimodal therapy aimed at improving local control is needed in RPS. Given the success of RT in extremity STS, several groups have evaluated whether such benefits can be extrapolated to RPS.

Early studies include two prospective nonrandomized studies of preoperative RT for RPS. In a study by the Toronto Sarcoma Program,[23] 55 patients with primary or locally recurrent RPS were treated with preoperative RT at 45 Gy followed by postoperative BT boost. In a separate phase I trial from the MD Anderson Cancer Center aiming to establish the maximum tolerated dose of preoperative RT when given concurrently with fixed-dose continuous infusion doxorubicin, 35 patients with intermediate-to-high-grade RPS were treated with preoperative EBRT (18.0–50.4 Gy) with concurrent chemotherapy, followed by surgery with intraoperative RT (IORT).[24] The results of the 72 patients with intermediate- or high-grade lesions enrolled in these two studies were subsequently combined to evaluate long-term relapse and survival.[25] At a median follow-up of 40.3 months, 37% of the 54 preoperatively treated patients that had macroscopically complete surgical resections (ie, R0 or R1) experienced local recurrences (three patients with local and distant recurrence).

Given these early promising findings, several groups have investigated whether the RT response can be augmented. In the Toronto Sarcoma Program's study, patients received adjuvant BT after preoperative RT and complete surgical resection.[23] BT was, however, associated with marked toxicity without disease control,[23,26], especially among patients receiving treatment to the upper abdomen. The German RETRO-WTS phase I/II trial evaluated the use of preoperative dose-escalated IMRT followed by surgery with IORT to provide a greater dose of radiation per fraction to primary or locally recurrent RPS while sparing adjacent organs and tissues.[27] The trial enrolled patients with $\geq$5 cm, localized, at least marginally resectable RPS. Primary endpoint was 5-year local control. An unplanned interim analysis was performed in

2014 due to slow accrual—at a median follow-up of 33 months, 26% and 30% of patients experienced local and distant failures, respectively. Grade 3 acute radiation-related toxicity occurred in 15%, primarily gastrointestinal and hematologic. The study was completed in February 2020; final results are awaited (NCT01566123). Preliminary results of a phase II trial investigating the use of preoperative image-guided intensity-modulated proton radiation therapy (IMPT) with simultaneously integrated boost (SIB) to the high-risk posterior margin have also been reported.[28] Among 60 patients treated with a 23-month median follow-up, two local recurrences have occurred. Recruitment for this trial is ongoing.

Administration of preoperative versus postoperative RT has many potential advantages for retroperitoneal STS, including reduced toxicity to adjacent organs (eg, small bowel) because of tumor displacement, more accurate radiation planning and delivery of higher doses to larger volumes, and the potential to sterilize the operative field of microscopic emboli.[23] Until recently, the only phase III trial evaluating the use of preoperative RT in retroperitoneal STS was the ACOSOG Z9031 study, which randomized patients with primary retroperitoneal or pelvic STS to treatment with surgery alone or preoperative RT followed by resection (NCT00091351). Projected enrollment was 370 patients; however, this study was closed prematurely because of slow accrual, demonstrating the difficulties in performing prospective studies of rare diseases.

The much-awaited STRASS trial,[29] published in 2020, represents the only phase III randomized study of preoperative RT plus surgery versus surgery alone for RPS. This global effort, involving 31 institutions across 13 countries, enrolled patients with localized, primary disease deemed operable and suitable for RT by institutional tumor boards. Patients were randomized to surgery alone or preoperative RT at a dose of 50.4 Gy over 28 fractions (3D conformal or IMRT) followed by surgery. Primary endpoint was abdominal recurrence-free survival (ARFS), a composite that included abdominal relapse (local or distant progressive disease during preoperative radiation, progression to inoperability, peritoneal metastases found at surgery, R2 resection, or local relapse after macroscopically complete resection) and death. Among the 266 patients randomized, with median follow-up 43.1 months, no differences in median or 3-year ARFS were found. Serious adverse events had occurred in 10% of patients in the surgery alone group as compared with 24% of patients in the RT plus surgery group. Thus, the authors concluded that preoperative radiation should not constitute standard of care for RPS.

Several caveats are important to highlight in interpretation of these results. One criticism of STRASS has been the likelihood of selection bias. STREXIT, a study of patients with RPS treated at the top 10 STRASS recruiting centers during the time period of trial enrollment but not enrolled in STRASS, demonstrated that 57% of unenrolled patients met eligibility criteria, yet 44% were not enrolled because of physician preferences.[30] In particular, there was an underrepresentation of high-risk patients with poor prognostic variables enrolled in STRASS. Another important consideration as to why results did not demonstrate a benefit to RT is the inclusion of all histologic subtypes. Following the design of STRASS, studies performed by the Transatlantic Australasian Retroperitoneal Sarcoma Working Group (TARPSWG) demonstrated histology-specific patterns of failure in RPS, primarily, predominance of local failures among liposarcomas (LPS) and distant failures among leiomyosarcomas (LMS).[31] Furthermore, subgroup analysis stratified by histology demonstrated a possible beneficial effect of RT among patients with LPS. In sensitivity analyses, where progression on RT was not considered an event if patients remained resectable, an 11% absolute difference in ARFS was demonstrated between patients with LPS who did and did not receive preoperative RT (3-year ARFS 60.4% vs 71.6%, respectively; HR 0.64, 95%CI:

0.40–1.01). Although promising for the treatment of LPS, the long-term results of STRASS are still awaited.

Systemic Treatment

Although chemotherapy is used in the advanced/metastatic disease setting (not reviewed here), there is no proven benefit for routine use of chemotherapy for localized disease, outside of the known chemosensitive histologies (ie, Ewing's sarcoma, rhabdomyosarcoma). The potential benefits of chemotherapy require balance against the adverse events associated with cytotoxic treatment. Below, we review the evidence basis for the use of chemotherapy in localized sarcoma and emerging directions for systemic treatment. Regional techniques will not be reviewed here.

Adjuvant chemotherapy has not consistently been shown to improve survival in soft-tissue sarcoma

Currently, there is no clear evidence in support of adjuvant chemotherapy for STS. Numerous randomized trials investigating the use of doxorubicin-based regimens have been conducted with conflicting results. A randomized trial by the Italian Sarcoma Group (ISG) initially produced some of the most compelling data in favor of adjuvant chemotherapy.[32] Patients with high-grade primary or recurrent STS in the extremities or girdle were randomized to no chemotherapy or 5 cycles of adjuvant doxorubicin and ifosfamide. This study was closed early after interim analysis demonstrated positive results—with a median follow-up of 59 months, disease-free survival (DFS) and OSwere significantly improved in patients treated with chemotherapy. The absolute OS benefit of chemotherapy was estimated at 13% at 2 years and 19% at 4 years. However, the intention-to-treat analysis of longer-term results was not statistically significant.[33]

An individual participant data meta-analysis conducted by the Sarcoma Meta-analysis Collaboration combined the results of 14 RCTs (n = 1,568) investigating the use of doxorubicin-based adjuvant chemotherapy across STS histologic subtypes and anatomic locations.[34] With a median follow-up of 9.4 years, a meta-analysis demonstrated improvements in local (HR 0.73; 95%CI: 0.56–0.94), distant (HR 0.70, 95%CI: 0.57–0.85), and overall (HR 0.75; 95%CI: 0.64–0.87) recurrence-free survival attributable to adjuvant chemotherapy. However, there was no significant difference in OS (HR 0.89, 95%CI: 0.76–1.03). The estimated absolute benefit on survival was only 4% at 10 years. Notably, in subgroup analysis, results varied by tumor location, with the strongest signal of benefit seen among patients with extremity STS (7% absolute OS benefit). The results of the meta-analysis were later updated with the addition of 4 RCTs that utilized regimens of doxorubin plus ifosfamide, rather than doxorubin alone, demonstrating a significant improvement in OS with chemotherapy.[35] However, the marginal improvements demonstrated need to be balanced against the significant toxicity of cytotoxic therapies and, as such, the results of these studies have not resulted in widespread routine adoption of chemotherapy for localized disease.

The need to weigh benefits against toxicities raises the question of whether subgroups can be identified who may benefit most from chemotherapy. The EORTC-STBSG 62931 randomized trial evaluated the use of doxorubicin, ifosfamide, and lenograstim in patients with intermediate-to high-grade STS at any site (n = 351, most with extremity or limb girdle STS), finding no differences in OS between patients treated and not treated with adjuvant chemotherapy (HR 0.94, 95%CI: 0.68–1.31).[36] In an unplanned subgroup analysis, participants were stratified into risk groups based on their 10-year predicted probability of OS, calculated using the Sarculator nomogram.[37] When stratified in this manner, the highest risk patients (predicted 10-year OS <60%) demonstrated significant DFS (HR 0.49, 95%CI: 0.28–0.85) and OS (HR 0.50; 95%CI: 0.30–0.90) benefits.

The routine use of neoadjuvant chemotherapy is not recommended; use of systemic treatment should be considered on a case-by-case basis

Based on the survival benefits demonstrated in the adjuvant ISG study and the observation of suboptimal dose intensity of the last two of five chemotherapy cycles administered, Gronchi and colleagues[38,39] conducted a phase III noninferiority study evaluating whether three cycles of preoperative chemotherapy with epirubicin and ifosfamide was non-inferior to three preoperative plus two postoperative cycles of the same regimen. Non-inferiority was successfully demonstrated, turning focus to neoadjuvant—which offers potential benefits, particularly in cases of unresectable or borderline resectable disease[6]—rather than adjuvant therapy.

Efficacy of neoadjuvant chemotherapy versus surgery alone was evaluated in a phase II trial, which randomized 150 patients with potentially resectable high-risk STS of various anatomic locations to surgery alone versus three cycles of doxorubin and ifosfamide.[40] No significant benefits were demonstrated in 5-year DFS (56% for chemotherapy group vs 52% for controls, $p = 0.35$) or OS (65% for chemotherapy group vs 64% for controls, $p = 0.22$). The study was not extended to the planned phase III component because of slow accrual.

Although these results argue against the use of neoadjuvant chemotherapy, further work demonstrates conflicting results. In a randomized trial investigating the use of histology-driven regimens of chemotherapy versus a generalized approach with epirubicin and ifosfamide, patients treated with histology-directed regimens did not demonstrate improved survival. However, of note, there was a >20% difference in DFS, favoring patients treated with epirubicin and ifosfamide, suggesting a potential benefit of the standard neoadjuvant chemotherapy regimen.[41] Given the conflicting results, current guidelines recognize the variability in practices and recommend against routine use of neoadjuvant or adjuvant chemotherapy but encourage discussion with high-risk patients about potential benefits and toxicities.[5]

The benefits of neoadjuvant chemotherapy for high-risk groups are being defined

STRASS2 (NCT04031677), an ongoing phase III randomized trial, aims to evaluate the efficacy of chemotherapy for retroperitoneal and pelvic STS, focusing on patients at the highest risk for metastatic disease (**Fig. 1**). Patients with resectable high-risk LMS (grade 2/3, size $\geq$5 cm) and dedifferentiated liposarcoma (grade 3, high-risk grade 2) are being randomized to surgery alone versus three cycles of preoperative histology-specific anthracycline-based chemotherapy (doxorubicin and ifosfamide for LPS; doxorubicin and dacarbazine for LMS) followed by surgery. Primary outcome is DFS. This study aims to evaluate the effect of preoperative chemotherapy on the rate and timing of disease failure among patients at the highest risk of distant failure and, secondarily, to assess the toxicity profile of neoadjuvant chemotherapy and evaluate tumor response. Recruitment is ongoing and enrollment is estimated at 250 patients. Study completion is projected for 2028.

Future directions: immunotherapy

Unlike other solid tumors that have demonstrated robust responses to immunotherapy, such as melanoma, STS exhibits a lower mutational burden, largely thought to render these tumors nonimmunogenic. Initial data on the efficacy of checkpoint inhibitors in sarcoma emerged from patients with metastatic or locally advanced unresectable tumors. Whereas response to immunotherapy can be negligible when

Schema

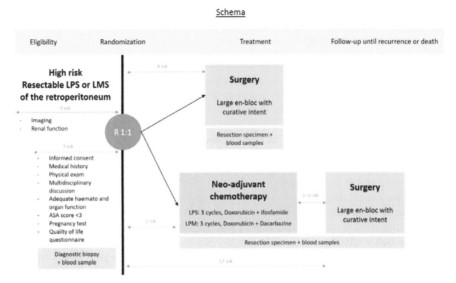

Fig. 1. *Study Schema for STRASS 2*: Neoadjuvant chemotherapy plus surgery vs surgery only for resectable LMS of the retroperitoneum.

administered to unselected patients with STS, the SARC028 phase II trial demonstrated histotype-specific responses to pembrolizumab in patients with advanced soft-tissue and bone sarcoma—objective response to treatment was demonstrated in 4 of 10 patients with undifferentiated pleomorphic sarcoma (UPS, 40%), 2 of 10 patients with dedifferentiated liposarcoma (DD-LPS, 20%), and none of the ten patients with LMS.[42] Results were attenuated in an expansion cohort of patients with UPS and DD-LPS (23% and 10% objective response, respectively)[43] but continue to suggest a possible role for immunotherapy in the treatment of patients with specific STS subtypes. Response rates of similar magnitude were seen in the Alliance A091401 phase II study, which randomized patients with the metastatic or unresectable disease to nivolumab alone versus nivolumab plus ipilimumab (objective response 5% and 16%, respectively). Subsequent studies have evaluated whether pairing checkpoint inhibitors with other systemic agents results in synergy. A phase II study of pembrolizumab plus the VEGF-inhibitor axitinib demonstrated durable responses in patients with alveolar soft-part sarcoma (median PFS 12.4 months, partial response 54.5%), with modest benefits in other subtypes.[44] In a phase II non-randomized trial of doxorubicin plus pembrolizumab in patients with advanced STS, partial response was seen in only 19%; however, two of three patients with UPS and two of four patients with DD-LPS demonstrated durable partial responses,[45] again highlighting a potential histotype-specific benefit to immunotherapy. Numerous ongoing clinical trials are similarly investigating the efficacy of cytotoxic chemotherapy with concurrent checkpoint blockade.

Germane to surgeons is the role of neoadjuvant immunotherapy in patients with resectable disease. Here too, histotype-specific responses are seen. In a phase II study of patients with resectable extremity/truncal UPS who received neoadjuvant RT plus immunotherapy (nivolumab or nivolumab + ipilimumab), median pathologic response was 95% and did not differ in the single versus dual immunotherapy arms.[46] In contrast, patients with DD-LPS receiving neoadjuvant immunotherapy (nivolumab or nivolumab + ipilimumab, without RT) had a 22.5% median pathologic response. The ongoing international SU2-SARC032 randomized phase II trial is evaluating the efficacy of neoadjuvant pembrolizumab with RT, followed by adjuvant pembrolizumab in patients with non-metastatic UPS or DD-LPS (grade 2 or 3) of the extremity and limb-girdle.[47] This trial is seeking to enroll 126 participants, with primary completion estimated for July 2024 (NCT03092323).

Future directions in immuno-oncology as it relates to STS include better identifying patients who may respond to immunotherapy and tailoring treatment regimens based on tumor biology. In a correlative analysis of the SARC028 trial, tumor microenvironments rich in activated T cells and tumor-associated macrophages were associated with a greater likelihood of response to pembrolizumab and improved PFS.[48] Similarly, a phase II study of durvalumab (anti-PD-L1) and tremelimumab (anti-CTLA-4) in patients with metastatic/advanced STS showed histotype-specific responses, and a correlation between clinical response and density of 3 categories of tumor-infiltrating lymphocytes (TIL).[49] Foundational work by Petitprez and colleagues[50] demonstrated that, independent of T cells, a tumor microenvironment rich in B cells is associated with both immunotherapy response and improved survival in patients with STS; 50% of patients enrolled in the SARC028 trial with pretreatment high expression of B lineage signatures exhibited objective responses to pembrolizumab. Together, these data suggest that, despite their historic classification as immunologically cold tumors, there likely exist immunogenic subtypes of STS that can be predicted based on histotype and tumor microenvironment. Such predictors may prove useful in the design of future clinical trials investigating the role of immunotherapy in STS.

GASTROINTESTINAL STROMAL TUMORS

GIST, which accounts for 0.2% of all GI cancers, represents the most common GI sarcoma. Although complete surgical resection remains the cornerstone of management for nonmetastatic disease, surgery alone achieves disease control in $\leq$50% of patients. GIST, however, illustrates the potential for molecular-driven targeted therapies in sarcoma. More than 90% of GIST harbor activating mutations in *KIT* or *PDGFRα*, which can be targeted by the tyrosine kinase inhibitor imatinib. With efficacy first demonstrated in the metastatic setting, where imatinib at doses of 400 mg or 600 mg daily was shown to induce a response in over 50% of patients[51] and improve survival,[52] use of imatinib has now been extended to the adjuvant and neoadjuvant settings for patients with high-risk disease.

Adjuvant Therapy

Adjuvant imatinib prolongs recurrence-free survival compared with surgery alone
Following the success of imatinib in the metastatic setting, the American College of Surgeons Oncology Group (ACOSOG) Z9000 single-arm phase II trial explored the use of adjuvant imatinib following complete gross resection of high-risk, localized, primary GIST (tumor >10 cm, intraperitoneal rupture, or up to 4 peritoneal implants).[53] Patients treated with imatinib at 400 mg/day for 1 year demonstrated 5-year OS of 83%, as compared with the 35% 5-year OS estimated for patients treated with surgery alone. Importantly, patients with *KIT* exon 9 mutations were demonstrated to have lower RFS and OS than those with exon 11 mutations.

The phase III, double-blind ACOSOG Z9001 study evaluated the efficacy of adjuvant imatinib in patients with localized, primary GIST.[54] In this trial, patients with *KIT* + tumors, $\geq$3 cm, were randomized to 1-year imatinib (400 mg/day) or placebo, with crossover to treatment at recurrence. This trial was stopped early because of interim evidence of efficacy. At 1-year, patients treated with imatinib demonstrated a 15% absolute improvement in recurrence-free survival (HR 0.35; 95%CI: 0.22–0.53) but no significant difference in OS (HR 0.66; 95%CI: 0.22–2.03). Subgroup analysis demonstrated benefits to imatinib across all tumor sizes, with increasing benefits with increasing size. Of note, although RFS remained significantly improved with imatinib in long-term follow-up,[55] absolute benefits of imatinib decreased over time, suggesting a delay in disease recurrence with imatinib.

Results of the EORTC 62024 trial,[56] which randomized patients with intermediate- or high-risk *KIT* + GIST to 2 years of imatinib (400 mg/day) versus no further therapy, also demonstrated benefits in RFS (84% vs 66% at 3 years for imatinib and surgery alone groups, respectively; log-rank p < 0.001), but not OS. Similar to the ACOSOG Z9001 trial, crossover to the treatment arm at the time of recurrence was permitted, which could, in part, explain these findings. Again, treatment with imatinib was shown to delay relapse, with RFS curves converging by 3 years after treatment cessation.

Current data support the use of adjuvant imatinib for three years post-resection

Evidence for recommendations on duration of adjuvant therapy comes from the Scandinavian XVIII/AIO phase III study, in which patients with surgically resected GIST at high risk of recurrence (as per modified NIH consensus criteria) were randomized to treatment with 400 mg of imatinib for 12 versus 36 months.[57] Patients treated for 36 months demonstrated improved RFS (HR 0.46; 95%CI: 0.32–0.65) and OS (HR 0.45; 95%CI: 0.22–0.89), with survival differences persisting at 5- and 10-year follow-up (10-year OS 79.0% vs 65.3% for 36-month and 12-month groups, respectively).[58,59]

Given the observation of delays in tumor recurrence attributable to imatinib, further protraction of treatment was explored in the PERSIST-5 phase II clinical trial, which evaluated 5 years of adjuvant imatinib in patients with complete macroscopic tumor resection.[60] Patients enrolled in this study demonstrated exceptional survival (5-year OS 95%; 5-year RFS 90%); only 1 recurrence was observed while patients were receiving treatment, occurring in a patient with an imatinib insensitive mutation (*PDGFRα D842 V*). However, nearly half of patients discontinued therapy before 5 years, with the majority being due to patient choice. Prolongation of treatment beyond 3 years is also being explored in the ImadGIST (NCT 02260505) and SSG XXII (NCT 02413736) trials.

Neoadjuvant Therapy

Neoadjuvant imatinib is safe and can result in objective tumor response

The potential for tumor downsizing, allowing for function-preserving, and oncologically superior resections, has led to the exploration of the utility of neoadjuvant imatinib.[61,62] Initial studies have focused on the safety of this approach, ensuring that neoadjuvant treatment would not lead to tumor rupture or bleeding. The RTOG 0132/ACRIN 6665 phase II study administered neoadjuvant imatinib (600 mg/day) to patients with primary ($\geq$5 cm) or operable metastatic ($\geq$2 cm) GIST for 8-12 weeks before surgical resection, followed by 2 years of adjuvant therapy.[63] Neoadjuvant treatment was well tolerated and no increases in postoperative complications were seen. In long-term follow-up, disease progression most commonly occurred after the cessation of adjuvant imatinib,[64] suggesting that preoperative treatment does not eliminate the need for adjuvant imatinib in intermediate-to high-risk patients. In a separate phase II study of patients with gastric GISTs $\geq$10 cm receiving 6-9 months of neoadjuvant imatinib, R0 resection was achieved in 91% of patients with minimal toxicity; objective best response rate by RECIST and Choi criteria were estimated at

62% and 98%, respectively.[65] McAuliffe and colleagues,[66] in a phase II trial where patients received 600 mg/day imatinib for 3, 5, or 7 days before surgery, followed by 2 years of adjuvant imatinib, demonstrated that radiographic response, as seen on FDG-PET and dynamic CT, can be detected as early as the first week of neoadjuvant therapy. However, the optimal duration of neoadjuvant treatment and patients for whom this approach is most efficacious has not been investigated in prospective trials. NCCN guidelines currently recommend consideration for neoadjuvant treatment where tumor downsizing can reduce surgical morbidity (eg, GIST requiring multivisceral resection; rectal or duodenal GIST; tumors close to esophagogastric junction).

IMPORTANCE OF GLOBAL COLLABORATIONS

The rarity of STS complicates the conduct of well-powered studies, particularly when limited to specific anatomic sites or histologic types. Global collaboration is therefore necessary to advance our understanding of fundamental tumor biology and to run trials seminal to the field.

Several examples of successful global collaboration exist. The most compelling of these is the completion of the STRASS trial. After the early closure of ACOSOG Z9031 (evaluating neoadjuvant RT in RPS) due to poor accrual, STRASS successfully enrolled 266 patients with resectable RPS at 31 centers to provide the first level I evidence for the treatment of RPS. The Transatlantic Australasian Retroperitoneal Sarcoma Working Group (TARPSWG) brings together international leaders in sarcoma research, generating expert-based consensus documents and establishing numerous international studies aimed at furthering our understanding of sarcoma tumor biology and response to treatment. The Retroperitoneal Sarcoma Registry (RESAR), established by TARPSWG in 2017, is one such initiative, prospectively collecting clinical, radiologic, and pathologic data from patients with RPS at participating centers. With enrollment to date of over 2,700 patients, these data will be used to examine patient outcomes, estimate the efficacy of various treatments (ie, surgery, chemotherapy, radiation), identify potential biomarkers of disease, run prospective clinical trials and hopefully share biologic materials for translational research. Ongoing global collaborations will be critical for further advancement of our understanding of these rare tumors.

SUMMARY

STS is not a single entity but, rather, a family of diseases with differing biologic behaviors and anatomic site- and histotype-specific responses to treatment. Whereas surgery remains the mainstay of treatment for primary, localized disease, evolving evidence is establishing the role of multimodality treatment for these tumors. This article summarizes prospective evidence to-date informing our treatment of STS. Key future directions will include advancing our understanding of fundamental tumor biology and mechanisms of response and recurrence, as well as defining the optimal provision of regional, systemic, and targeted therapies, including the role of immunotherapy. Ongoing global collaborations will be integral to progress in treating these rare tumors.

REFERENCES

1. World Health Organization Publication. WHO classification of tumours: soft-tissue and bone tumours. Geneva, Switzerland: International Agency for Research on Cancer; 2020.

2. Catton CN, O'Sullivan B, Kotwall C, et al. Outcome and prognosis in retroperitoneal soft-tissue sarcoma. Int J Radiat Oncol Biol Phys 1994;29(5):1005–10.

3. Cancer Care Ontario. Adult sarcoma management in ontario. Expert Panel Rep 2009 2009.

4. Ray-Coquard I, Thiesse P, Ranchère-Vince D, et al. Conformity to clinical practice guidelines, multidisciplinary management and outcome of treatment for soft-tissue sarcomas. Ann Oncol 2004;15(2):307–15.

5. Gronchi A, Miah A, Dei Tos A, et al. Soft-tissue and visceral sarcomas: ESMO–EURACAN–GENTURIS Clinical Practice Guidelines for diagnosis, treatment and follow-up. Ann Oncol 2021;32(11):1348–65.

6. Swallow CJ, Strauss DC, Bonvalot S, et al. Management of primary retroperitoneal sarcoma (RPS) in the adult: an updated consensus approach from the transatlantic australasian RPS working group. Ann Surg Oncol 2021;28(12):7873–88.

7. Rosenberg SA, Tepper J, Glatstein E, et al. The treatment of soft-tissue sarcomas of the extremities: prospective randomized evaluations of (1) limb-sparing surgery plus radiation therapy compared with amputation and (2) the role of adjuvant chemotherapy. Ann Surg 1982;196(3):305.

8. Ghert MA, Abudu A, Driver N, et al. The indications for and the prognostic significance of amputation as the primary surgical procedure for localized soft-tissue sarcoma of the extremity. Ann Surg Oncol 2005;12(1):10–7.

9. Smith HG, Thomas JM, Smith MJ, et al. Major amputations for extremity soft-tissue sarcoma. Ann Surg Oncol 2018;25(2):387–93.

10. Karakousis C, Proimakis C, Walsh D. Primary soft-tissue sarcoma of the extremities in adults. J Br Surg 1995;82(9):1208–12.

11. Raut CP, Swallow CJ. Are radical compartmental resections for retroperitoneal sarcomas justified? Ann Surg Oncol 2010;17(6):1481–4.

12. Cantin J, McNeer GP, Chu FC, et al. The problem of local recurrence after treatment of soft-tissue sarcoma. Ann Surg 1968;168(1):47.

13. Pisters PW, Harrison LB, Leung DH, et al. Long-term results of a prospective randomized trial of adjuvant brachytherapy in soft-tissue sarcoma. J Clin Oncol 1996;14(3):859–68.

14. Beane JD, Yang JC, White D, et al. Efficacy of adjuvant radiation therapy in the treatment of soft-tissue sarcoma of the extremity: 20-year follow-up of a randomized prospective trial. Ann Surg Oncol 2014;21(8):2484–9.

15. O'Sullivan B, Davis AM, Turcotte R, et al. Preoperative versus postoperative radiotherapy in soft-tissue sarcoma of the limbs: a randomised trial. The Lancet 2002;359(9325):2235–41.

16. Davis AM, O'Sullivan B, Turcotte R, et al. Late radiation morbidity following randomization to preoperative versus postoperative radiotherapy in extremity soft-tissue sarcoma. Radiother Oncol 2005;75(1):48–53.

17. Wang D, Zhang Q, Eisenberg BL, et al. Significant reduction of late toxicities in patients with extremity sarcoma treated with image-guided radiation therapy to a reduced target volume: results of Radiation Therapy Oncology Group RTOG-0630 trial. J Clin Oncol 2015;33(20):2231.

18. O'Sullivan B, Griffin AM, Dickie CI, et al. Phase 2 study of preoperative image-guided intensity-modulated radiation therapy to reduce wound and combined modality morbidities in lower extremity soft-tissue sarcoma. Cancer 2013; 119(10):1878–84.

19. Lansu J, Bovée JV, Braam P, et al. Dose reduction of preoperative radiotherapy in myxoid liposarcoma: a nonrandomized controlled trial. JAMA Oncol 2021;7(1): e205865.

20. Karakousis CP, Gerstenbluth R, Kontzoglou K, et al. Retroperitoneal sarcomas and their management. Arch Surg 1995;130(10):1104–9.
21. Jaques DP, Coit DG, Hajdu SI, et al. Management of primary and recurrent soft-tissue sarcoma of the retroperitoneum. Ann Surg 1990;212(1):51–9.
22. Mäkelä J, Kiviniemi H, Laitinen S. Prognostic factors predicting survival in the treatment of retroperitoneal sarcoma. Eur J Surg Oncol 2000;26(6):552–5.
23. Jones JJ, Catton CN, O'Sullivan B, et al. Initial results of a trial of preoperative external-beam radiation therapy and postoperative brachytherapy for retroperitoneal sarcoma. Ann Surg Oncol 2002;9(4):346–54.
24. Pisters PW, Ballo MT, Fenstermacher MJ, et al. Phase I trial of preoperative concurrent doxorubicin and radiation therapy, surgical resection, and intraoperative electron-beam radiation therapy for patients with localized retroperitoneal sarcoma. J Clin Oncol 2003;21(16):3092–7.
25. Pawlik TM, Pisters PW, Mikula L, et al. Long-term results of two prospective trials of preoperative external beam radiotherapy for localized intermediate-or high-grade retroperitoneal soft-tissue sarcoma. Ann Surg Oncol 2006;13(4):508–17.
26. Smith MJ, Ridgway PF, Catton CN, et al. Combined management of retroperitoneal sarcoma with dose intensification radiotherapy and resection: long-term results of a prospective trial. Radiother Oncol 2014;110(1):165–71.
27. Roeder F, Ulrich A, Habl G, et al. Clinical phase I/II trial to investigate preoperative dose-escalated intensity-modulated radiation therapy (IMRT) and intraoperative radiation therapy (IORT) in patients with retroperitoneal soft-tissue sarcoma: interim analysis. BMC cancer 2014;14(1):1–12.
28. DeLaney TF, Mullen JT, Chen Y-L, et al. Preliminary results of phase 2 trial of preoperative image guided intensity modulated proton radiation therapy (IMPT) with simultaneously integrated boost (SIB) to the high-risk margin for retroperitoneal sarcomas (RPS). Philadelphia, PA: Wolters Kluwer Health; 2021.
29. Bonvalot S, Gronchi A, Le Péchoux C, et al. Preoperative radiotherapy plus surgery versus surgery alone for patients with primary retroperitoneal sarcoma (EORTC-62092: STRASS): a multicentre, open-label, randomised, phase 3 trial. Lancet Oncol 2020;21(10):1366–77.
30. Callegaro D, RC AT, Strauss D, et al. Preoperative radiotherapy in patients with primary retroperitoneal sarcoma: trial (STRASS) versus off-trial (STREXIT) results. Paper presented at: CTOS Annual Meeting2020.
31. Gronchi A, Strauss DC, Miceli R, et al. Variability in patterns of recurrence after resection of primary retroperitoneal sarcoma (RPS): a report on 1007 patients from the multi-institutional collaborative RPS working group. Ann Surg 2016; 263(5):1002–9.
32. Frustaci S, Gherlinzoni F, De Paoli A, et al. Adjuvant chemotherapy for adult soft-tissue sarcomas of the extremities and girdles: results of the Italian randomized cooperative trial. J Clin Oncol 2001;19(5):1238–47.
33. Frustaci S, De Paoli A, Eea B, et al. Ifosfamide in the adjuvant therapy of soft-tissue sarcomas. Oncology 2003;65(Suppl. 2):80–4.
34. Collaboration SM-a. Adjuvant chemotherapy for localised resectable soft-tissue sarcoma of adults: meta-analysis of individual data. The Lancet 1997; 350(9092):1647–54.
35. Pervaiz N, Colterjohn N, Farrokhyar F, et al. A systematic meta-analysis of randomized controlled trials of adjuvant chemotherapy for localized resectable soft-tissue sarcoma. Cancer 2008;113(3):573–81.

36. Woll PJ, Reichardt P, Le Cesne A, et al. Adjuvant chemotherapy with doxorubicin, ifosfamide, and lenograstim for resected soft-tissue sarcoma (EORTC 62931): a multicentre randomised controlled trial. Lancet Oncol 2012;13(10):1045–54.

37. Pasquali S, Pizzamiglio S, Touati N, et al. The impact of chemotherapy on survival of patients with extremity and trunk wall soft-tissue sarcoma: revisiting the results of the EORTC-STBSG 62931 randomised trial. Eur J Cancer 2019;109:51–60.

38. Gronchi A, Ferrari S, Quagliuolo V, et al. sarcoma Full-dose neoadjuvant anthracycline+ ifosfamide chemotherapy is associated with a relapse free survival (RFS) and overall survival (OS) benefit in localized high-risk adult soft-tissue sarcomas (STS) of the extremities and trunk wall: Interim analysis of a prospective randomized trial. Ann Oncol 2016;27:vi587.

39. Gronchi A, Frustaci S, Mercuri M, et al. Short, full-dose adjuvant chemotherapy in high-risk adult soft-tissue sarcomas: a randomized clinical trial from the Italian Sarcoma Group and the Spanish Sarcoma Group. J Clin Oncol 2012;30(8):850–6.

40. Gortzak E, Azzarelli A, Buesa J, et al. A randomised phase II study on neoadjuvant chemotherapy for 'high-risk'adult soft-tissue sarcoma. Eur J Cancer 2001;37(9):1096–103.

41. Gronchi A, Ferrari S, Quagliuolo V, et al. Histotype-tailored neoadjuvant chemotherapy versus standard chemotherapy in patients with high-risk soft-tissue sarcomas (ISG-STS 1001): an international, open-label, randomised, controlled, phase 3, multicentre trial. Lancet Oncol 2017;18(6):812–22.

42. Tawbi HA, Burgess M, Bolejack V, et al. Pembrolizumab in advanced soft-tissue sarcoma and bone sarcoma (SARC028): a multicentre, two-cohort, single-arm, open-label, phase 2 trial. Lancet Oncol 2017;18(11):1493–501.

43. Burgess MA, Bolejack V, Schuetze S, et al. Clinical activity of pembrolizumab (P) in undifferentiated pleomorphic sarcoma (UPS) and dedifferentiated/pleomorphic liposarcoma (LPS): Final results of SARC028 expansion cohorts. J Clin Oncol 2019;37(15_suppl):11015.

44. Wilky BA, Trucco MM, Subhawong TK, et al. Axitinib plus pembrolizumab in patients with advanced sarcomas including alveolar soft-part sarcoma: a single-centre, single-arm, phase 2 trial. Lancet Oncol 2019;20(6):837–48.

45. Pollack SM, Redman MW, Baker KK, et al. Assessment of doxorubicin and pembrolizumab in patients with advanced anthracycline-naive sarcoma: a phase 1/2 nonrandomized clinical trial. JAMA Oncol 2020;6(11):1778–82.

46. Roland CL, Keung EZ-Y, Lazar AJ, et al. Preliminary results of a phase II study of neoadjuvant checkpoint blockade for surgically resectable undifferentiated pleomorphic sarcoma (UPS) and dedifferentiated liposarcoma (DDLPS). Am J Clin Oncol 2020;38(15_suppl):11505.

47. Mowery YM, Ballman KV, Riedel RF, et al. SU2C-SARC032: a phase II randomized controlled trial of neoadjuvant pembrolizumab with radiotherapy and adjuvant pembrolizumab for high-risk soft-tissue sarcoma. J Clin Oncol 2018; 36(15_suppl):TPS11588.

48. Keung EZ, Burgess M, Salazar R, et al. Correlative analyses of the SARC028 trial reveal an association between sarcoma-associated immune infiltrate and response to pembrolizumabsarcoma-associated immune infiltrate and Anti-PD1 therapy. Clin Cancer Res 2020;26(6):1258–66.

49. Somaiah N, Conley AP, Lin HY, et al. A phase II multi-arm study of durvalumab and tremelimumab for advanced or metastatic sarcomas. Am J Clin Oncol 2020;38(15_suppl):11509.

50. Petitprez F, de Reyniès A, Keung EZ, et al. B cells are associated with survival and immunotherapy response in sarcoma. Nature 2020;577(7791):556–60.

51. Demetri GD, Von Mehren M, Blanke CD, et al. Efficacy and safety of imatinib mesylate in advanced gastrointestinal stromal tumors. N Engl J Med 2002;347(7): 472–80.

52. Blanke CD, Demetri GD, Von Mehren M, et al. Long-term results from a randomized phase II trial of standard-versus higher-dose imatinib mesylate for patients with unresectable or metastatic gastrointestinal stromal tumors expressing KIT. J Clin Oncol 2008;26(4):620–5.

53. DeMatteo RP, Ballman KV, Antonescu CR, et al. Long-term results of adjuvant imatinib mesylate in localized, high-risk, primary gastrointestinal stromal tumor (GIST): ACOSOG Z9000 (Alliance) intergroup phase 2 trial. Ann Surg 2013; 258(3):422.

54. DeMatteo RP, Ballman KV, Antonescu CR, et al. Adjuvant imatinib mesylate after resection of localised, primary gastrointestinal stromal tumour: a randomised, double-blind, placebo-controlled trial. Lancet 2009;373(9669):1097–104.

55. Corless CL, Ballman KV, Antonescu CR, et al. Pathologic and molecular features correlate with long-term outcome after adjuvant therapy of resected primary GI stromal tumor: the ACOSOG Z9001 trial. J Clin Oncol 2014;32(15):1563.

56. Casali P, Cesne AL, Velasco AP, et al. Time to definitive failure to the first tyrosine kinase inhibitor in localized gi stromal tumors treated with imatinib as an adjuvant: a european organisation for research and treatment of cancer soft-tissue and bone sarcoma group intergroup randomized trial in collaboration with the australasian gastro-intestinal trials group, UNICANCER, french sarcoma group, italian sarcoma group, and spanish group for research on sarcomas. J Clin Oncol 2015;33:4276–83.

57. Joensuu H, Eriksson M, Hall KS, et al. One vs three years of adjuvant imatinib for operable gastrointestinal stromal tumor: a randomized trial. JAMA 2012;307(12): 1265–72.

58. Joensuu H, Eriksson M, Hall KS, et al. Survival outcomes associated with 3 years vs 1 year of adjuvant imatinib for patients with high-risk gastrointestinal stromal tumors: an analysis of a randomized clinical trial after 10-year follow-up. JAMA Oncol 2020;6(8):1241–6.

59. Joensuu H, Eriksson M, Sundby Hall K, et al. Adjuvant imatinib for high-risk GI stromal tumor: analysis of a randomized trial. J Clin Oncol 2016;34(3):244–50.

60. Raut CP, Espat NJ, Maki RG, et al. Efficacy and tolerability of 5-year adjuvant imatinib treatment for patients with resected intermediate-or high-risk primary gastrointestinal stromal tumor: the PERSIST-5 clinical trial. JAMA Oncol 2018; 4(12):e184060.

61. Andtbacka RH, Ng CS, Scaife CL, et al. Surgical resection of gastrointestinal stromal tumors after treatment with imatinib. Ann Surg Oncol 2007;14(1):14–24.

62. Sjölund K, Andersson A, Nilsson E, et al. Downsizing treatment with tyrosine kinase inhibitors in patients with advanced gastrointestinal stromal tumors improved resectability. World J Surg 2010;34(9):2090–7.

63. Eisenberg BL, Harris J, Blanke CD, et al. Phase II trial of neoadjuvant/adjuvant imatinib mesylate (IM) for advanced primary and metastatic/recurrent operable gastrointestinal stromal tumor (GIST): early results of RTOG 0132/ACRIN 6665. J Surg Oncol 2009;99(1):42–7.

64. Wang D, Zhang Q, Blanke CD, et al. Phase II trial of neoadjuvant/adjuvant imatinib mesylate for advanced primary and metastatic/recurrent operable gastrointestinal stromal tumors: long-term follow-up results of Radiation Therapy Oncology Group 0132. Ann Surg Oncol 2012;19(4):1074–80.

65. Kurokawa Y, Yang HK, Cho H, et al. Phase II study of neoadjuvant imatinib in large gastrointestinal stromal tumours of the stomach. Br J Cancer 2017; 117(1):25–32.
66. McAuliffe JC, Hunt KK, Lazar AJ, et al. A randomized, phase II study of preoperative plus postoperative imatinib in GIST: evidence of rapid radiographic response and temporal induction of tumor cell apoptosis. Ann Surg Oncol 2009;16(4):910–9.

The Evolving Landscape of Neuroendocrine Tumors

Ashley Russo, MD, Alexandra Gangi, MD*

KEYWORDS

- Neuroendocrine tumor • Carcinoid • Pancreatic • Small bowel • Liver metastases
- Somatostatin

KEY POINTS

- Neuroendocrine tumors (NETs) can originate in the foregut, midgut, or hindgut and can be associated with functional syndromes when accompanied by hormone hypersecretion.
- On the basis of retrospective data, surgery is the mainstay of treatment for patients with NETs to improve symptoms and survival.
- In the case of hepatic metastatic disease in both symptomatic and asymptomatic patients, there is a role for hepatic cytoreduction if >70% hepatic disease can be debulked.
- Several prospective randomized clinical trials have shown improved progression-free survival associated with the use of various medical therapies in the management of advanced, metastatic, and unresectable NETs.

INTRODUCTION

Neuroendocrine tumors (NETs) represent a heterogenous group of tumors that arise from enterochromaffin cells that are distributed throughout the body. NETs can originate in the foregut (bronchial, gastric, duodenal, and pancreatic), midgut (jejunal, ileal, appendiceal, and proximal colon), or hindgut (distal colon and rectum) and can be associated with functional syndromes when resulting in hormone hypersecretion. The most common NETs are found in the lung, followed by small bowel (jejunal and ileal), rectal, and pancreatic.[1] Owing to the indolent nature of NETs, approximately 40%–45% of patients are initially diagnosed with distant metastases, which most frequently occur in the liver.[2,3] In the metastatic setting, NETs are one of the few tumor types in which cytoreductive surgery is recommended in appropriately selected patients.

Neuroendocrine neoplasms are divided into two categories: well-differentiated NETs and poorly differentiated neuroendocrine carcinomas (NECs). The European Neuroendocrine Tumor Society (ENETS) and World Health Organization (WHO) have

Department of Surgery, Cedars-Sinai Medical Center, 8700 Beverly Boulevard, Los Angeles, CA 90048, USA
* Corresponding author.
E-mail address: alexandra.gangi@cshs.org

Surg Oncol Clin N Am 32 (2023) 185–198
https://doi.org/10.1016/j.soc.2022.08.003
1055-3207/23/© 2022 Elsevier Inc. All rights reserved.

surgonc.theclinics.com

classified well-differentiated NETs as grade 1 if they have <2 mitoses/10 high-power field (HPF) and <3% Ki-67 index, grade 2 if they have 2–20 mitoses/10 HPF or 3% to 20% Ki-67 index, and grade 3 if they have >20 mitoses/10 HPF or >20% Ki-67 index. Poorly differentiated NECs have >20 mitoses/10 HPF or >20% Ki-67 and are similar in behavior and histology to adenocarcinoma. Up to one-third of patients can present with typical signs and symptoms of carcinoid syndrome, which include flushing, watery diarrhea, wheezing, and abdominal pain. For patients with long-term carcinoid syndrome, carcinoid heart disease can develop, which presents as right-sided heart failure. Carcinoid crisis is an extreme manifestation of carcinoid syndrome and can result in hemodynamic instability, bronchoconstriction, and refractory shock.

Regardless of the site of origin, surgery is the mainstay of treatment for most gastro-enteropancreatic (GEP)-NETs for both symptom control and to improve survival. Owing to the low incidence, variability in presentation, and indolent nature of NETs, there are no randomized control trials (RCT) to help guide principles of and indications for surgical resection, and current clinical practices and society guidelines rely largely on retrospective and single-institution studies, as well as expert opinion. On the contrary, there are several high-quality prospective RCTs to support the use of different medical therapies in the management of patients with NETs, particularly in patients with advanced metastatic and unresectable NETs. The goal of this review is to provide background on the commonly encountered types of NETs in general surgical oncology practice, namely small-bowel neuroendocrine tumors (SBNETs) and pancreatic neuroendocrine tumors (PNETs), discuss the management of NET liver metastases (NETLM), and to summarize the best available evidence that has shaped the most current guidelines for both the surgical and medical management of patients with NETs.

BACKGROUND: SMALL-BOWEL NEUROENDOCRINE TUMORS

SBNETs have been slowly increasing in incidence and are now the most common primary tumor of the small bowel.[1,4] SBNETs primarily refer to NETs arising in the jejunum and ileum, with over 70% arising within 100 cm of the ileocecal valve.[5] Current literature estimates that anywhere from 20% to 56% of patients with SBNET present with multi-focal disease and up to 60% of patients will present with lymph node (LN) metastases.[6]

SURGICAL PRINCIPLES FOR SMALL-BOWEL NEUROENDOCRINE TUMORS

Surgery consisting of resection of the primary tumor and associated LNs is the mainstay of treatment of SBNETS as it can improve both symptoms and survival.[7,8] Surgical resection also decreases the risk of complications associated with disease progression, namely metastatic disease and progression of disease resulting in obstruction or bleeding complications.[9–12] Even in patients with advanced metastatic disease, primary tumor resection (PTR) with or without cytoreduction can improve survival and alleviate symptoms associated with hormone hypersecretion, bleeding, and intestinal obstruction.[13–16]

Open surgery is the gold standard for resection of SBNETs to facilitate manual palpation of the entire small bowel to detect small, multifocal lesions. As lesions can be as small as a few millimeters, the use of minimally invasive surgery (MIS) is controversial in the management of SBNETs as MIS instruments provide limited haptic feedback. Studies that have described successful MIS resection of SBNETs use of routine manual palpation of the small bowel by either exteriorization of the bowel or by the placement of a hand-assist port.[17] A study by Kasai and colleagues[18] identified factors that may predict conversion to open: namely mesenteric masses ≤ 2 cm from the ileocolic artery and vein (39% vs 9% when >2 cm away) and the presence of mesenteric masses that involve the superior mesenteric artery (SMA)/superior mesenteric vein (SMV) or proximal to the origin of the ileocolic artery and vein (80% conversion to open). On the basis of these and other studies, consensus guidelines agree that hand-assisted laparoscopy may be a reasonable approach if the surgeon is confident that the entire small bowel can be adequately assessed and if cytoreduction can be achieved via the laparoscopic approach.[7,8]

In terms of the extent of surgery, current guidelines recommend routine resection of regional LNs and mesenteric masses during PTR for patients with SBNETs.[7,8] Surgical clearance of regional LNs and masses should be achieved by performing a resection of the involved bowel and a wedge of associated mesentery down to the segmental vessels coming from the SMA and SMV, with the caveat that complete resection of masses that involve or encase the SMA and SMV may not be possible.[19,20] Rationale for resection of regional LNs is supported largely by retrospective data. A large, retrospective study from the Surveillance, Epidemiology, and End Results (SEER) database was performed to evaluate the impact of mesenteric LN resection. On multivariate analysis, removal of >7 LNs (hazard ratio [HR] 0.73, $p = 0.05$) and an LN ratio (LNR, positive-to-negative node ratio) of <0.29 was associated with improved overall survival (OS) (HR 1.65 for LNR >0.29, $p = 0.0019$).[21]

In patients with metastatic disease, the role of PTR in asymptomatic patients is controversial. Multiple studies have shown improvement in OS with PTR, whereas others have shown no difference. A study by Ahmed and colleagues[16] from 2009 found an improved OS from 4.7 to 6.7 years to 9.9 years when patients underwent PTR (relative risk [RR] 0.26) and found that PTR was an independent predictor of survival on multivariate analysis ($p = 0.015$). A later National Cancer Database (NCDB) analysis by Gangi and colleagues[15] from 2020 showed an improvement in 5-year OS (49% vs 66%, $p < 0.001$) in patients with SBNETs with unresectable liver-only metastases who underwent PTR. Looking at slightly different outcomes, Bennett and colleagues[14] performed a 2:1 propensity-matched analysis of upfront small-bowel resection (USBR) compared with no surgery in patients with SBNETs and synchronous metastases and showed that USBR was associated with a lower 3-year risk of admission (72.6% vs 86.4%, $p < 0.001$, HR 0.72) and lower risk of subsequent small-bowel surgery (15.4% vs 40.3%, $p < 0.001$, HR 0.44). Conversely, Daskalakis and colleagues found no survival benefit to prophylactic surgery within 6 months of diagnosis compared with nonsurgical or delayed surgical management in patients with asymptomatic stage-IV SBNETs. Propensity-score matching between these two groups found no significant difference in median OS (7.9 vs 7.6 years, $p = 0.93$) or median cancer-specific survival (7.7 vs 7.6 years, $p = 0.99$).[22] It is worth noting; however, that most of the patients in the nonsurgical or delayed surgery group (>6 months after diagnosis) ultimately required surgery, which may have been prevented with a prophylactic surgery. A recent review by Hallet and colleagues[23] suggested that PTR should be strongly considered for patients with SBNET to avoid future locoregional complications and potentially improve survival.

On the basis of the available retrospective and observational data, NANETS and ENETS recommend evaluation and consideration of PTR for patients with metastatic SBNETs to alleviate symptoms, minimize future symptoms or complications, and improve both progression-free survival (PFS) and OS.[7,8]

BACKGROUND: PANCREATIC NEUROENDOCRINE TUMORS

PNETs arise from pancreatic islet cells and are primarily classified according to their grade and whether they are functional. Although still a relatively rare entity, due to both increased use of cross-sectional imaging and endoscopic ultrasound, the incidence of PNETs is increasing.[1] Functional PNETs can secrete hormones and are often associated with well-described clinical syndromes. These tumors can be sporadic or may occur as part of a genetic syndrome, most commonly Multiple Endocrine Neoplasia type 1 (MEN1). (**Table 1**).

SURGICAL PRINCIPALS FOR PANCREATIC NEUROENDOCRINE TUMORS

Like SBNETs, there is a paucity of randomized clinical evidence to guide the surgical management of PNETs. Nonetheless, surgery remains the mainstay of treatment for most PNETs. For small (<1 cm), well-differentiated, low-grade, nonfunctional (NF) tumors, observation can be recommended. This is based on several single institutions and multicenter retrospective studies that have shown that the risk of LN metastasis or distant metastasis increases based on tumor size.[24–26] There are also several retrospective studies that have compared active surveillance to surgical resection for small, asymptomatic, NF-PNETs that did not show any disease-specific survival (DSS) or OS benefit in patients who underwent surgical resection, with the caveat that these studies used slightly difference size cutoffs ranging from 2 to 4 cm and were all retrospective in nature.[27–33] (**Table 2**) For resected PNETs, Zaidi and colleagues[34] performed an internal validation of a recurrence risk score (RRS) which can be used to stratify recurrence-free survival for patients with resected PNET into low-, intermediate-, or high-risk groups. This can, in turn, be used to help guide a surveillance strategy to minimize radiation exposure and optimize the utilization of resources.

For any tumor that is functional, >2 cm, grade 2 or higher, or any tumor with clinical concern for regional LN involvement, surgical resection is recommended. Given the propensity of these tumors to metastasize to regional LNs, a formal pancreatectomy with regional lymphadenectomy is the recommended operation for most PNETs. There are no prospective randomized data to support regional lymphadenectomy at the time of PNET resection, but studies have shown a propensity of spread to regional LNs and that LN positivity is a consistent poor prognostic factor for survival and recurrence; therefore, regional lymphadenectomy is recommended.[35–40] Despite this recommendation, several studies, including large population-based studies have failed to show a therapeutic benefit of performing a regional lymphadenectomy.[41,42] For tumors <2 cm, there is retrospective data to support the use of LN risk scores to stratify the risk of LN metastases and help guide management strategies.[43]

It may be reasonable to omit a formal lymphadenectomy and perform a parenchymal-preserving pancreatic resection for smaller tumors when suspicion of regional LN metastasis is low. Insulinomas are the most common functional PNET and given their extremely low malignant potential, can typically be treated with a parenchymal-preserving pancreatic resection (enucleation) and do not require routine lymphadenectomy.[44] For 1–2 cm tumors, clinicians are encouraged to make a patient-specific decision regarding active surveillance versus resection depending on the patient's surgical risk and clinicopathologic features of their tumor.[25,45] For patients with MEN1, the indication for surgical resection has a slightly higher size threshold of 2 to 3 cm due to the multiplicity of MEN1-associated PNETs.[46] In addition, given the likelihood of recurrence, parenchymal-preserving approaches are favored in MEN1 patients.

In contrast to SBNETs, there are prospective randomized data to support the use of MIS when feasible for patients with PNETs, especially distal pancreatic lesions. The LEOPARD trial is a prospective randomized trial that compared MIS versus open distal pancreatectomy.[47] Patients undergoing MIS resection had decreased time to functional recovery, decreased blood loss, and improved quality of life, but longer

Table 1
Functional PNETs, associated syndromes, and association with MEN1

Type	Syndrome	Malignancy Risk (%)	Association with MEN1 (%)
Insulinoma	Hypoglycemia	<10	4–5
Gastrinoma	Peptic ulcer disease and diarrhea	60–90	20–25
VIPoma	Watery diarrhea, hypokalemia, achlorhydria, and dehydration	40–70	6
Glucagonoma	Diabetes and necrolytic migratory erythema	50–80	1–20
Somatostatinoma	Diabetes, cholestasis, steatorrhea, and diarrhea	>70	10

operative times when compared with open distal pancreatectomy. There is currently no data to support the use of the laparoscopic platform over the robotic platform, and the decision should be based on surgeon experience. The benefit of using MIS techniques in the management of pancreatic head lesions is less clear and is currently only recommended for patients being treated at high-volume centers.[35] The role of laparoscopy for these lesions has not been shown, as the LEOPARD-2 trial comparing laparoscopic versus open pancreaticoduodenectomy, closed early due to increased mortality in the laparoscopic group.[48] There is some data to support the use of the robotic platform for pancreatic head lesions but again, should only be performed at high-volume centers.[49,50]

With respect to pancreatic preservation via either enucleation or central pancreatectomy, these options should only be offered to patients with small ≤2 cm NF-PNETs or insulinomas, especially those which are exophytic or peripheral, as these have the lowest risk of regional LN metastases. Although some studies have shown parenchyma-preserving approaches are associated with reduced endocrine and exocrine insufficiency, shorter operations, and decreased blood loss, others have shown higher rates of postoperative complications, including postoperative fistulas, and longer length of stay.[51–54]

Similar to the data in support of PTR for patients with metastatic SBNETs, there is also retrospective data to support PTR for patients with metastatic PNETs. A SEER database study by Keutgen and colleagues showed an improvement in OS (10 months vs 65 months, $p < 0.001$) for patients with metastatic NF-PNETs who underwent PTR. Multivariate analysis showed that tumor location influenced survival as well, specifically that tumors of the body/tail were associated with improved OS.[55]

BACKGROUND: NEUROENDOCRINE CARCINOMAS

NECs are poorly differentiated, high-grade neoplasms that are characterized by a high mitotic rate and Ki-67 index and are behaviorally similar to adenocarcinomas. NECs are aggressive tumors with a poor median OS of 7.7 months.[56] The management of NEC is typically multimodal with some combination of surgery, chemotherapy, and radiation. In patients with localized disease, surgical resection can be offered, but for patients with unresectable locoregional or metastatic disease, the mainstay of treatment is chemotherapy with or without radiation. Several cytotoxic chemotherapy regimens have been evaluated as first-line agents for patients with resectable, locoregional unresectable, and metastatic diseases that include cisplatin/etoposide, carboplatin/

Table 2
Retrospective studies comparing surgical resection to active surveillance for small asymptomatic, NF-PNETs

Authors, Year	Setting	Resection, Patients (N)	Active Surveillance, Patients (N)	Size Cutoff (cm)	Findings
Sadot et al.[27] 2016	Single-institution	77	104	<3	No difference in DSS
Lee et al.[29] 2012	Single-institution	56	77	<4	No difference in DSS
Kurita et al.[30] 2020	Single-institution	52	23	≤2	No difference in OS
Barenboim et al.[31] 2020	Single-institution	55	44	<2	No difference in DSS
Rosenberg et al.[32] 2016	Single-institution	8	10	<2	No difference in DSS
Regenet et al.[33] 2016	Multi-Institution	66	14	≤2	No difference in disease-free survival (DFS)

etoposide, FOLOFOX, FOLFIRI, and temozolomide with or without capecitabine.[39] For patients who progress on cytotoxic chemotherapy, consideration of combination immunotherapy with ipilimumab and nivolumab may be appropriate, as the phase II DART SWOG 1609 basket trial showed an objective response rate (ORR) of 44% in patients with non-pancreatic NECs treated with this combination therapy.[57] There are several ongoing clinical trials evaluating the safety and efficacy of different chemotherapy and immune therapy regimens for patients with NEC.

BACKGROUND: NEUROENDOCRINE TUMOR LIVER METASTASES

Up to 40% to 45% of patients present with distant metastatic disease, most commonly in the liver, at the time of initial NET diagnosis.[2,3] In the metastatic setting, NETs are one of the few tumor types in which cytoreductive surgery is recommended in appropriately selected patients if >70% of the disease burden can be safely cleared, as debulking improves survival and controls symptoms related to hormone hypersecretion.[12,58,59] NETLM are known to be a negative prognostic factors for OS.[10,12,16,60]

SURGICAL PRINCIPLES FOR NEUROENDOCRINE TUMOR LIVER METASTASES

For patients with metastatic disease to the liver, studies have shown that a survival benefit and symptom management can be achieved if >70% of hepatic disease burden is resected. Importantly, the studies that have evaluated thresholds of cytoreduction for patients with NETLM did not show any improvements in PFS or OS when the threshold of >70% was compared with thresholds of 90% to 99% and 100%.[13,61,62] Factors that have been identified as negative predictive factors for PFS and OS in patients with NETLM are age <50, liver metastases ≥ 5 cm, the presence of synchronous disease at the primary site, extrahepatic disease at the time of liver resection, and NF hormone status.[10,59,63] Scott and colleagues[61] validated the debulking threshold of 70% and showed that aggressive debulking can be achieved even in patients with >10 liver metastases. It is critical to note that even with complete debulking, liver metastasis recurrence rates are quite high, >80% at 5 years and approximately 100% at 10 years.[10,12]

LIVER-DIRECTED THERAPIES FOR NEUROENDOCRINE TUMOR LIVER METASTASES

Hepatic cytoreduction can be achieved by several different modalities including surgical resection (which may include enucleation or intraoperative thermal ablation), hepatic arterial embolization, including bland embolization, chemoembolization (TACE), and radioembolization, cryotherapy, irreversible electroporation, and percutaneous thermal ablation. There is an ongoing prospective, open-label, multicenter RCT (RETNET) that is being conducted to determine the optimal embolization strategy in patients with progressive or symptomatic unresectable NETLM, with a primary endpoint of hepatic PFS.[64] The first safety report of the trial indicated severe hepatobiliary complications with drug-eluting beads (DEB)-TACE and therefore this arm of the trial has been halted. Despite the lack of mature data comparing different intra-arterial therapies, there have been several studies comparing intra-arterial strategies to surgical resection. A multi-center international analysis by Mayo and colleagues[65] compared surgical resection to intra-arterial therapy in matched patients with >25% liver involvement with and without carcinoid symptoms. Using propensity score matching, this study found that patients with low-volume or symptomatic disease derived more of a benefit from surgical resection compared with those with a large burden of disease or who were asymptomatic.

Table 3
Clinical trials for medical management of advanced and unresectable NETs

Trial	Patient Population	Trial Arms	Primary Endpoint	Results
PROMID[71]	Metastatic SBNETs (midgut)	Octreotide LAR vs placebo	PFS	14.3 vs 6 months, HR 0.34, p < 0.001
CLARINET[67]	Metastatic GEP-NETs	Lanreotide vs placebo	PFS	Not reached vs 18 months, HR 0.47, p < 0.001
NETTER-1[68]	Metastatic SBNETs (midgut)	177Lu-Dotatate with octreotide LAR vs octreotide LAR	PFS	Not reached vs 8.4 months, HR 0.21, p < 0.001
RADIANT-4[72]	Advanced NF-NETs of lung and GI tract	Everolimus vs placebo	PFS	11 vs 3.9 months, HR 0.48, p < 0.001
Sunitinib[73]	Advanced PNETs	Sunitinib vs placebo	PFS	11.4 vs 5.5 months, HR 0.58, p = 0.023
ECOG 2211[74]	Advanced PNETs	Temozolomide vs temozolomide plus capecitabine	PFS	14.4 vs 22.7 months, HR 0.21, p < 0.001

MEDICAL MANAGEMENT FOR NEUROENDOCRINE TUMORS

As an alternative to cytoreduction, there is randomized data to support the use of medical therapies in the management of patients with advanced disease, which include somatostatin analogs (SSA), peptide receptor radionuclide therapy (PRRT), and targeted therapies. Several of these treatment advances have been shown to improve PFS.[66–70] It should be noted that it is unlikely that a comparison of the survival benefit between surgical cytoreduction and medical therapy can be determined via RCT given the low incidence of NETs, the long duration of follow-up that would be required, and the need for equipoise related to treatment. With that in mind, there are several high-quality RCTs that support the use of medical therapies in the management of patients with advanced and unresectable NETs (**Table 3**).

SUMMARY

NETs are a heterogeneous group of tumors with variable clinical presentations. Surgery remains the mainstay of treatment for most NETs. Multiple society guidelines recommend that a regional lymphadenectomy be performed at the time of PTR as several retrospective studies have shown the increased risk of LN metastases with increasing tumor size and the prognostic significance of LN metastases. The presence of distant metastases at the time of initial diagnosis is common among patients with NETs, which most frequently occur in the liver. Whether by surgical resection, intraoperative or percutaneous ablation, or intra-arterial liver-directed therapies, hepatic cytoreduction of >70% is recommended for patients with NETLM to improve both symptoms and survival. For patients with metastatic, advanced, or unresectable disease, there have been several RCTs that support the use of medical therapies, including SSA, PRRT, and targeted therapies in this patient population. Keeping in mind the available evidence along with its inherent limitations, decisions regarding an individual patient's care should ultimately be made in a multidisciplinary setting with consideration for the patient's risk factors, disease biology, available treatment options, and experience of the treating surgeon to best optimize patient outcomes.

FUTURE DIRECTIONS

There are currently several trials evaluating adjuvant therapies for patients with high-risk or metastatic neuroendocrine tumors. There is an actively enrolling phase II SWOG trial that is evaluating the role of postoperative treatment with capecitabine and temozolomide (CAPTEM) versus observation alone for patients with high-risk well-differentiated PNETs (Ki-67 $\geq$ 3% and $\leq$ 55%, tumor >2 cm, symptomatic tumor, or positive LN) (ClinicalTrials.gov Identifier: NCT05040360). The primary endpoint is PFS, and the secondary endpoints are OS and the safety and tolerability of the CAPTEM regimen compared with observation alone. There is also an actively enrolling phase 1 pilot study of perioperative PRRT in patients with metastatic GEP-NET who are candidates for surgical cytoreduction (ClinicalTrials.gov Identifier: NCT04609592). The primary objective of this trial was to evaluate the safety and feasibility of the combination of perioperative PRRT and surgical cytoreduction, and secondary outcomes measures will assess response rates, recurrence-free survival, and OS of the overall treatment strategy. The results of these and other trials are anxiously awaited and will ultimately help to inform future multimodal treatment strategies for patients with NET.

CLINICS CARE POINTS

- Resection of small-bowel neuroendocrine tumors (SBNETs) requires manual palpation of the small bowel to detect small, multifocal lesions. If minimally invasive surgery techniques are employed, a hand-assist port or small incision to eviscerate the small bowel for inspection should be considered.

- Most pancreatic neuroendocrine tumors (PNETs) require anatomic resection; however, for small (<2 cm), nonfunctional-PNETs or insulinomas, parenchymal sparing approaches with or without lymphadenectomy may be considered in appropriately selected patients.

- Regional lymphadenectomy should be performed for most neuroendocrine tumors at the time of surgery due to the increasing incidence of lymph node (LN) metastases with increasing tumor size and the prognostic value of positive LNs.

- Primary tumor resection should be considered in patients with metastatic SBNETs to alleviate symptoms, minimize future symptoms or complications, and improve both progression-free survival (PFS) and overall survival.

- Hepatic cytoreduction should be done if >70% of hepatic disease burden can be treated to improve both symptoms and survival.

- For patients with advanced, unresectable, or metastatic disease, there is a robust body of data that supports the use of somatostatin analogs, peptide receptor radionuclide therapy, and targeted therapy to improve PFS.

DISCLOSURE

The authors have nothing to disclose.

REFERENCES

1. Dasari A, Shen D, Halperin B, et al. Trends in the incidence, prevalence, and survival outcomes in patients with neuroendocrine tumors in the united states. JAMA Oncol 2017;3(10):1335–42.

2. Frilling A, Modlin IM, Kidd M, et al. Recommendations for management of patients with neuroendocrine liver metastases. Lancet Oncol 2014;15(1):e8–21.

3. Pavel M, Baudin E, Couvelard A, et al. ENETS Consensus Guidelines for the management of patients with liver and other distant metastases from neuroendocrine neoplasms of foregut, midgut, hindgut, and unknown primary. Neuroendocrinology 2012;95(2):157–76.

4. Bilimoria KY, Bentrem DJ, Wayne JD, et al. Small bowel cancer in the United States: changes in epidemiology, treatment, and survival over the last 20 years. Ann Surg 2009;249(1):63–71.

5. Keck KJ, Maxwell JE, Utria AF, et al. The distal predilection of small bowel neuroendocrine tumors. Ann Surg Oncol 2018;25(11):3207–13.

6. Kuiper DH, Gracie WA Jr, Pollard HM. Twenty years of gastrointestinal carcinoids. Cancer 1970;25(6):1424–30.

7. Howe JR, Cardona K, Fraker DL, et al. The surgical management of small bowel neuroendocrine tumors: consensus guidelines of the north american neuroendocrine tumor society. Pancreas 2017;46(6):715–31.

8. Niederle B, Pape UF, Costa F, et al. ENETS consensus guidelines update for neuroendocrine neoplasms of the jejunum and ileum. Neuroendocrinology 2016;103(2):125–38.

9. Tierney JF, Chivukula SV, Wang X, et al. Resection of primary tumor may prolong survival in metastatic gastroenteropancreatic neuroendocrine tumors. Surgery 2019;165(3):644–51.

10. Mayo SC, de Jong MC, Pulitatno C, et al. Surgical management of hepatic neuro-endocrine tumor metastasis: results from an international multi-institutional analysis. Ann Surg Oncol 2010;17(12):3129–36.

11. Givi B, Pommier SJ, Thompson AK, et al. Operative resection of primary carcinoid neoplasms in patients with liver metastases yields significantly better survival. Surgery 2006;140(6):891–7 [discussion: 897-8].

12. Sarmiento JM, Heywood G, Rubin J, et al. Surgical treatment of neuroendocrine metastases to the liver: a plea for resection to increase survival. J Am Coll Surg 2003;197(1):29–37.

13. Chambers AJ, Pasieka JL, Dixon E, et al. The palliative benefit of aggressive sur-gical intervention for both hepatic and mesenteric metastases from neuroendo-crine tumors. Surgery 2008;144(4):645–51 [discussion: 651-3].

14. Bennett S, Coburn N, Law C, et al. Upfront small bowel resection for small bowel neuroendocrine tumors with synchronous metastases: a propensity-score matched comparative population-based analysis. Ann Surg 2020. Online ahead of print.

15. Gangi A, Manguso N, Gong J, et al. Midgut neuroendocrine tumors with liver-only metastases: benefit of primary tumor resection. Ann Surg Oncol 2020;27(11): 4525–32.

16. Ahmed A, Turner G, King B, et al. Midgut neuroendocrine tumours with liver me-tastases: results of the UKINETS study. Endocr Relat Cancer 2009;16(3):885–94.

17. Wang SC, Parekh JR, Zuraek MB, et al. Identification of unknown primary tumors in patients with neuroendocrine liver metastases. Arch Surg 2010;145(3):276–80.

18. Kasai Y, Mahuron K, Hirose K, et al. A novel stratification of mesenteric mass involvement as a predictor of challenging mesenteric lymph node dissection by minimally invasive approach for ileal neuroendocrine tumors. J Surg Oncol 2020;122(2):204–11.

19. Ohrvall U, Eriksson B, Juhlin C, et al. Method for dissection of mesenteric metas-tases in mid-gut carcinoid tumors. World J Surg 2000;24(11):1402–8.

20. Tran CG, Sherman SK, Howe JR. Small bowel neuroendocrine tumors. Curr Probl Surg 2020;57(12):100823.

21. Landry CS, Lin HY, Phan A, et al. Resection of at-risk mesenteric lymph nodes is associated with improved survival in patients with small bowel neuroendocrine tu-mors. World J Surg 2013;37(7):1695–700.

22. Daskalakis K, Karakatsanis A, Hessman O, et al. Association of a prophylactic surgical approach to stage iv small intestinal neuroendocrine tumors with sur-vival. JAMA Oncol 2018;4(2):183–9.

23. Hallet J, Law C, Commonwealth S. Neuroendocrine tumours research collabora-tive surgical, role of primary tumor resection for metastatic small bowel neuroen-docrine tumors. World J Surg 2021;45(1):213–8.

24. Poultsides GA, Huang LC, Chen Y, et al. Pancreatic neuroendocrine tumors: radiographic calcifications correlate with grade and metastasis. Ann Surg Oncol 2012;19(7):2295–303.

25. Dong DH, Zhang XF, Poultisides G, et al. Impact of tumor size and nodal status on recurrence of nonfunctional pancreatic neuroendocrine tumors </=2 cm after curative resection: A multi-institutional study of 392 cases. J Surg Oncol 2019; 120(7):1071–9.

26. Cherenfant J, Stocker SJ, Gage MK, et al. Predicting aggressive behavior in nonfunctioning pancreatic neuroendocrine tumors. Surgery 2013;154(4):785–91 [discussion: 791-3].

27. Sadot E, Reidy-Lagunes L, Tang LH, et al. Observation versus resection for small asymptomatic pancreatic neuroendocrine tumors: a matched case-control study. Ann Surg Oncol 2016;23(4):1361–70.

28. Gaujoux S, Partelli S, Maire F, et al. Observational study of natural history of small sporadic nonfunctioning pancreatic neuroendocrine tumors. J Clin Endocrinol Metab 2013;98(12):4784–9.

29. Lee LC, Grant CS, Salomao DR, et al. Small, nonfunctioning, asymptomatic pancreatic neuroendocrine tumors (PNETs): role for nonoperative management. Surgery 2012;152(6):965–74.

30. Kurita Y, Hara K, Kuwahara T, et al. Comparison of prognosis between observation and surgical resection groups with small sporadic non-functional pancreatic neuroendocrine neoplasms without distant metastasis. J Gastroenterol 2020; 55(5):543–52.

31. Barenboim A, Lahat G, Nachmany I, et al. Resection versus observation of small asymptomatic nonfunctioning pancreatic neuroendocrine tumors. J Gastrointest Surg 2020;24(6):1366–74.

32. Rosenberg AM, Friedmann P, Del Rivero J, et al. Resection versus expectant management of small incidentally discovered nonfunctional pancreatic neuroendocrine tumors. Surgery 2016;159(1):302–9.

33. Regenet N, Carrere N, Boulanger G, et al. Is the 2-cm size cutoff relevant for small nonfunctioning pancreatic neuroendocrine tumors: a French multicenter study. Surgery 2016;159(3):901–7.

34. Zaidi MY, Lopez-Aguiar AG, Switchenko JM, et al. A novel validated recurrence risk score to guide a pragmatic surveillance strategy after resection of pancreatic neuroendocrine tumors: an international study of 1006 patients. Ann Surg 2019; 270(3):422–33.

35. Howe JR, Merchant NB, Conrad C, et al. The north american neuroendocrine tumor society consensus paper on the surgical management of pancreatic neuroendocrine tumors. Pancreas 2020;49(1):1–33.

36. Falconi M, Erikkson B, Kaltsas G, et al. ENETS consensus guidelines update for the management of patients with functional pancreatic neuroendocrine tumors and non-functional pancreatic neuroendocrine tumors. Neuroendocrinology 2016;103(2):153–71.

37. Falconi M, Bartsch DK, Erikkson B, et al. ENETS Consensus Guidelines for the management of patients with digestive neuroendocrine neoplasms of the digestive system: well-differentiated pancreatic non-functioning tumors. Neuroendocrinology 2012;95(2):120–34.

38. Mansour JC, Chavin K, Morris-Stiff G, et al. Management of asymptomatic, well-differentiated PNETs: results of the Delphi consensus process of the Americas Hepato-Pancreato-Biliary Association. HPB (Oxford) 2019;21(5):515–23.

39. NCCN Clinical Practice Guidelines in Oncology (NCCN Guidelines®) for Guideline Name V.X.202X. © National Comprehensive Cancer Network, Inc. 202X. NCCN.org. Accessed April 1, 2022.

40. Tanaka M, Heckler M, Mihaljevic AL, et al. Systematic review and metaanalysis of lymph node metastases of resected pancreatic neuroendocrine tumors. Ann Surg Oncol 2021;28(3):1614–24.

41. Mao R, Zhao H, Li K, et al. Outcomes of lymph node dissection for non-metastatic pancreatic neuroendocrine tumors: a propensity score-weighted analysis of the National Cancer Database. Ann Surg Oncol 2019;26(9):2722–9.

42. Conrad C, Kutlu OC, Dasari A, et al. Prognostic value of lymph node status and extent of lymphadenectomy in pancreatic neuroendocrine tumors confined to and extending beyond the pancreas. J Gastrointest Surg 2016;20(12):1966–74.

43. Lopez-Aguiar AG, Ethun CG, Zaidi MY, et al. The conundrum of < 2-cm pancreatic neuroendocrine tumors: a preoperative risk score to predict lymph node metastases and guide surgical management. Surgery 2019;166(1):15–21.

44. Mehrabi A, Fischer L, Hafezi M, et al. A systematic review of localization, surgical treatment options, and outcome of insulinoma. Pancreas 2014;43(5):675–86.

45. Partelli S, Cirocchi R, Crippa S, et al. Systematic review of active surveillance versus surgical management of asymptomatic small non-functioning pancreatic neuroendocrine neoplasms. Br J Surg 2017;104(1):34–41.

46. Sadowski SM, Pieterman CRC, Perrier ND, et al. Prognostic factors for the outcome of nonfunctioning pancreatic neuroendocrine tumors in MEN1: a systematic review of literature. Endocr Relat Cancer 2020;27(6):R145–61.

47. de Rooij T, van Hilst J, van Santvoort H, et al. Minimally invasive versus open distal pancreatectomy (LEOPARD): a multicenter patient-blinded randomized controlled trial. Ann Surg 2019;269(1):2–9.

48. van Hilst J, de Rooij T, Bosscha K, et al. Laparoscopic versus open pancreatoduodenectomy for pancreatic or periampullary tumours (LEOPARD-2): a multicentre, patient-blinded, randomised controlled phase 2/3 trial. Lancet Gastroenterol Hepatol 2019;4(3):199–207.

49. Boone BA, Zenati M, Hogg ME, et al. Assessment of quality outcomes for robotic pancreaticoduodenectomy: identification of the learning curve. JAMA Surg 2015;150(5):416–22.

50. Ricci C, Casadei R, Taffurelli G, et al. Minimally Invasive Pancreaticoduodenectomy: What is the Best "Choice"? A Systematic Review and Network Meta-analysis of Non-randomized Comparative Studies. World J Surg 2018;42(3):788–805.

51. Huttner FJ, Koessler-Ebbs J, Hackert T, et al. Meta-analysis of surgical outcome after enucleation versus standard resection for pancreatic neoplasms. Br J Surg 2015;102(9):1026–36.

52. Dragomir MP, Sabo AA, Petrescu GED, et al. Central pancreatectomy: a comprehensive, up-to-date meta-analysis. Langenbecks Arch Surg 2019;404(8):945–58.

53. Dalla Valle R, Cremaschi E, Lamecchi L, et al. Open and minimally invasive pancreatic neoplasms enucleation: a systematic review. Surg Endosc 2019;33(10):3192–9.

54. Wakabayashi T, Felli E, Cherkaoui Z, et al. Robotic Central Pancreatectomy for Well-Differentiated Neuroendocrine Tumor: Parenchymal-Sparing Procedure. Ann Surg Oncol 2019;26(7):2121.

55. Keutgen XM, Nilubol N, Glanville J, et al. Resection of primary tumor site is associated with prolonged survival in metastatic nonfunctioning pancreatic neuroendocrine tumors. Surgery 2016;159(1):311–8.

56. Dasari A, Mehta K, Byers LA, et al. Comparative study of lung and extrapulmonary poorly differentiated neuroendocrine carcinomas: A SEER database analysis of 162,983 cases. Cancer 2018;124(4):807–15.

57. Patel SP, Othus M, Chae YK, et al. A Phase II Basket Trial of Dual Anti-CTLA-4 and Anti-PD-1 Blockade in Rare Tumors (DART SWOG 1609) in Patients with Nonpancreatic Neuroendocrine Tumors. Clin Cancer Res 2020;26(10):2290–6.

58. Bagante F, Spolverato G, Merath K, et al. Neuroendocrine liver metastasis: The chance to be cured after liver surgery. J Surg Oncol 2017;115(6):687–95.

59. Graff-Baker AN, Sauer DA, Pommier SJ, et al. Expanded criteria for carcinoid liver debulking: maintaining survival and increasing the number of eligible patients. Surgery 2014;156(6):1369–76 [discussion: 1376-7].

60. Panzuto F, Boninsegna L, Fazio N, et al. Metastatic and locally advanced pancreatic endocrine carcinomas: analysis of factors associated with disease progression. J Clin Oncol 2011;29(17):2372–7.

61. Scott AT, Breheny PJ, Keck KJ, et al. Effective cytoreduction can be achieved in patients with numerous neuroendocrine tumor liver metastases (NETLMs). Surgery 2019;165(1):166–75.

62. Gangi A, Howe JR. The Landmark Series: Neuroendocrine Tumor Liver Metastases. Ann Surg Oncol 2020;27(9):3270–80.

63. Morgan RE, Pommier SJ, Pommier RF. Expanded criteria for debulking of liver metastasis also apply to pancreatic neuroendocrine tumors. Surgery 2018; 163(1):218–25.

64. Chen JX, Wileyto EP, Soulen MC. Randomized Embolization Trial for NeuroEndocrine Tumor Metastases to the Liver (RETNET): study protocol for a randomized controlled trial. Trials 2018;19(1):390.

65. Mayo SC, de Jong MC, Bloomston M, et al. Surgery versus intra-arterial therapy for neuroendocrine liver metastasis: a multicenter international analysis. Ann Surg Oncol 2011;18(13):3657–65.

66. Yao JC, Fazio N, Singh S, et al. Everolimus for the Treatment of Advanced Pancreatic Neuroendocrine Tumors: Overall Survival and Circulating Biomarkers From the Randomized, Phase III RADIANT-3 Study. J Clin Oncol 2016;34(32):3906–13.

67. Caplin ME, Pavel M, Cwikla A, et al. Lanreotide in metastatic enteropancreatic neuroendocrine tumors. N Engl J Med 2014;371(3):224–33.

68. Strosberg J, El-Haddad G, Wolin E, et al. Phase 3 Trial of (177)Lu-Dotatate for Midgut Neuroendocrine Tumors. N Engl J Med 2017;376(2):125–35.

69. Rinke A, Wittenberg M, Schade-Brittinger C, et al. Placebo-Controlled, Double-Blind, Prospective, Randomized Study on the Effect of Octreotide LAR in the Control of Tumor Growth in Patients with Metastatic Neuroendocrine Midgut Tumors (PROMID): Results of Long-Term Survival. Neuroendocrinology 2017;104(1): 26–32.

70. Kaderli RM, Spanjol M, Kollar A, et al. Therapeutic options for neuroendocrine tumors: a systematic review and network meta-analysis. JAMA Oncol 2019;5(4): 480–9.

71. Rinke A, Muller HH, Schade-Brittinger C, et al. Placebo-controlled, double-blind, prospective, randomized study on the effect of octreotide LAR in the control of tumor growth in patients with metastatic neuroendocrine midgut tumors: a report from the PROMID Study Group. J Clin Oncol 2009;27(28):4656–63.

72. Yao JC, Fazio N, Singh S, et al. Everolimus for the treatment of advanced, nonfunctional neuroendocrine tumours of the lung or gastrointestinal tract (RADIANT-4): a randomised, placebo-controlled, phase 3 study. Lancet 2016; 387(10022):968–77.

73. Raymond E, Dahan L, Raoul JL, et al. Sunitinib malate for the treatment of pancreatic neuroendocrine tumors. N Engl J Med 2011;364(6):501–13.

74. Kunz PL, Catalano PJ, Nimeiri H, et al. A randomized study of temozolomide or temozolomide and capecitabine in patients with advanced pancreatic neuroendocrine tumors: A trial of the ECOG-ACRIN Cancer Research Group (E2211). J Clin Oncol 2018;36(15_suppl):4004.

Advances in Endocrine Surgery

Michael S. Lui, MD, Aditya S. Shirali, MD, Bernice L. Huang, MD,
Sarah B. Fisher, MD[1], Nancy D. Perrier, MD[1],*

KEYWORDS

- Papillary thyroid cancer • Thyroid lobectomy • Lymph node dissection
- Hyperparathyroidism • Parathyroid carcinoma • Adrenocortical carcinoma
- Pheochromocytoma • Cushing's syndrome

KEY POINTS

- Well-selected patients with low-risk papillary thyroid carcinoma can be adequately treated with thyroid lobectomy. Identification of available radiologic, pathologic, and molecular risk factors can help identify those at higher risk of disease recurrence who are better served with total thyroidectomy.
- Prophylactic central lymph node dissection for patients with papillary thyroid carcinoma should not be routinely performed but should be considered for selected patients with large primary tumors considered to be at risk for clinically significant occult nodal disease.
- Advancements in multiple imaging modalities and localization adjuncts have allowed for more directed surgical approaches in the management of primary hyperparathyroidism.
- Management of localized parathyroid carcinoma involves parathyroidectomy with en bloc resection of directly involved tissue, whereas the management of locally advanced or distantly metastatic parathyroid carcinoma requires multidisciplinary care including well-selected surgical resection, antiresorptive therapies, and calcimimetics to control hypercalcemia, with immunotherapy and/or targeted therapy showing promise as potential therapeutics.
- A minimally invasive approach to adrenalectomy should be considered for benign and/or functional adrenal tumors, whereas an open approach is preferred when there is a concern for potential primary malignancy.

ADVANCES IN THE MANAGEMENT OF PAPILLARY THYROID CARCINOMA

Introduction

Differentiated thyroid cancer (DTC) is the most common endocrine malignancy with an estimated incidence of 43,800 people in the United States alone in 2022 (**Table 1**).[1] Survival is favorable, with 5-year survival greater than 98%.[2] Thyroid cancer

Department of Surgical Oncology, The University of Texas MD Anderson Cancer Center, 1515 Holcombe Boulevard, Houston, TX 77030, USA
[1] Co-senior authorship.
* Corresponding author. Unit 1484, 1515 Holcombe Boulevard, Houston, TX 77030.
E-mail address: Nperrier@mdanderson.org

Surg Oncol Clin N Am 32 (2023) 199–220
https://doi.org/10.1016/j.soc.2022.08.004
1055-3207/23/© 2022 Elsevier Inc. All rights reserved.

Table 1
Summary of 5 randomized control trials looking at outcomes of thyroid surgery with prophylactic central lymph node dissection for patients with papillary thyroid cancer without preoperative evidence of nodal disease (cN0)

Authors, Year	Randomized Groups	n	Ages	Primary Tumor Size (cm)[c]	Follow-up (months)	Nodal Disease (n,%)	Recurrence (n)	Endpoint Outcomes	Complications
Lee et al,[44] (2015)	TT	104	51.6	1.6	49.2	n/a	4	No mortality in either group	TT/pCLND had higher transient hypocalcemia (36.6% vs 20.3%, $P = 0.043$)
	TT/pCLND	153	52.3	1.7	55.2	35 (22.8%)	5	*Recurrence Rate ($P = .780$)* TT: 3.9% ‖ TT/pCLND: 3.3%	No difference in transient/ permanent vocal cord paralysis and postoperative bleeding ($P = NS$)
Viola et al,[45] (2015)	TT	88	41	1.6		6 (6.8%)	7	*Persistent/Recurrence ($P = 0.9$)* TT: 8.0% ‖ TT/pCLND: 7.5%	TT/pCLND had higher permanent hypoparathyroidism (19.4% vs 8%, $P = 0.02$)
	TT/pCLND	93	45.5	1.6	60 (median)	43 (46.2%)	7		No difference in recurrent laryngeal nerve palsy ($P = NS$)
[a]Kim et al,[46] (2020)	Lobectomy	82	47.9	0.6	72.6	n/a	1	*Recurrence Rate ($P > 0.99$)* Lobectomy: 1.2% Lobectomy/pCLND:3.6	No difference in vocal cord paralysis (1.2% vs 0%, $P = 0.49$)
	Lobectomy pCLND	82	48.5	0.68	74.2	41 (50%)	3	No difference in recurrence free survival ($P = .929$)	No patients developed hypocalcemia. No reported mortality
[b]Sippel et al,[47] (2020)	TT	30	46.1	2.45	12	10%	1	1 y Tg < 0.2 ($P = 1.00$) TT: 88.9%, ‖ TT/pCLND 90.0%	No difference in hypoparathyroidism or recurrent laryngeal nerve paralysis at 2-wk and 6-mo after surgery ($P = NS$)
	TT/pCLND	30	50.1	1.91	12	27.6%	1	*1 y negative-US ($P = 0.7$)* TT: 85.7% ‖ TT/pCLND: 85.1% *Indeterminate US/Tg data ($P = 0.70$)* TT: 10.7% ‖ TT/pCLND 14.8%	No difference in QOL based on the thyroid cancer-specific QOL measures between groups

| Ahn et al,[48] (2022) | TT | 50 | 51.8 | 1.1 | 46.3 | 3 (6%) | 1 | No patients developed structural recurrence | No difference in hypoparathyroidism or recurrent laryngeal nerve paralysis after surgery (P = NS). |
| | TT/pCLND | 51 | 53.6 | 1.0 | 46.8 | 14 (27.5%) | 1 | No difference local recurrence rates (2% vs 2%, P = 0.945) | All postoperative symptoms resolved at 6-mo follow-up |

Abbreviations: ATA, American Thyroid Association; *pCLND*, prophylactic central lymph node dissection; *US*, ultrasound; *TT*, total thyroidectomy; *Tg*, thyroglobulin, QOL, quality of life

[a] Kim et al looked at patients with microcarcinomas with an intention to treat protocol.

[b] Sippel et al categorized oncologic outcomes at 1 year based on 2016 ATA definition for *Response to Initial Therapy*.[20]

[c] Tumor sizes recorded as mean unless otherwise labeled.

management focuses on 3 strategies: (1) surgical resection, (2) radioactive iodine ablation (RAI), and (3) thyroid-stimulating hormone suppression. Total thyroidectomy (TT) was traditionally the recommended surgical approach for all patients with DTC greater than 1 cm as it removes disease, facilitates adjuvant therapy with RAI, and allows for thyroglobulin monitoring for long-term surveillance. More recently, this paradigm has shifted as studies have shown similar survival and recurrence rates for patients with low-risk cancers undergoing lobectomy alone. Thyroid lobectomy, when oncologically appropriate, preserves native thyroid hormone function and further reduces already low risks of complications.[3] The following sections will discuss the studies that have shaped current guidelines in the surgical management of papillary thyroid cancer (PTC).

Extent of Surgical Intervention for Papillary Thyroid Cancer

Survival and recurrence data stratified by operative extent

Staging for DTC is unique in that while it incorporates the traditional tumor-node-metastasis classification, it also incorporates age, with all patients aged younger than 55 years classified as stage I unless distant metastases are present (and then classified as stage II).[4] Although recent modifications to the eighth edition better risk stratify patients than previous editions,[5] additional meaningful prognostic factors described in prognostic scoring systems (ie, MACIS: metastasis, age, completeness of resection, invasion, size) may better predict cancer-specific survival,[6,7] and allow stratification into "low-risk" and "high-risk" categories.[8–10] Early studies using risk-stratification scoring systems suggested that in patients with low-risk disease, TT did not improve disease-specific survival (DSS) over lobectomy.[11,12] In 2007, Bilimoria and colleagues[13] published a large retrospective study using the National Cancer Database (NCDB), which showed that patients who underwent TT for tumors greater than 1 cm had higher 10-year overall survival (OS), and lower recurrence rates than those that had lobectomy. This robust study was the cornerstone of the 2009 American Thyroid Association (ATA) recommendation for TT for tumors greater than 1 cm.[14] However, others point out that other important prognostic factors such as extrathyroidal extension (ETE), patient comorbidities, and multifocality were not included into the analysis. Follow-up studies using the Surveillance, Epidemiology, and End Results (SEER) database stratified patients by tumor size (in 1 cm increments) and found, after controlling for confounding variables, no difference in OS or DSS when comparing TT to lobectomy.[15,16] This was further confirmed by the now largest study combining both NCDB and SEER data which showed no significant difference in OS between TT and lobectomy when adjusting for patient-specific and tumor-specific factors, highlighting the importance of appropriate patient selection.[17–19] In light of these findings, the current ATA guidelines now recognize that lobectomy is sufficient for well-selected patients with cancers less than 4 cm in size without clinical evidence of nodal metastasis or adverse histopathologic factors (multifocality, ETE, tall cell/columnar/hobnail variants, BRAF p.V600 E mutation), provided they have no family history of thyroid cancer or personal history of excess exposure to radiation.[20] It is important to note that while molecular testing on fine needle aspiration specimens can sometimes preoperatively identify mutations (ie, *BRAF* and *TERT*), the role of mutational status in guiding extent of surgical therapy remains unclear (see "Role of Molecular Testing" section). The decision between lobectomy and TT should incorporate all available objective data as well as patient values and preferences to allow for individualized management.

Role of Molecular Testing

The BRAF p.V600 E mutation is identified in up to 70% of PTC[21] and is associated with more aggressive disease biology with increased rates of ETE,[21] lymph node metastasis,[21,22] distant metastasis,[22] and recurrence.[21,23] However, establishing a direct relationship between *BRAF*-mutation status and survival remains challenging because it requires prohibitively long prospective studies because OS in these patients remains high compared with other malignancies.[20,22,24] It is likely that *BRAF*-mutation status, in combination with other clinicopathologic factors informs risk stratification, and further research is necessary to evaluate the optimal combination of risk factors that should guide decisions regarding the extent of surgery.

Recently, the *TERT* promoter mutation has been identified as a marker in predicting clinically aggressive behavior in PTC and has been associated with worse disease-free survival (odds ratio 4.68, 95% confidence interval 1.54–14.27).[25] Xing and colleagues[26] showed that individuals with a *TERT* mutation in conjunction with a *BRAF*-mutation had higher recurrence rates (68.6% vs 8.7%, $P < .001$) compared with those that had neither mutation. The ATA has incorporated *BRAF*-mutation and *TERT*-mutation status into their risk stratification system with either conferring a higher risk for recurrence.[20]

Molecular testing is designed to identify mutations in cytologically indeterminate thyroid nodules, with the goal of selecting those nodules at higher risk of malignancy and thus decreasing the number diagnostic lobectomies for ultimately benign pathologic condition. Two common tests, an RNA-based gene analyzer[27] and a DNA-based and RNA-based next generation sequencing[28] were found to have sensitivities of 92% and 70% to 96%, and specificities of 52% and 77% to 92%, respectively.[29] A recent randomized control trial (RCT) comparing these tests found no statistical difference between the modalities with both having 97% to 100% sensitivities and 80% to 85% specificities.[29] Although molecular testing may be helpful in risk stratifying patients with indeterminate cytology, the role of molecular testing in deciding the extent of surgery for known malignancy continues to be an area of research. Routine testing of patients with early stage/resectable thyroid cancers remains controversial and is not universally adopted or recommended in the setting of a clear indication for thyroidectomy.[20] Future studies evaluating the impact of molecular profiling of thyroid cancer on surgical decision-making are needed.

Active Surveillance

Active surveillance (AS) as a management strategy for papillary thyroid microcarcinoma (typically tumor size <1 cm) was first proposed by Ito and colleagues[30] in 2003 in which patients without unfavorable features (tumors adjacent to the trachea, tumors potentially invading the recurrent laryngeal nerve, lymph node suggestive of metastasis) were surveilled regularly for signs of progression rather than treated surgically. At 5-year and 10-year follow-up, 6.4% and 15.9% of patients demonstrated tumor enlargement, respectively, defined as growth of at least 3 mm, whereas 1.4% and 3.4% of patients developed nodal metastases, respectively.[31] In addition, there were no cases of recurrence or mortality in patients that were later selected for surgery, suggesting the ability to salvage patients who progressed without an impact on DSS. Brito and Ito and colleagues[32] developed a risk-stratification system incorporating patient, tumor, and medical team factors to best identify the ideal candidate for AS. Although the 2015 ATA guidelines acknowledge that AS may have a role in low-risk, well-selected patients with PTC, this management strategy requires appropriate counseling, patient motivation and compliance, and an experienced multidisciplinary team.[20]

Impact of Patient Preferences

Survivorship for patients with well DTC is excellent, yet many report an impaired quality of life similar to that of other cancer survivors.[33,34] The decision between lobectomy and TT, when such a choice is oncologically appropriate, should incorporate individual patient preference and relative value placed on preserving native thyroid hormone function versus concern for recurrence. For example, one recent study examined psychological factors influencing patient decision-making regarding surveillance or completion thyroidectomy after lobectomy for low-risk DTC. Fear of taking lifelong thyroid hormone supplementation most frequently swayed patients to choose surveillance, whereas fear of disease progression was associated with preference for completion surgery.[35] Thyroid hormone supplementation may still be required after lobectomy, and this possibility should be clearly communicated preoperatively and factored in to decision-making to avoid a negative impact on the physician–patient relationship. Pairing patient preferences and priorities with appropriate therapy when oncologically reasonable is essential for developing a personalized management plan.

Lymph Node Dissection for Papillary Thyroid Cancer

Therapeutic compartmental lymph node dissection is appropriate for patients with clinically evident lymph node metastases (LNM). The management of clinically negative regional lymph nodes within the central neck is more controversial, with rates of occult LNM ranging from 20% to 90% depending on the extent of dissection performed.[20,36,37] Current ATA recommendations support consideration of a prophylactic central LN dissection (pCLND) in patients with advanced primary tumors (T3/T4) or in patients with clinically involved lateral neck lymph nodes.[20] Proponents of pCLND cite better disease clearance, lower postoperative thyroglobulin levels,[38] potential decrease of local recurrence rates,[39] and no increased risk of permanent morbidity in expert hands.[40] In contrast, the identification of occult micro-LNM found during pCLND no longer upstages patients in the eighth edition American Joint Committee on Cancer guidelines,[41] and others argue that there is no conclusive evidence that pCLND improves long-term outcomes,[42] with several studies demonstrating higher morbidity.[39,43]

To date, there are 5 RCTs published studying the impact of pCLND on locoregional recurrence (LRR) and complication rates in patients with low-risk PTC.[44–48] Four of these studies included patients who had low-risk PTCs originally scheduled for TT,[44,45,47,48] whereas Kim and colleagues[46] focused on patients with papillary thyroid microcarcinoma undergoing lobectomy. Most of these studies had extended median follow-up of 5 years with average primary tumor sizes less than 2 cm. Sippel and colleagues[47] reported a follow-up time of 12 months as their study was specifically powered to look at short-term predictors of recurrence. The incidence of occult LNM ranged from 23% to 43%. No study found differences in LRR rates although there was heterogeneity in indications for and application of adjuvant RAI. No study identified any difference in recurrent laryngeal nerve palsy rates. Two of the studies found that patients who had pCLND had higher transient (36.6% vs 20.3%)[44] and permanent hypoparathyroidism (19.4% vs 8.0%).[45] A recent meta-analysis of these 5 RCTs calculated that the number of patients needed to treat with pCLND was 500, whereas the number of patients needed to harm was 33.[49] In patients undergoing lobectomy, concomitant pCLND may place the recurrent laryngeal nerve at risk of injury while doing little to prevent recurrence as structural recurrence is frequently seen on the contralateral lobe.[50] The decision for pCLND with concomitant TT should be a shared decision after balancing clinical risk factors and patients' preferences.

ADVANCES IN THE MANAGEMENT OF PARATHYROID DISEASE
Introduction

The management of parathyroid disease has evolved during the past decade with emerging technologies to guide surgical decision-making and changes in treatment of advanced malignancy. In 2016, the American Association of Endocrine Surgeons published guidelines for the diagnosis, management, and surveillance of primary hyperparathyroidism (PHPT) based on years of available evidence.[51] Since then, advancements in radiographic studies, our understanding of parathyroid biology, and molecular profiling have moved the management of parathyroid disease forward.

Preoperative Localization Strategies

Preoperative radiographic studies for parathyroid localization commonly include ultrasonography (US), parathyroid scintigraphy using technetium (^{99}Tc) sestamibi-single photon emission computed tomography/computed tomography (sestamibi-SPECT/CT), and four-dimensional computed tomography (4D-CT; **Fig. 1**). Minimally invasive parathyroidectomy (MIP) requires localization of a single abnormal gland on at least one imaging modality, with accuracy increasing with multiple concordant studies.[52,53] Sestamibi-SPECT/CT and US individually have a sensitivity of between 72% and 79% with false-positive results frequently related to benign or malignant thyroid pathologic condition or lymphadenopathy.[54] Four-dimensional CT is up to 97% accurate for lateralization of single gland disease and up to 87% accurate for quadrant localization.[55] When 4D-CT was combined with sestamibi-SPECT/CT, quadrant localization increased to 94% and was superior to sestamibi-SPECT/CT alone.[55] Despite accuracy in localization with 4D-CT, this study has been only slowly adopted by surgeons throughout the United States. In a study of more than 7000 patients at 14 different

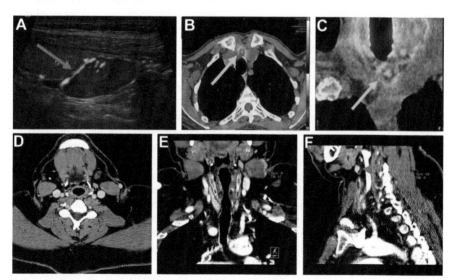

Fig. 1. (*A*) Ultrasonography of a suspected hyperfunctioning parathyroid gland with a polar feeding vessel (*blue arrow*). (*B, C*) Technetium sestamibi-SPECT/CT fused axial (*B*) and coronal (*C*) showing persistent activity within the right suprasternal region (*yellow arrow*) and activity within the left thyroid. (*D–F*) Four-dimensional computed tomography of an undescended left superior parathyroid gland seen in axial (*D*), coronal (*E*), and sagittal (*F*) images showing a suspected left superior parathyroid gland inferior and medial to the left submandibular gland in an undescended position (*red arrowhead*).

institutions, Kuo and colleagues[56] found that 4D-CT was used in only 20.4% of patients with institutional rates of use ranging from 0.1% to 88.7% despite previous studies demonstrating the association of 4D-CT with increased utilization of MIP and decreased length of stay.[57] Cost–utility analysis of preoperative localization strategies for PHPT found that while institutional differences in localization sensitivity exist, analyses have pointed to the selective utility of 4D-CT as being the most cost-effective strategy in parathyroidectomy due to decreased rates of bilateral cervical exploration.[58,59]

Imaging with ^{11}C-labeled and ^{18}F-labeled choline analogs and PET/CT, although limited to a few centers in the United States, has shown promise in parathyroid adenoma localization with high sensitivity (89%) and specificity (96%),[60] with particular utility in the reoperative setting. Latge and colleagues[61] showed 95% sensitivity and 88% detection rate for ^{18}F-fluorocholine PET/CT compared with 4D-CT in patients with persistent or recurrent PHPT with no increase in detection after combining the 2 modalities. Although significant advancements in imaging modalities have been made in the detection of parathyroid disease, the most important aspect of preoperative imaging is that the surgeon understands the institution-specific strengths and weaknesses of each technique.

Intraoperative Adjuncts

During parathyroidectomy most surgeons use intraoperative adjuncts to localize a suspicious hyperfunctioning gland, confirm the histology of a resected parathyroid specimen, and/or confirm operative completion. The most commonly used adjunct is the use of intraoperative parathyroid hormone assay (ioPTH), which relies on the rapid rate of decay of PTH to quantitatively detect a decline following excision of a suspected hyperfunctioning parathyroid gland. The most common ioPTH protocols anticipate a greater than 50% PTH drop at 10 minutes from either the highest preincision or preexcision (before the parathyroid vascular pedicle is ligated) ioPTH level in a peripheral blood sample to conclude parathyroidectomy; and some also require the final PTH to decrease to the normal range. Both criteria have a positive predictive value of 97% for postoperative eucalcemia and cure rates of 97% to 99%.[62] Yet the ioPTH process requires laboratory expertise and equipment and may add variable operative time. Recently, some groups have advocated for MIP without ioPTH guidance, particularly *in well-selected cases with suspected single gland disease* with at least 2, but especially 3, concordant imaging studies. The combination of a functional isotope study (sestamibi) combined with anatomic cross-sectional study with perfusion (4D-CT) and sonographic evaluation of surrounding structures (US) is particularly sensitive. A recent single-institution study of more than 2400 parathyroidectomies performed without ioPTH compared bilateral cervical exploration with MIP, indicated for suspected single-gland disease with concordant imaging, and found similar combined persistence and recurrence rates of 2.2% on intention-to-treat analysis.[63] Although few studies exist comparing MIP with and without ioPTH, it is clear that successful MIP hinges on a combination of high-quality preoperative localization studies, intraoperative findings, and surgeon experience.

Due to variability in the location and appearance of parathyroid glands, adjuncts may be used to confirm in vivo localization and ex vivo tissue confirmation apart from intraoperative frozen section or parathyroid aspiration. The discovery of parathyroid glands exhibiting strong autofluorescence under near-infrared light has led to the use of near-infrared autofluorescence (NIRAF) for intraoperative identification of parathyroid glands using 2 Food and Drug Administration-approved products: PTeye (probe-based; AiBiomed, Santa Barbara, CA) and Fluobeam-800 (image-based;

Fluoptics, France).[64] These fluorescence-based products were found to be accurate in detecting parathyroid tissue, with abnormal parathyroid glands showing different autofluorescence intensity compared with normal parathyroid tissue.[65,66] An early prospective feasibility trial of 59 patients undergoing parathyroidectomy by 2 experienced endocrine surgeons showed that NIRAF utilization led to an increase in surgeon confidence of adequate resection compared with visual inspection of the specimen with a 20% improvement in in vivo localization.[67] For surgeons with less experience identifying parathyroid tissue, NIRAF may be a useful tool to aid with localization of suspected parathyroid glands during both thyroid and parathyroid surgery. This technology may be particularly helpful in identifying and preserving parathyroid tissue in the setting of bulky lymphadenopathy while performing a central neck dissection for thyroid cancer, which has a risk of transient hypoparathyroidism of 15% to 30%.[39,68] Although further research is needed to examine its utility in identifying parathyroid disease, NIRAF may have the ability to replace intraoperative frozen section analysis or gland aspiration for PTH, which may help decrease operative time.

Treatment of Parathyroid Carcinoma

Surgical management of parathyroid carcinoma (PC) is the principal initial treatment strategy for patients with localized disease. The extent of surgery depends on the level of local invasion and includes parathyroidectomy and en bloc resection of directly involved tissue.[69] The presence of nodal metastases is rare (3%)[70] and performance of prophylactic central neck dissection is not correlated with DSS.[71,72] Patients with locally advanced or distantly metastatic PC often require multiple surgical resections and a combination of antiresorptive therapies and calcimimetics to control hypercalcemia, which is the primary factor impacting survival in this disease. Although multimodality therapy in the form of chemotherapy and/or external beam radiation with calcimemetics has been shown to improve control of hypercalcemia in select patients, no definitive impact on OS or DSS has been observed.[73] Tyrosine kinase inhibitors have shown efficacy in suppressing the proliferative and bone resorptive properties of PC as demonstrated by several case studies from various institutions with the use of cabozantinib, sorafenib, lenvatinib, and everolimus.[74,75] The use of next generation sequencing and germline testing in PC has paved the way for therapies targeted against patient-specific mutation pathways.[74] Recent studies examining the PC tumor microenvironment and mutational burden have identified increased programmed death ligand I and tumor-infiltrating expression in surrounding microenvironment of some tumors as well as high mutational tumor burdens with microsatellite instability and DNA mismatch repair, suggesting a potential role for immunotherapy in some patients with PC.[75,76] Two reports describe the use of pembrolizumab to achieve biochemical and radiographic regression in patients with metastatic PC.[77,78] Due to the rarity of the disease, clinical trials are lacking for both treatment approaches and prognostication of patients with advanced parathyroid PC. As the pendulum swings toward the use of liquid biopsy to guide treatment and prognostication of solid tumors, multi-institutional collaborations and consolidation of databases and tumor banks are of utmost importance.

ADVANCES IN THE MANAGEMENT OF ADRENAL DISEASE
Introduction

Adrenalectomy is indicated for patients with symptomatic large benign tumors, functional tumors, primary malignancy (when technically feasible and oncologically appropriate), metastatic disease (in conjunction with multidisciplinary management for well-selected patients), and in certain palliative situations to control secondary hormonal excess.

Surgical Approach

Minimally Invasive Surgery

For small benign and/or functional adrenal tumors a minimally invasive approach is appropriate[79] and is associated with decreased operative time, length-of-stay, and lower 30-day morbidity rates when compared with open adrenalectomy.[80–82]

Generally, the choice between laparoscopic transabdominal and retroperitoneal approaches is based on surgeon preference and experience, although certain patient and tumor characteristics may favor a particular approach. A retroperitoneoscopic approach is preferential for bilateral disease and may be preferred in a patient with multiple prior abdominal surgeries, whereas operative times for the retroperitoneoscopic approach may be longer in patients with greater posterior adiposity.[83] Several RCTs have attempted to compare both minimally invasive approaches. Chai and colleagues[84] found similar mean operative times, blood loss, postoperative pain, and overall complication rates in a study of 83 patients, whereas Barczynski and colleagues[85] noted shorter surgery duration, less operative blood loss, and lower postoperative pain, and Kozlowski and colleagues[86] also noted less postoperative pain and shorter length-of-stay with the retroperitoneal approach despite similar safety and efficacy.

Robotic adrenalectomy has also been increasingly performed. Ma and colleagues[87] conducted an RCT with 140 patients with pheochromocytoma, which compared robotic-assisted laparoscopic adrenalectomy with laparoscopic adrenalectomy and concluded, although both approaches were similarly safe and effective, select patients with higher catecholamine excess may benefit from the reduced blood loss and shorter operative time with the robotic approach although it was associated with higher overall cost. The benefits of the chosen operative approach will depend on surgeon choice, determination of time spent versus benefits, familiarity, and expertise.

Surgical Approach for Malignancy

Open adrenalectomy is generally reserved for larger tumors or if there is concern for malignancy. The oncologic success of all treatment is largely based on complete surgical resection because there are no proven systemic therapies for recurrence of metastatic disease, which portends such a poor prognosis. Patient outcomes in adrenocortical carcinoma (ACC), including recurrence rates and OS, are highly dependent on a complete margin negative resection without tumor spillage.[88] This can be challenging to achieve from a minimally invasive surgery (MIS) approach, particularly in large or locally invasive tumors, with retrospective studies demonstrating decreased OS with the laparoscopic approach due to higher incidence of incomplete resection and need for conversion to open procedure; en bloc resection remains the standard of care.[89–91] Although a few experienced adrenal surgeons use MIS approaches for highly selected patients with small ACCs,[92] the preference for surgical approach remains open resection with complete clearance using palpation and manual dexterity as key technical indicators.

In contrast to ACC, MIS approaches to adrenalectomy for patients with metastatic disease are technically feasible and oncologically appropriate for highly selected patients. Retrospective series of patients with adrenal metastases from lung, melanoma, renal, and other primary malignancies demonstrated prolonged survival as compared with medical therapy alone, which is most likely a function of multimodality therapy and patient selection rather than surgery alone.[82,93–96] Factors associated with decreased survival after metastectomy include larger metastasis size, synchronous presentation, and incomplete resection of adrenal disease, with primary tumor histology also likely impacting prognosis. Interestingly, the presence of extra-adrenal oligo-metastatic disease in well-selected patients may not affect prognosis.[97] Biopsy confirmation of a suspected metastatic adrenal lesion is not required but may be considered if the results would affect the treatment plan and only after appropriate hormonal workup has been completed. The utilization of radiation therapy and other ablative technologies should not be performed without multidisciplinary discussion with surgical inclusion due to the complexity of adrenalectomy after tumor progression following these techniques.

Clinical Trials in the Surgical Management of Functional Tumors

Localization in Primary Aldosteronism

Primary aldosteronism (PA) occurs in 5% to 10% of all hypertensive patients[98] and up to 14% to 21% of patients with medically resistant hypertension.[99] Laparoscopic adrenalectomy is the treatment-of-choice for PA due to a unilateral aldosterone-producing adenoma or unilateral adrenal hyperplasia. There is generally no role for surgery in PA due to bilateral adrenal hyperplasia, which is managed medically with mineralocorticoid antagonists.

Adrenal vein sampling (AVS) is used to identify patients with unilateral PA through cannulation of bilateral adrenal veins and comparison of serum aldosterone levels sampled from each side while using cortisol levels as a control. Although the addition of AVS to cross-sectional imaging is thought to improve accuracy in lateralization of PA and is generally low-risk when performed by experienced hands, it is still an invasive and resource intensive procedure. Part of the challenge of studying AVS and a potential reason for the many discordant findings is the variations in techniques and interpretation of results. Previously, most guidelines recommended the routine use of AVS in addition to CT or MRI in all patients undergoing adrenalectomy because aldosterone-producing adenomas tend to be small in size and may not be seen on cross-sectional imaging. In 2016, the SPARTACUS trial showed similar clinical outcomes 1 year after surgery between patients who underwent surgery based on CT findings alone as compared with universal application of CT and AVS together, although concerns have been raised about the study design including selection bias toward patients with florid PA, primary endpoint of intensity of antihypertensive drug treatment instead of cure of PA, and the confounding impact of use of mineralocorticoid receptor antagonists in the study.[100] Several small retrospective studies have demonstrated greater than 90% concordance between CT and AVS findings in young patients (age <35 years) with clear unilateral adenoma greater than 1 cm with normal contralateral adrenal gland on CT imaging.[101–103] Recent guidelines state that AVS may be deferred in this particular population based on the risk–benefit ratio of cannulating the contralateral gland and causing negative sequalae.[98]

Preoperative Blockade in Pheochromocytoma

Preoperative alpha (with or without beta) blockade is recommended to minimize the risk of perioperative hemodynamic instability for patients with pheochromocytoma or functional paragangliomas (PPGL). Historically, phenoxybenzamine, a nonselective α-adrenergic blocker, was the medication of choice. Patient tolerance of phenoxybenzamine is limited by its associated reflex tachycardia and orthostatic hypotension and drug availability. Selective α_1-receptor antagonists such as doxazosin, prazosin, and terazosin and calcium channel blockers have been used increasingly in place of phenoxybenzamine, with overall similar rates of intraoperative hemodynamic stability and no significant difference in postoperative outcomes such as length of stay, need for vasopressor support or rate of postoperative complications.[104–106]

Calcium channel blockers can be used in conjunction with α-blockers for preoperative blockade in PPGL patients, with a few small-scale studies directly comparing their use alone.[107,108] One retrospective review of 155 patients demonstrated similar rates of intraoperative hemodynamic instability between patients blocked with phenoxybenzamine versus nicardipine (39% vs 35%, $P = .609$), with a greater number and duration of severe hypertensive and hypotensive episodes and increased use of intraoperative vasoactive agents in patients on phenoxybenzamine, although this may be influenced by selection bias toward phenoxybenzamine for more active PPGLs.[108]

Given overall similar clinical outcomes among the different options, the choice of preoperative blockade still depends on surgeon preference, drug availability, and patient-specific factors. Select studies performed in predominantly normotensive patients at high-volume adrenal centers have demonstrated safe outcomes without preoperative blockade.[109] While preoperative blockage protocols will vary between institutions and providers, the most important part of managing these patients is having constant communication between the surgeon and anesthesiologist throughout the pre-, peri- and postoperative course to prevent, identify and treat signs of hemodynamic instability.

Management of Metastatic Pheochromocytoma or Functional Paragangliomas

Surgical resection or debulking of primary tumor, although rarely curative even when combined with complete resection of metastases, is appropriate in select patients with metastatic PPGL and may prevent local complications and improving quality of life from compression and, lowering rates of hormonal morbidity and potentially improving survival.[110,111] There is no clear consensus on the use of adjuvant or neoadjuvant therapy in metastatic PPGL.

Targeted radionuclide therapies (TRT), immunotherapy, and tyrosine kinase inhibitors, either alone or in combination play a role in multimodality therapy. The North American Neuroendocrine Tumor Society (NANETs) 2021 guidelines[111] recommend cytotoxic therapy as first-line for patients with symptomatic, bulky, or rapidly progressive disease with limited data, suggesting potential partial radiographic and partial biochemical response in 37% and 40% of patients, respectively.[112] Tyrosine kinase inhibitors were also described as potential treatment, particularly for meta-iodobezylguanidine (MIBG) nonavid tumors or rapid progression. TRT with high specific activity (HSA) I-131 MIBG has been shown in a single-arm phase II trial to improve symptom control with 25% of patients achieving the primary endpoint of reduction in antihypertensive medication and 69% of patients demonstrating stable disease at 12 months.[113] NANETs guidelines recommend consideration of HSA I-131 MIBG in patients with MIBG avid tumors who require systemic therapy. Additionally, peptide receptor radionuclide therapy Lu-177 DOTATATE, which targets somatostatin receptor, has been approved for use in treatment of gastroenteropancreatic neuroendocrine tumors. It has been shown to result in longer median OS in metastatic PPGL when compared with an alternative somatostatin receptor targeted radionuclide therapy Y-90 DOTATOC,[114] although it has not been compared with HSA I-131 MIBG. NANETs guidelines suggest consideration of Lu-177 DOTATATE therapy through clinical trials for patients with MIBG nonavid and somatostatin receptor PET-avid disease. Although a recent phase II trial of pembrolizumab for metastatic PPGL demonstrated a nonprogression rate of 40% and an objective response rate of 9%,[115] NANETs guidelines also recommends immunotherapy to be limited to clinical trials while further data is obtained. In the metastatic setting, radiotherapy can provide local control and pain relief from symptomatic metastatic lesions while also preventing pathologic fractures.[113]

Genetic Testing in Pheochromocytoma or Functional Paragangliomas

All patients with PPGL should undergo genetic testing, as up to 40% of cases are associated with an identifiable hereditary syndrome, including Von Hippel-Lindau (VHL) disease, multiple endocrine neoplasia type 2 (MEN 2), neurofibromatosis 1 (NF1), and familial PPGL syndrome that occur secondary to *VHL*, *RET*, *NF1*, and *SDHA/B/C/D* (*SDHx*) germline gene mutations, respectively. These genes may also be implicated in sporadic PPGL. Use of molecular profiling has increased understanding of the mechanisms driving tumorigenesis in PPGL, although there remains much to learn. SDHB germline mutations have been most strongly associated with metastatic PPGL but may have better response to cytotoxic chemotherapy and sunitinib therapy.[116–118] Somatic ATRX mutations and MAML3 fusions are additional molecular prognosticators associated with increased risk of aggressive disease.[119]

Patients with VHL, MEN 2, or NF1 are at increased risk of bilateral tumors that should prompt consideration of cortical sparing adrenalectomy if technically feasible, particularly in younger patients. Although cortical sparing adrenalectomy is associated with an increased risk of recurrence in remnant adrenal tissue (recurrence rates 9%–30%), the recurrence is that of a benign tumor and patients at high risk for needing contralateral adrenalectomy may still benefit overall from preservation of endogenous steroid production, reducing dependence on chronic steroid hormone replacement and risk of adrenal crisis.[120,121]

Management of Hypercortisolism Related to Benign Adrenal Pathology

Adrenalectomy is appropriate for patients with Cushing's syndrome (CS) due to adrenocorticotropic hormone (ACTH) independent cortisol-secreting adrenal tumors. Mild autonomous cortisol secretion (MACS), formerly known as subclinical CS, is also an indication for adrenalectomy. Patients with MACS demonstrate evidence of nonsuppressed cortisol (>1.8–5 mcg/dL after low-dose dexamethasone suppression test) without the typical physical stigmata of CS (round face, dorsal fat deposition, hirsutism, pronounced skin striae, bruising). These patients often display increased rates of obesity, hypertension, dyslipidemia, type 2 diabetes mellitus, and metabolic bone disease,[122–124] with improvement in blood pressure, glycemic control, and body mass index after adrenalectomy.[125–127]

Bilateral ACTH-independent CS can be due to micronodular or macronodular hyperplasia. Primary bilateral macronodular adrenal hyperplasia (PBMAH) is characterized by bilateral adrenal nodules greater than 1 cm in diameter with variable levels of excess cortisol secretion, and accounts for less than 2% of all endogenous CS. Recent guidelines recommend consideration of unilateral laparoscopic adrenalectomy for CS due to PBMAH in order to achieve control of hypercortisolism without causing permanent adrenal insufficiency, as would result from bilateral adrenalectomy. Unilateral adrenalectomy of the largest gland may be sufficient for palliation of hypercortisolism and improvement in obesity, diabetes mellitus, and hypertension,[128–130] although recurrence has been observed in up to two-thirds of patients.[131,132]

Nearly all patients with CS and approximately 60% of patients with MACS experience adrenal insufficiency related to contralateral suppression following adrenalectomy and require exogenous steroid support. The duration of steroid requirement is shorter for patients with MACS as compared with those with CS.[133,134] Cosyntropin stimulation testing on postoperative day one may identify patients at higher risk of adrenal insufficiency to allow for selective use of glucocorticoid replacement in patients with MACS.[135]

SUMMARY

In summary, the past two decades have greatly influenced our understanding and management of thyroid, parathyroid, and adrenal disease. Utilization of large database studies has allowed for the de-escalation of thyroid resection for well-selected patients with low-risk thyroid cancers. Similarly, improved localization imaging and intraoperative testing have paved the way for more minimally invasive parathyroidectomies for benign parathyroid disease. Improved understanding of molecular pathogenesis has increased the ability to risk stratify patients with thyroid cancer, identified potential therapeutic targets for patients with parathyroid cancer, and modified guidelines for surveillance of patients with familial adrenal disease.

CLINICS CARE POINTS

- The extent of surgery for thyroid cancer should incorporate all available objective data as well as patient values and preferences to allow for personalized management.
- Although molecular testing may provide prognostic information in select circumstances, there is currently no evidence to support its use in guiding extent of surgery for known malignancy.
- There are no reliable tools to help one recognize parathyroid cancer preoperatively. Apart from extreme PTH and calcium levels, surgeons must recognize the presence and extent of malignant parathyroid disease intraoperatively.
- Outcomes in adrenocortical carcinoma are highly dependent on a complete negative resection margin without tumor spillage, which can be challenging to achieve from a minimally invasive approach. The preferred surgical approach for a suspected adrenocortical carcinoma is open resection.

DISCLOSURE

The authors have no disclosures

REFERENCES

1. Siegel RL, Miller KD, Fuchs HE, et al. Cancer statistics. CA Cancer J Clin 2022; 72(1):7–33.
2. Surveillance, Epidemiology, and End Results (SEER) Program Populations (1969-2019). National Cancer Institute, DCCPS. Available at: www.seer.cancer.gov/popdata.
3. Shaha AR. Extent of surgery for papillary thyroid carcinoma: the debate continues: comment on "surgery for papillary thyroid carcinoma. Arch Otolaryngol Head Neck Surg 2010;136(11):1061–3.
4. Perrier ND, Brierley JD, Tuttle RM. Differentiated and anaplastic thyroid carcinoma: Major changes in the American Joint Committee on Cancer eighth edition cancer staging manual. CA Cancer J Clin 2018;68(1):55–63.

5. Tam S, Boonsripitayanon M, Amit M, et al. Survival in Differentiated Thyroid Cancer: Comparing the AJCC Cancer Staging Seventh and Eighth Editions. Thyroid 2018;28(10):1301–10.

6. Lang BH, Lo CY, Chan WF, et al. Staging systems for papillary thyroid carcinoma: a review and comparison. *Ann Surg* Mar 2007;245(3):366–78.

7. Dwamena S, Patel N, Egan R, et al. Impact of the change from the seventh to eighth edition of the AJCC TNM classification of malignant tumours and comparison with the MACIS prognostic scoring system in non-medullary thyroid cancer. BJS Open 2019;3(5):623–8.

8. Hay ID, Grant CS, Taylor WF, et al. Ipsilateral lobectomy versus bilateral lobar resection in papillary thyroid carcinoma: a retrospective analysis of surgical outcome using a novel prognostic scoring system. Surgery 1987;102(6):1088–95.

9. Cady B, Rossi R. An expanded view of risk-group definition in differentiated thyroid carcinoma. Surgery 1988;104(6):947–53.

10. Hay ID, Bergstralh EJ, Goellner JR, et al. Predicting outcome in papillary thyroid carcinoma: development of a reliable prognostic scoring system in a cohort of 1779 patients surgically treated at one institution during 1940 through 1989. Surgery 1993;114(6):1050–7 ; discussion 1057-8.

11. Shah JP, Loree TR, Dharker D, et al. Lobectomy versus total thyroidectomy for differentiated carcinoma of the thyroid: a matched-pair analysis. Am J Surg 1993;166(4):331–5.

12. Hay ID, Grant CS, Bergstralh EJ, et al. Unilateral total lobectomy: is it sufficient surgical treatment for patients with AMES low-risk papillary thyroid carcinoma? Surgery 1998;124(6):958–64 [discussion: 964-6].

13. Bilimoria KY, Bentrem DJ, Ko CY, et al. Extent of surgery affects survival for papillary thyroid cancer. Ann Surg 2007;246(3):375–81 [discussion: 381-4].

14. David S, Cooper GMD, Haugen Bryan R, Kloos Richard T, et al. Tuttle. Revised American Thyroid Association Management Guidelines for Patients with Thyroid Nodules and Differentiated Thyroid Cancer. Thyroid 2009;19(11):1167–214.

15. Barney BM, Hitchcock YJ, Sharma P, et al. Overall and cause-specific survival for patients undergoing lobectomy, near-total, or total thyroidectomy for differentiated thyroid cancer. Head Neck 2011;33(5):645–9.

16. Mendelsohn AH, Elashoff DA, Abemayor E, et al. Surgery for papillary thyroid carcinoma: is lobectomy enough? Arch Otolaryngol Head Neck Surg 2010;136(11):1055–61.

17. Nixon IJ, Ganly I, Patel SG, et al. Thyroid lobectomy for treatment of well differentiated intrathyroid malignancy. Surgery 2012;151(4):571–9.

18. Adam MA, Pura J, Gu L, et al. Extent of surgery for papillary thyroid cancer is not associated with survival: an analysis of 61,775 patients. Ann Surg 2014;260(4):601–5 [discussion: 605-7].

19. Adam MA, Pura J, Goffredo P, et al. Impact of extent of surgery on survival for papillary thyroid cancer patients younger than 45 years. J Clin Endocrinol Metab 2015;100(1):115–21.

20. Haugen BR, Alexander EK, Bible KC, et al. 2015 American Thyroid Association Management Guidelines for Adult Patients with Thyroid Nodules and Differentiated Thyroid Cancer: The American Thyroid Association Guidelines Task Force on Thyroid Nodules and Differentiated Thyroid Cancer. Thyroid : official J Am Thyroid Assoc 2016;26(1):1–133.

21. Tufano RP, Teixeira GV, Bishop J, et al. BRAF mutation in papillary thyroid cancer and its value in tailoring initial treatment: a systematic review and meta-analysis. Medicine (Baltimore) 2012;91(5):274–86.

22. Xing M, Alzahrani AS, Carson KA, et al. Association between BRAF V600E mutation and mortality in patients with papillary thyroid cancer. Jama 2013;309(14): 1493–501.

23. Chen Y, Sadow PM, Suh H, et al. BRAF(V600E) Is Correlated with Recurrence of Papillary Thyroid Microcarcinoma: A Systematic Review, Multi-Institutional Primary Data Analysis, and Meta-Analysis. Thyroid 2016;26(2):248–55.

24. Niederer-Wüst SM, Jochum W, Förbs D, et al. Impact of clinical risk scores and BRAF V600E mutation status on outcome in papillary thyroid cancer. Surgery 2015;157(1):119–25.

25. Melo M, da Rocha AG, Vinagre J, et al. TERT promoter mutations are a major indicator of poor outcome in differentiated thyroid carcinomas. J Clin Endocrinol Metab 2014;99(5):E754–65.

26. Xing M, Liu R, Liu X, et al. BRAF V600E and TERT promoter mutations cooperatively identify the most aggressive papillary thyroid cancer with highest recurrence. J Clin Oncol 2014;32(25):2718–26.

27. Alexander EK, Kennedy GC, Baloch ZW, et al. Preoperative diagnosis of benign thyroid nodules with indeterminate cytology. N Engl J Med 2012;367(8):705–15.

28. Nikiforov YE, Carty SE, Chiosea SI, et al. Impact of the Multi-Gene ThyroSeq Next-Generation Sequencing Assay on Cancer Diagnosis in Thyroid Nodules with Atypia of Undetermined Significance/Follicular Lesion of Undetermined Significance Cytology. Thyroid 2015;25(11):1217–23.

29. Livhits MJ, Zhu CY, Kuo EJ, et al. Effectiveness of Molecular Testing Techniques for Diagnosis of Indeterminate Thyroid Nodules: A Randomized Clinical Trial. JAMA Oncol 2021;7(1):70–7.

30. Ito Y, Uruno T, Nakano K, et al. An observation trial without surgical treatment in patients with papillary microcarcinoma of the thyroid. Thyroid 2003;13(4):381–7.

31. Ito Y, Miyauchi A, Inoue H, et al. An observational trial for papillary thyroid microcarcinoma in Japanese patients. World J Surg 2010;34(1):28–35.

32. Brito JP, Ito Y, Miyauchi A, et al. A Clinical Framework to Facilitate Risk Stratification When Considering an Active Surveillance Alternative to Immediate Biopsy and Surgery in Papillary Microcarcinoma. Thyroid 2016;26(1):144–9.

33. Applewhite MK, James BC, Kaplan SP, et al. Quality of Life in Thyroid Cancer is Similar to That of Other Cancers with Worse Survival. World J Surg 2016;40(3): 551–61.

34. Mongelli MN, Giri S, Peipert BJ, et al. Financial burden and quality of life among thyroid cancer survivors. Surgery 2020;167(3):631–7.

35. Sawka AM, Ghai S, Rotstein L, et al. A Quantitative Analysis Examining Patients' Choice of Active Surveillance or Surgery for Managing Low-Risk Papillary Thyroid Cancer. Thyroid 2022. https://doi.org/10.1089/thy.2021.0485.

36. Noguchi S, Noguchi A, Murakami N. Papillary carcinoma of the thyroid. II. Value of prophylactic lymph node excision. Cancer 1970;26(5):1061–4.

37. Kouvaraki MA, Shapiro SE, Fornage BD, et al. Role of preoperative ultrasonography in the surgical management of patients with thyroid cancer. Surgery 2003; 134(6):946–54.

38. Popadich A, Levin O, Lee JC, et al. A multicenter cohort study of total thyroidectomy and routine central lymph node dissection for cN0 papillary thyroid cancer. Surgery 2011;150(6):1048–57.

39. Hughes DT, Rosen JE, Evans DB, et al. Prophylactic Central Compartment Neck Dissection in Papillary Thyroid Cancer and Effect on Locoregional Recurrence. Ann Surg Oncol 2018;25(9):2526–34.
40. Wang TS, Cheung K, Farrokhyar F, et al. A meta-analysis of the effect of prophylactic central compartment neck dissection on locoregional recurrence rates in patients with papillary thyroid cancer. Ann Surg Oncol 2013;20(11):3477–83.
41. Tuttle M, Morris L, Haugen B, et al. Thyroid-differentiated and anaplastic carcinoma (Chapter 73). Springer International Publishing; 2017.
42. Nixon IJ, Wang LY, Palmer FL, et al. The impact of nodal status on outcome in older patients with papillary thyroid cancer. Surgery 2014;156(1):137–46.
43. Shen WT, Ogawa L, Ruan D, et al. Central neck lymph node dissection for papillary thyroid cancer: the reliability of surgeon judgment in predicting which patients will benefit. Surgery 2010;148(2):398–403.
44. Lee DY, Oh KH, Cho JG, et al. The Benefits and Risks of Prophylactic Central Neck Dissection for Papillary Thyroid Carcinoma: Prospective Cohort Study. Int J Endocrinol 2015;2015:571480.
45. Viola D, Materazzi G, Valerio L, et al. Prophylactic central compartment lymph node dissection in papillary thyroid carcinoma: clinical implications derived from the first prospective randomized controlled single institution study. J Clin Endocrinol Metab 2015;100(4):1316–24.
46. Kim BY, Choi N, Kim SW, et al. Randomized trial of prophylactic ipsilateral central lymph node dissection in patients with clinically node negative papillary thyroid microcarcinoma. Eur Arch Otorhinolaryngol 2020;277(2):569–76.
47. Sippel RS, Robbins SE, Poehls JL, et al. A Randomized Controlled Clinical Trial: No Clear Benefit to Prophylactic Central Neck Dissection in Patients With Clinically Node Negative Papillary Thyroid Cancer. Ann Surg 2020;272(3):496–503.
48. Ahn JH, Kwak JH, Yoon SG, et al. A prospective randomized controlled trial to assess the efficacy and safety of prophylactic central compartment lymph node dissection in papillary thyroid carcinoma. Surgery 2022;171(1):182–9.
49. Sanabria A, Betancourt C, Sanchez JG, et al. Prophylactic Central Neck Lymph Node Dissection in Low-Risk Thyroid Carcinoma Patients Does not Decrease the Incidence of Locoregional Recurrence: A Meta-Analysis of Randomized Trials. Ann Surg 2022. https://doi.org/10.1097/SLA.0000000000005388.
50. Song E, Han M, Oh HS, et al. Lobectomy Is Feasible for 1-4 cm Papillary Thyroid Carcinomas: A 10-Year Propensity Score Matched-Pair Analysis on Recurrence. Thyroid 2019;29(1):64–70.
51. Wilhelm SM, Wang TS, Ruan DT, et al. The American Association of Endocrine Surgeons Guidelines for Definitive Management of Primary Hyperparathyroidism. JAMA Surg 2016;151(10):959–68.
52. Kebebew E, Hwang J, Reiff E, et al. Predictors of single-gland vs multigland parathyroid disease in primary hyperparathyroidism: a simple and accurate scoring model. Arch Surg 2006;141(8):777–82 [discussion: 782].
53. Broome DT, Naples R, Bailey R, et al. Use of Preoperative Imaging in Primary Hyperparathyroidism. J Clin Endocrinol Metab 2021;106(1):e328–37.
54. Cheung K, Wang TS, Farrokhyar F, et al. A meta-analysis of preoperative localization techniques for patients with primary hyperparathyroidism. Ann Surg Oncol 2012;19(2):577–83.
55. Vu TH, Schellingerhout D, Guha-Thakurta N, et al. Solitary Parathyroid Adenoma Localization in Technetium Tc99m Sestamibi SPECT and Multiphase Multidetector 4D CT. AJNR Am J Neuroradiol 2019;40(1):142–9.

56. Kuo LE, Bird SH, Lubitz CC, et al. Four-dimensional computed tomography (4D-CT) for preoperative parathyroid localization: A good study but are we using it? Am J Surg 2022;223(4):694–8.

57. Abbott DE, Cantor SB, Grubbs EG, et al. Outcomes and economic analysis of routine preoperative 4-dimensional CT for surgical intervention in de novo primary hyperparathyroidism: does clinical benefit justify the cost? J Am Coll Surg 2012;214(4):629–37 [discussion: 637-9].

58. Lubitz CC, Stephen AE, Hodin RA, et al. Preoperative localization strategies for primary hyperparathyroidism: an economic analysis. Ann Surg Oncol 2012; 19(13):4202–9.

59. Wang TS, Cheung K, Farrokhyar F, et al. Would scan, but which scan? A cost-utility analysis to optimize preoperative imaging for primary hyperparathyroidism. Surgery 2011;150(6):1286–94.

60. Graves CE, Hope TA, Kim J, et al. Superior sensitivity of (18)F-fluorocholine: PET localization in primary hyperparathyroidism. Surgery 2022;171(1):47–54.

61. Latge A, Riehm S, Vix M, et al. (18)F-Fluorocholine PET and 4D-CT in Patients with Persistent and Recurrent Primary Hyperparathyroidism. Diagnostics (Basel) 2021;11(12).

62. Chiu B, Sturgeon C, Angelos P. Which intraoperative parathyroid hormone assay criterion best predicts operative success? A study of 352 consecutive patients. Arch Surg May 2006;141(5):483–7 [discussion: 487-8].

63. Di Marco A, Mechera R, Glover A, et al. Focused parathyroidectomy without intraoperative parathyroid hormone measurement in primary hyperparathyroidism: Still a valid approach? Surgery 2021;170(5):1383–8.

64. McWade MA, Paras C, White LM, et al. A novel optical approach to intraoperative detection of parathyroid glands. Surgery 2013;154(6):1371–7 [discussion: 1377].

65. McWade MA, Sanders ME, Broome JT, et al. Establishing the clinical utility of autofluorescence spectroscopy for parathyroid detection. Surgery 2016;159(1): 193–202.

66. Akbulut S, Erten O, Kim YS, et al. Development of an algorithm for intraoperative autofluorescence assessment of parathyroid glands in primary hyperparathyroidism using artificial intelligence. Surgery 2021;170(2):454–61.

67. Squires MH, Jarvis R, Shirley LA, et al. Intraoperative Parathyroid Autofluorescence Detection in Patients with Primary Hyperparathyroidism. Ann Surg Oncol 2019;26(4):1142–8.

68. Kim DH, Kim SW, Kang P, et al. Near-Infrared Autofluorescence Imaging May Reduce Temporary Hypoparathyroidism in Patients Undergoing Total Thyroidectomy and Central Neck Dissection. Thyroid 2021;31(9):1400–8.

69. Cetani F, Pardi E, Marcocci C. Parathyroid Carcinoma. Front Horm Res 2019;51: 63–76.

70. Silva-Figueroa AM, Hess KR, Williams MD, et al. Prognostic Scoring System to Risk Stratify Parathyroid Carcinoma. J Am Coll Surg 2017. https://doi.org/10.1016/j.jamcollsurg.2017.01.060.

71. Asare EA, Silva-Figueroa A, Hess KR, et al. Risk of Distant Metastasis in Parathyroid Carcinoma and Its Effect on Survival: A Retrospective Review from a High-Volume Center. Ann Surg Oncol 2019;26(11):3593–9. https://doi.org/10.1245/s10434-019-07451-3.

72. Hsu KT, Sippel RS, Chen H, et al. Is central lymph node dissection necessary for parathyroid carcinoma? Surgery 2014;156(6):1336–41. https://doi.org/10.1016/j.surg.2014.08.005 ; discussion 1341.

73. Salcuni AS, Cetani F, Guarnieri V, et al. Parathyroid carcinoma. Best Pract Res Clin Endocrinol Metab 2018;32(6):877–89. https://doi.org/10.1016/j.beem. 2018.11.002.
74. Kutahyalioglu M, Nguyen HT, Kwatampora L, et al. Genetic profiling as a clinical tool in advanced parathyroid carcinoma. J Cancer Res Clin Oncol 2019;145(8): 1977–86. https://doi.org/10.1007/s00432-019-02945-9.
75. Kang H, Pettinga D, Schubert AD, et al. Genomic Profiling of Parathyroid Carcinoma Reveals Genomic Alterations Suggesting Benefit from Therapy. Oncologist 2019;24(6):791–7.
76. Silva-Figueroa A, Villalobos P, Williams MD, et al. Characterizing parathyroid carcinomas and atypical neoplasms based on the expression of programmed death-ligand 1 expression and the presence of tumor-infiltrating lymphocytes and macrophages. *Surg* Nov 2018;164(5):960–4.
77. Park D, Airi R, Sherman M. Microsatellite instability driven metastatic parathyroid carcinoma managed with the anti-PD1 immunotherapy, pembrolizumab. BMJ Case Rep 2020;(9):13. https://doi.org/10.1136/bcr-2020-235293.
78. Lenschow C, Fuss CT, Kircher S, et al. Case Report: Abdominal Lymph Node Metastases of Parathyroid Carcinoma: Diagnostic Workup, Molecular Diagnosis, and Clinical Management. Front Endocrinol (Lausanne) 2021;12:643328.
79. Kebebew E, Siperstein AE, Duh QY. Laparoscopic adrenalectomy: the optimal surgical approach. J Laparoendosc Adv Surg Tech A 2001;11(6):409–13. https://doi.org/10.1089/10926420152761941.
80. Lee J, El-Tamer M, Schifftner T, et al. Open and laparoscopic adrenalectomy: analysis of the National Surgical Quality Improvement Program. J Am Coll Surg 2008;206(5):953–9 [discussion: 959-61].
81. Elfenbein DM, Scarborough JE, Speicher PJ, et al. Comparison of laparoscopic versus open adrenalectomy: results from American College of Surgeons-National Surgery Quality Improvement Project. J Surg Res 2013;184(1):216–20.
82. Romero Arenas MA, Sui D, Grubbs EG, et al. Adrenal metastectomy is safe in selected patients. World J Surg 2014;38(6):1336–42.
83. Lindeman B, Gawande AA, Moore FD Jr, et al. The Posterior Adiposity Index: A Quantitative Selection Tool for Adrenalectomy Approach. J Surg Res 2019;233: 26–31.
84. Chai YJ, Yu HW, Song RY, et al. Lateral Transperitoneal Adrenalectomy Versus Posterior Retroperitoneoscopic Adrenalectomy for Benign Adrenal Gland Disease: Randomized Controlled Trial at a Single Tertiary Medical Center. Ann Surg 2019;269(5):842–8.
85. Barczyński M, Konturek A, Nowak W. Randomized clinical trial of posterior retroperitoneoscopic adrenalectomy versus lateral transperitoneal laparoscopic adrenalectomy with a 5-year follow-up. *Ann Surg* Nov 2014;260(5):740–7 ; discussion 747-8.
86. Kozłowski T, Choromanska B, Wojskowicz P, et al. Laparoscopic adrenalectomy: lateral transperitoneal versus posterior retroperitoneal approach - prospective randomized trial. Wideochir Inne Tech Maloinwazyjne 2019;14(2): 160–9.
87. Ma W, Mao Y, Zhuo R, et al. Surgical outcomes of a randomized controlled trial compared robotic versus laparoscopic adrenalectomy for pheochromocytoma. Eur J Surg Oncol 2020;46(10 Pt A):1843–7.
88. Margonis GA, Kim Y, Prescott JD, et al. Adrenocortical Carcinoma: Impact of Surgical Margin Status on Long-Term Outcomes. Ann Surg Oncol 2016;23(1): 134–41.

89. Delozier OM, Stiles ZE, Deschner BW, et al. Implications of Conversion during Attempted Minimally Invasive Adrenalectomy for Adrenocortical Carcinoma. Ann Surg Oncol 2021;28(1):492–501.

90. Huynh KT, Lee DY, Lau BJ, et al. Impact of Laparoscopic Adrenalectomy on Overall Survival in Patients with Nonmetastatic Adrenocortical Carcinoma. J Am Coll Surg 2016;223(3):485–92.

91. Grubbs EG, Callender GG, Xing Y, et al. Recurrence of adrenal cortical carcinoma following resection: surgery alone can achieve results equal to surgery plus mitotane. Ann Surg Oncol 2010;17(1):263–70.

92. Fassnacht M, Dekkers OM, Else T, et al. European Society of Endocrinology Clinical Practice Guidelines on the management of adrenocortical carcinoma in adults, in collaboration with the European Network for the Study of Adrenal Tumors. Eur J Endocrinol 2018;179(4):G1–46.

93. Wachtel H, Roses RE, Kuo LE, et al. Adrenalectomy for Secondary Malignancy: Patients, Outcomes, and Indications. Ann Surg 2021;274(6):1073–80.

94. Mittendorf EA, Lim SJ, Schacherer CW, et al. Melanoma adrenal metastasis: natural history and surgical management. Am J Surg Mar 2008;195(3):363–8 [discussion: 368-9].

95. Vazquez BJ, Richards ML, Lohse CM, et al. Adrenalectomy improves outcomes of selected patients with metastatic carcinoma. World J Surg 2012;36(6):1400–5.

96. Vlk E, Ebbehoj A, Donskov F, et al. Outcome and prognosis after adrenal metastasectomy: nationwide study. BJS Open 2022;(2):6. https://doi.org/10.1093/bjsopen/zrac047.

97. Russo AE, Untch BR, Kris MG, et al. Adrenal Metastasectomy in the Presence and Absence of Extraadrenal Metastatic Disease. Ann Surg Aug 2019;270(2):373–7.

98. Funder JW, Carey RM, Mantero F, et al. The Management of Primary Aldosteronism: Case Detection, Diagnosis, and Treatment: An Endocrine Society Clinical Practice Guideline. J Clin Endocrinol Metab 2016;101(5):1889–916.

99. Clark D 3rd, Ahmed MI, Calhoun DA. Resistant hypertension and aldosterone: an update. Can J Cardiol 2012;28(3):318–25.

100. Dekkers T, Prejbisz A, Kool LJS, et al. Adrenal vein sampling versus CT scan to determine treatment in primary aldosteronism: an outcome-based randomised diagnostic trial. Lancet Diabetes Endocrinol 2016;4(9):739–46.

101. Lim V, Guo Q, Grant CS, et al. Accuracy of adrenal imaging and adrenal venous sampling in predicting surgical cure of primary aldosteronism. J Clin Endocrinol Metab 2014;99(8):2712–9.

102. Zhu L, Zhang Y, Zhang H, et al. Comparison between adrenal venous sampling and computed tomography in the diagnosis of primary aldosteronism and in the guidance of adrenalectomy. Medicine (Baltimore) 2016;95(39):e4986.

103. Umakoshi H, Ogasawara T, Takeda Y, et al. Accuracy of adrenal computed tomography in predicting the unilateral subtype in young patients with hypokalaemia and elevation of aldosterone in primary aldosteronism. Clin Endocrinol (Oxf) 2018;88(5):645–51.

104. Liu C, Lv Q, Chen X, et al. Preoperative selective vs non-selective α-blockade in PPGL patients undergoing adrenalectomy. Endocr Connect 2017;6(8):830–8.

105. Buitenwerf E, Osinga TE, Timmers H, et al. Efficacy of α-Blockers on Hemodynamic Control during Pheochromocytoma Resection: A Randomized Controlled Trial. J Clin Endocrinol Metab 2020;105(7):2381–91.

106. Kong H, Li N, Yang XC, et al. Nonselective Compared With Selective α-Blockade Is Associated With Less Intraoperative Hypertension in Patients With Pheochromocytomas and Paragangliomas: A Retrospective Cohort Study With Propensity Score Matching. Anesth Analg 2021;132(1):140–9.

107. Siddiqi HK, Yang HY, Laird AM, et al. Utility of oral nicardipine and magnesium sulfate infusion during preparation and resection of pheochromocytomas. Surgery 2012;152(6):1027–36.

108. Brunaud L, Boutami M, Nguyen-Thi PL, et al. Both preoperative alpha and calcium channel blockade impact intraoperative hemodynamic stability similarly in the management of pheochromocytoma. Surgery 2014;156(6):1410–7 [discussion: 1417-8].

109. Groeben H, Nottebaum BJ, Alesina PF, et al. Perioperative α-receptor blockade in phaeochromocytoma surgery: an observational case series. *Br J Anaesth* Feb 2017;118(2):182–9.

110. Roman-Gonzalez A, Zhou S, Ayala-Ramirez M, et al. Impact of Surgical Resection of the Primary Tumor on Overall Survival in Patients With Metastatic Pheochromocytoma or Sympathetic Paraganglioma. Ann Surg 2018;268(1):172–8.

111. Fishbein L, Del Rivero J, Else T, et al. The North American Neuroendocrine Tumor Society Consensus Guidelines for Surveillance and Management of Metastatic and/or Unresectable Pheochromocytoma and Paraganglioma. Pancreas 2021;50(4):469–93.

112. Niemeijer ND, Alblas G, van Hulsteijn LT, et al. Chemotherapy with cyclophosphamide, vincristine and dacarbazine for malignant paraganglioma and pheochromocytoma: systematic review and meta-analysis. Clin Endocrinol (Oxf) 2014;81(5):642–51.

113. Pryma DA, Chin BB, Noto RB, et al. Efficacy and Safety of High-Specific-Activity (131)I-MIBG Therapy in Patients with Advanced Pheochromocytoma or Paraganglioma. J Nucl Med 2019;60(5):623–30.

114. Severi S, Bongiovanni A, Ferrara M, et al. Peptide receptor radionuclide therapy in patients with metastatic progressive pheochromocytoma and paraganglioma: long-term toxicity, efficacy and prognostic biomarker data of phase II clinical trials. ESMO Open 2021;6(4):100171.

115. Jimenez C, Subbiah V, Stephen B, et al. Phase II Clinical Trial of Pembrolizumab in Patients with Progressive Metastatic Pheochromocytomas and Paragangliomas. Cancers (Basel) 2020;(8):12. https://doi.org/10.3390/cancers12082307.

116. Fishbein L, Ben-Maimon S, Keefe S, et al. SDHB mutation carriers with malignant pheochromocytoma respond better to CVD. Endocr Relat Cancer 2017;24(8):L51–5.

117. Hadoux J, Favier J, Scoazec JY, et al. SDHB mutations are associated with response to temozolomide in patients with metastatic pheochromocytoma or paraganglioma. Int J Cancer 2014;135(11):2711–20.

118. Ayala-Ramirez M, Chougnet CN, Habra MA, et al. Treatment with sunitinib for patients with progressive metastatic pheochromocytomas and sympathetic paragangliomas. J Clin Endocrinol Metab 2012;97(11):4040–50.

119. Fishbein L, Leshchiner I, Walter V, et al. Comprehensive Molecular Characterization of Pheochromocytoma and Paraganglioma. Cancer Cell 2017;31(2):181–93.

120. Neumann HPH, Tsoy U, Bancos I, et al. Comparison of Pheochromocytoma-Specific Morbidity and Mortality Among Adults With Bilateral Pheochromocytomas Undergoing Total Adrenalectomy vs Cortical-Sparing Adrenalectomy. JAMA Netw Open 2019;2(8):e198898.

121. Grubbs EG, Rich TA, Ng C, et al. Long-term outcomes of surgical treatment for hereditary pheochromocytoma. J Am Coll Surg 2013;216(2):280–9.
122. Rossi R, Tauchmanova L, Luciano A, et al. Subclinical Cushing's syndrome in patients with adrenal incidentaloma: clinical and biochemical features. J Clin Endocrinol Metab 2000;85(4):1440–8.
123. Prete A, Subramanian A, Bancos I, et al. Cardiometabolic Disease Burden and Steroid Excretion in Benign Adrenal Tumors : A Cross-Sectional Multicenter Study. Ann Intern Med 2022;175(3):325–34.
124. Athimulam S, Delivanis D, Thomas M, et al. The Impact of Mild Autonomous Cortisol Secretion on Bone Turnover Markers. J Clin Endocrinol Metab 2020; 105(5):1469–77.
125. Iacobone M, Citton M, Viel G, et al. Adrenalectomy may improve cardiovascular and metabolic impairment and ameliorate quality of life in patients with adrenal incidentalomas and subclinical Cushing's syndrome. Surgery 2012;152(6): 991–7.
126. Pisano G, Calò PG, Erdas E, et al. Adrenal incidentalomas and subclinical Cushing syndrome: indications to surgery and results in a series of 26 laparoscopic adrenalectomies. Ann Ital Chir 2015;86:406–12.
127. Toniato A, Merante-Boschin I, Opocher G, et al. Surgical versus conservative management for subclinical Cushing syndrome in adrenal incidentalomas: a prospective randomized study. Ann Surg 2009;249(3):388–91.
128. Iacobone M, Albiger N, Scaroni C, et al. The role of unilateral adrenalectomy in ACTH-independent macronodular adrenal hyperplasia (AIMAH). World J Surg 2008;32(5):882–9.
129. Debillon E, Velayoudom-Cephise FL, Salenave S, et al. Unilateral Adrenalectomy as a First-Line Treatment of Cushing's Syndrome in Patients With Primary Bilateral Macronodular Adrenal Hyperplasia. J Clin Endocrinol Metab 2015; 100(12):4417–24.
130. Xu Y, Rui W, Qi Y, et al. The role of unilateral adrenalectomy in corticotropin-independent bilateral adrenocortical hyperplasias. World J Surg 2013;37(7): 1626–32.
131. Osswald A, Quinkler M, Di Dalmazi G, et al. Long-Term Outcome of Primary Bilateral Macronodular Adrenocortical Hyperplasia After Unilateral Adrenalectomy. J Clin Endocrinol Metab 2019;104(7):2985–93.
132. Zhang Y, Li H. Classification and surgical treatment for 180 cases of adrenocortical hyperplastic disease. Int J Clin Exp Med 2015;8(10):19311–7.
133. Foster T, Bancos I, McKenzie T, et al. Early assessment of postoperative adrenal function is necessary after adrenalectomy for mild autonomous cortisol secretion. Surgery 2021;169(1):150–4.
134. Di Dalmazi G, Berr CM, Fassnacht M, et al. Adrenal function after adrenalectomy for subclinical hypercortisolism and Cushing's syndrome: a systematic review of the literature. J Clin Endocrinol Metab 2014;99(8):2637–45.
135. DeLozier OM, Dream SY, Findling JW, et al. Selective Glucocorticoid Replacement Following Unilateral Adrenalectomy for Hypercortisolism and Primary Aldosteronism. J Clin Endocrinol Metab 2022;107(2):e538–47.

Diversity, Equity, and Inclusion in Clinical Trials

Grace Keegan, BS[a], Angelena Crown, MD[b], Kathie-Ann Joseph, MD, MPH[c,d],*

KEYWORDS

- Minority groups • Vulnerable populations • Diversity • Equity • Inclusion
- Clinical trials

KEY POINTS

- Despite higher cancer mortality rates, Black/African American patients are underrepresented in clinical trials.
- Representation in clinical trials varies across different races/ethnicities, sociodemographic status, and age groups.
- Physicians can play a role in improving clinical trial enrollent and retention among underrepresented groups.

INTRODUCTION

According to the American Cancer Society's report on the status of cancer disparities in 2021, the overall mortality rate from cancer in both Black men and women is significantly higher (19% and 12%, respectively) than in White men and women.[1] This reflects a difference in cancer mortality rates of 178.6 deaths per 100,000 people among non-Hispanic Blacks and 157.2 deaths per 100,000 people among non-Hispanic Whites. This is startling when weighed against the fact that overall rates of cancer are higher among non-Hispanic Whites (476.3 cases per 100,000 people) than non-Hispanic Blacks (459.0 cases per 100,000 people), Hispanics (354.3 cases per 100,000 people), and Asian/Pacific Islanders (308.3 cases per 100,000 people).[2] Black women, in particular, have an 8% lower incidence of cancer than White women despite these overall higher mortality rates.[1] The National Comprehensive Cancer Network (NCCN) maintains that clinical trials provide some of the best treatment options to eligible patients; as a result, ensuring equitable access and participation in

[a] Keegan-University of Chicago, Pritzker School of Medicine, 924 E. 57th Street, Chicago, IL 60637, USA; [b] Breast Surgery, True Family Women's Cancer Center, Swedish Cancer Institute, Seattle, WA, USA; [c] Department of Surgery, New York University Grossman School of Medicine, NYC Health and Hospitals/Bellevue, New York, NY, USA; [d] NYU Langone Health's Institute for Excellence in Health Equity, 180 Madison Avenue, New York, NY, USA
* Corresponding author. Department of Surgery, NYU Grossman School of Medicine, 424 East 34th Street, Kimmel Pavilion, KP-3 Room 3-102, New York, NY 10016.
E-mail address: Kathie-Ann.Joseph@nyulangone.org

Surg Oncol Clin N Am 32 (2023) 221–232
https://doi.org/10.1016/j.soc.2022.08.005
1055-3207/23/© 2022 Elsevier Inc. All rights reserved.

surgonc.theclinics.com

clinical trials across diverse populations is critical for reducing disparities in cancer outcomes.

When studying the benefits of a drug, the demographic composition of clinical trial enrollees should be proportional to the number of patients in each category (race, gender, and sexual identity) affected by the disease. Clinical trials have historically included a disproportionately low percentage of minority groups, although many of the cancers or subtypes targeted by the trial affect these populations at a greater rate, including triple-negative breast cancer (TNBC) in women and prostate cancer in men.[3] Expanding accessibility of clinical trials to proportionately include diverse patient populations has proved challenging as the range of clinical trials has expanded, and these disparities persist.

DISPARITIES AND ACCESSIBILITY OF CLINICAL TRIALS TO DIVERSE POPULATIONS

On both a national and international scale, the lack of racial and ethnic representation in clinical trials precludes the generalizability and effectiveness of applying clinical findings to these populations. Although approximately 40% of people in the United States identify as a racial or ethnic minority, one study describing the representation of minorities in oncology clinical trials from 2003 to 2016 found that people of color as a group represent only 14% of clinical trials participants.[4,5] Another report on clinical trials supporting the US Food and Drug Administration (FDA) approval of drugs in the year 2019 cited overall an inclusion of 8% Black/African American, 6% Asian, and 11% Hispanic or Latinx participants.[6] Although this is representative of the Asian population in the United States, these numbers underrepresent both the Black/African American population, which is 13.4% of the US population, and the Hispanic or Latinx population, which is 18.5% of the total.[7] For Black/African American populations specifically, this lack of representation has been particularly striking. In a review of FDA-approved proposals from 1997 to 2014, the median percentage of African and African American participants per trial ranged from 1.8% to 3.5%.[8] In pharmaceutical company-sponsored trials, there is a poor representation of Black patients on a similar scale, as only 2.9% of participants in these trials overall identified as African American or Black.[9]

The equity concerns implicated by these disparities are important to highlight, given that clinical trials often give patients an opportunity to treat their disease when other options have failed. Ensuring that members of racial and ethnic minority groups have access to clinical trials may help improve disparities in health outcomes and promote just distribution of health resources. In addition, one review found that 20% of drugs approved in clinical trials show different clinical responses across racial and ethnic groups. This finding underscores the importance of enrolling a diverse population of patients within clinical trials to better understand drug toxicity and efficacy across populations.[10]

Oncology clinical trials are no exception to this overall pattern. In a study of oncology trials since 2000, non-Hispanic Whites were more likely to be enrolled in trials, representing 120% of their percentage in the population overall, whereas Black/African American participants were represented at 70% and Hispanic or Latinx participants at 40% of their proportion of the overall population.[4] Another review of clinical trials leading to cancer drug approvals from 2008 to 2018 examined racial and ethnic representation in trial participants compared with demographic proportions in US cancer incidence and found that representation among Black patients was only 22% of expected, and representation among Hispanic patients was only 44% of expected. Asian patients were overrepresented in clinical trials when weighted to cancer incidence rates.[11]

These disparities are even more drastic in trials for particular cancers and drugs. Specifically, in immunotherapy trials, Black patients constitute less than 4% of patients enrolled.[12] A study in breast cancer clinical trial enrollment found that Black and Hispanic patients were significantly less likely to be aware of clinical trials than White patients.[13] A lack of knowledge of clinical trials prevents patients from actively seeking out trials or choosing to get care at an institution offering the trial, contributing to the disparities in trial enrollment that exist.

An illustrative example of this inequitable phenomenon is the recent Keynote 522 trial for TNBC. TNBC is highly aggressive and has few viable therapeutic options. Although TNBC comprises 15% of breast cancers in the United States, this rate is estimated to be twice as high among Black women and makes up 39% of breast cancers among premenopausal Black women.[14–16] Although TNBC is remarkably heterogeneous at the molecular level, it is typically associated with an aggressive clinical course, including higher rates of brain and lung metastases and shorter disease-free intervals compared with other subtypes.[17–19] The Keynote 522 study was a Phase III trial that showed improved disease-free survival with the addition of pembrolizumab to standard chemotherapy for high-risk early-stage TNBC.[20] Given the increased prevalence of TNBC among Black women and the high rate of side effects in the study, the fact that only 4.5% of trial participants were Black women is highly concerning and highlights the importance of recruiting underrepresented minorities into clinical trials. This level of representation of Black women in breast cancer trials is consistent with recent studies evaluating the Oncotype DX (Genomic Health) recurrence score, which is widely used to determine chemotherapy benefit in luminal type breast cancers. Indeed, Black women made up 4% of women in the recent TAILORx study, which provided data to support the omission of chemotherapy for women >50 years with mid-range recurrence scores.[21] Given that Black women have worse outcomes relative to White women at each recurrence score range and Black women were underrepresented in the studies that validated the recurrence score, it raises questions of whether the test is as accurate in estimating prognosis and predicting chemotherapy benefit for Black women with breast cancer.[22]

Disparities in clinical trial representation also exist within socioeconomic strata and across age groups. The Centers for Disease Control and Prevention Behavioral Risk Factor Surveillance System Survey found that higher income and lower age correlated with greater participation in cancer clinical trials from 2011 to 2021. Educational attainment, however, was not correlated with enrollment.[23] A study of gastrointestinal cancer surgical patients found patients with public health insurance were significantly less likely to participate in clinical trials.[24] In this study, Medicaid patients were 51% as likely to enroll in clinical trials than people with private insurance. The same trial identified interactions between race and income in clinical trial participation. Both high-income (odds ratio [OR] 0.67) and low-income (OR 0.75) Blacks were less likely to participate in clinical trials than low-income and high-income Whites.[25] Low income, and people of color, is more likely to get their health care at a community center where they are likely to receive their cancer diagnosis and treatment options. Cancer clinical trial enrollment at community centers is extremely low (7%). The national percentage of patients with cancer enrolled in clinical trials is already low at 8%, so the number of patients seeking care at community centers who have access to clinical trials is exceptionally small.[26] This presents a formidable structural barrier to trial enrollment for patients of low socioeconomic status (SES) with burdensome logistical challenges, including needing to travel large distances to access trials and receive investigational medications.

Linguistic minorities are also unrepresented in oncology clinical trials and may be misrepresented in trials that rely on patient-reported outcome measures (PROMs) for obtaining data. Indeed, one review of oncology trials reported that the majority of trials using a PROM as a primary endpoint did not offer trial materials with a validated Spanish or Chinese language translation.[27] Health literacy is known to be lower in ethnic minorities; moreover, limited knowledge of research opportunities or understanding of the consent process in linguistically diverse patients are implicated in the underrepresentation of this population among clinical trial participants.[28] Measures that assess the quality of informed consent in clinical trials are lower in patients with limited English proficiency (LEP).[29] Furthermore, requirements of English language competence in trial recruitment and factors of the research setting that foment mistrust of the consenting process have been identified as major barriers to recruitment of linguistically diverse populations.[30]

Finally, physician attitudes and structural racism also contribute to the low accessibility of oncology clinical trials to diverse populations. Physician attitudes about patient adherence to trial protocols were cited as a major inhibitor to offering trial enrollment opportunities to underrepresented populations in 61% of trials included in a systematic review.[31] These disparities in access to oncology clinical trials, which lead to inequitable enrollment, require intervention at individual and institutional levels.

Increasing Enrollment of Diverse Patient Populations

The persisting disparities within oncology clinical trial accessibility warrant further exploration into strategies for increasing enrollment of diverse patient populations. Here we will further explore misconceptions about trial enrollment in various underrepresented groups and identify strategies that have shown to be effective in increasing access and enrollment in these populations.

A perception of lack of interest and a higher rate of declining enrollment in clinical trials is often incorrectly cited as the cause of lower rates of participation of racial and ethnic minorities in clinical trials.[13] However, a breast cancer clinical trial patient survey found no significant difference in patient interest in trial participation or rates of patients declining to participate in clinical trials based on race or ethnicity.[13] Therefore, strategies for promoting enrollment of racial and ethnic minorities must focus on structural barriers to access trials rather than regarding it as a natural process of patient autonomy. These findings do not ignore the presence of trust barriers that exist in the relationship between racial and ethnic minorities and the health care system, related to historical exclusion and exploitation of these populations in the medical field.

An investigation into the recruitment of racial and ethnic minorities used an interventional mapping approach based on health behavior theories and conducting needs-assessments within specialty clinics and found this strategy to be an effective way for health centers to identify population-specific barriers and influence minority recruitment.[32] In addition, the multistakeholder approach has been suggested as an effective way to increase enrollment of racial and ethnic minorities given that referring physicians, trial sponsors, and trial coordinators or recruiters all play a large role in the enrollment of ethnic and racial minorities in studies.[33] Together, these studies suggest that strategies to increase enrollment of ethnic and racial minorities must be intersectional and based on the specific barriers identified within populations under-enrolled in clinical trials.

Increasing enrollment of linguistic minorities is very important given the increasing linguistic diversity in the US population. 21.5% of people living in the United States (67.8 million) speak a language other than English at home.[34] Enrollment of linguistically diverse populations in clinical research currently requires special prepa-rations indicated by many study sponsors and institutional review boards (IRBs). These requirements contribute to under-enrollment of these populations. IRBs should reduce unnecessary effort related to including patients with LEP in research.[35] Lan-guage barriers also bring to question the quality of informed consent and health liter-acy in patients with LEP. Therefore, enrollment of patients with LEP can only increase after better translation standards are developed to improve the transmission of high-quality information about health care, especially in providing consent for trials.[36] The use of multimedia tools that aim to improve linguistic and cultural inclusion in medical interactions and trial recruitment, such as animations, could also help increase enroll-ment for this population. This specific strategy also encourages patients to ask ques-tions about health research and promotes a more thorough conversation about trials before consent and enrollment to protect this vulnerable population.[28]

Increasing the representation of patients of low SES in clinical trials is essential for improving equity in medical care. There are numerous requirements of the clinical trial identification and enrollment process that present barriers to patients of low SES, which contribute to the low rate of enrollment among these patients. Patients at com-munity care centers are less likely to have doctors that offer clinical trial opportunities or are connected with academic medical centers. One study reported that 30% of pa-tient responses to a survey question on barriers to participation involved logistical concerns related to low SES, including the inability to pay for childcare or transporta-tion or to afford time off from work.[13] These barriers can also contribute to incomplete follow-up, which highlights the difficulties associated with both recruitment and reten-tion of diverse populations in clinical trials. A randomized control trial studying preterm birth found that offering financial incentives, assistance with transportation, and su-pervised childcare services to all patients desiring to enroll resulted in proportionate follow-up rates across race and ethnicity, SES, and marital status.[37] Providing these services, which reduce the burden of enrollment, particularly for patients with low SES, should be more widely applied. Rural populations may also benefit from these improvements. Because SES and race/ethnicity are often associated, strategies to reduce this formidable barrier to clinical trial enrollment for already medically vulner-able populations can promote equity across multiple underrepresented groups.

Recognizing that most cancer-related clinical trials and research traditionally have been conducted in academic settings, yet 85% of patients with cancer receive their care in the community, the National Cancer Institute (NCI) has sponsored initiatives and programs for community-based clinical research and cancer trials such as the Community Clinical Oncology Program (CCOP), NCI Community Cancer Centers Pro-gram (NCCCP) and the NCI Community Oncology Research Program (NCORP). These programs support clinical trials and research in community-based settings. Although these programs have helped to promote diversity and access to clinical trials, there remain barriers to conducting trials in the community setting. Even with NCI support, funding remains an issue for these smaller programs and maintaining an adequate infrastructure to conduct cancer trials. More importantly, efforts need to be made to increase awareness of the importance of clinical trials at the hospital leadership level to support these efforts.

Elderly patients are the largest consumers of health care in the United States. Increasing age is the most significant risk factor associated with cancer incidence rates in the United States.[38] Consequently, drugs studied in clinical trials have the po-tential to provide significant benefits for this elderly population with complex health conditions. However, this population is largely underrepresented in clinical trials. This is often an effect of trial design, which often excludes elderly populations due to concerns about comorbidities and toxicities. Most data on toxicity in clinical trials are reported up to the 75–80 age group, and with our aging population, this needs to be expanded.[39,40] Trial unavailability or ineligibility was reported as the major reason for non-enrollment in research for elderly patients, with 60% of respondents in this survey indicating this barrier.[41] The physician also plays a role in the underrepresentation of elderly patients. In a study on physician involvement in patient recruitment, a discussion about clinical trial participation was reported in interactions with 76% of eligible patients younger than 65 but only 58% of eligible patients over 65.[41] The poor understanding of response to treatment in older patients resulting from low enrollment in clinical trials is of high concern because these drugs are often prescribed to elderly patients.[42] It is imperative that clinical research leadership takes steps to improve the understanding of toxicity in older patients by enrolling more older patients in trials specifically focused on the elderly.

Sexual and gender minorities are particularly hard to reach for clinical trial recruitment and are consequently underrepresented in trial participants. Demographic information on sexual orientation and gender identity is often omitted from health care system data collection or results of clinical research.[43,44] Clinical trial sponsors and investigators should encourage the reporting of sexual orientation and gender identity, as patients are willing to disclose, to better understand the degree of underrepresentation of this population in trials. The application of a mobile app for engagement and recruitment of underrepresented populations, specifically sexual and gender minorities, has shown to be a cost-effective way of increasing the representation of this vulnerable population in clinical research.[45] Digital engagement strategies may help reduce stigma or avoid the effects of bias in interpersonal interactions with health care professionals. Further research should work to identify strategies for improving recruitment and retention in this population.

Greater enrollment of these underrepresented populations as a whole could be achieved through fundamental changes to clinical trial design. Clinical trial leadership should work to broaden and more universally apply recommendations published by the FDA that encourage the modernization of eligibility criteria. Critically evaluating and implementing more inclusive eligibility criteria, in turn, may prevent unnecessary exclusion of patients from trials and specifically address unfair criteria that particularly disadvantage minority populations.[26,46] Inclusion of patients with chronic conditions should be encouraged whenever possible, particularly in later phase trials in which existing therapies are being tested for new indications and safety has been established. Indeed, most trials that restrict eligibility based on language ability or chronic diseases often disproportionately exclude marginalized and minority patients.[13] Consequently, these measures may increase enrollment of various minority groups and greatly improve the generalizability of research findings as new drugs are often prescribed to patients with chronic comorbidities. Strategies that target underrepresented groups with multifaceted approaches have the highest potential to be effective.

Overcoming Barriers to Patient Enrollment

Barriers to enrollment of minority groups must be addressed in strategies to increase recruitment and retention of these populations. Both logistical barriers, including engagement with community-based health centers and integration of these centers with academic medical centers, and interpersonal barriers, including patient-provider trust and attitudes, are important considerations in clinical trial design. Efforts to overcome these barriers may be pursued from a system, individual provider, and patient-focused perspective.

Although strategies to address logistical barriers that offer financial reimbursement, transportation, and child care can effectively enroll and retain minority groups, a large percentage of patients from underrepresented minorities receive health care at community centers and cannot take advantage of these initiatives.[37] At the system level, strategies to increase engagement of community health centers in clinical trials have proven to be effective at targeting both racial and ethnic minorities, people of low SES, and people from rural communities. Basic community outreach performed by clinical trial personnel at community centers, churches, and neighborhood schools increases knowledge of trials in low-income and minority populations.[13] In addition, increasing awareness of clinical trials among community-based health providers is key to improving enrollment among underrepresented populations receiving care at community centers. Increased contact between community-based and academic center providers through a streamlined referral system can bridge the gap between trial access for these populations.[13]

Conducting substudies or developing a study arm in a specific geographic area or health center with a greater percentage of a target minority population that is difficult to recruit at main study centers can also be an effective way to engage these communities.[8] By designing online and printed clinical trial information at eighth-grade reading level or lower, researchers can make materials more accessible at community health centers.[13] Effectively engaging patients and providers at community-based health centers, when applied in combination with other strategies such as providing assistance with travel and childcare, may help to increase enrollment of these underrepresented populations.

It is also important that these strategies that target underrepresented populations are culturally sensitive and that providers set aside their biases and offer clinical trial enrollment to all eligible patients equitably. One study of oncology cancer trials found that when patients with cancer are offered the opportunity to participate in clinical trials, 50% do, yet only 8% of these eligible patients are enrolled.[47] Though these numbers may reflect some degree of logistical barriers, this finding also suggests that discrimination may play a role in the under-enrollment of underrepresented minority patients. Patients also look to their physicians as the key source for information about trials, above online resources, so it is crucial that doctors offer trials to all eligible patients.[48] Physicians can play a key role in reducing the knowledge barrier to enrollment for underrepresented patients.

At the level of the patient, some studies report that mistrust among ethnic minorities is commonly cited as a barrier to inclusion in research, and awareness of a history of unethical practices in the medical field contributes to low enrollment of these patients.[49] Other researchers have further explored this idea and found that beliefs about the institution of medicine as elitist and not truly committed to promoting health for vulnerable and ethnic minority communities contribute to mistrust.[50] Building trust between a patient and researcher becomes more natural when the individuals share a similar background, so recruiting more culturally diverse research coordinators and physicians is important for addressing this challenge.[51] Engagement within communities at health centers and the development of referral systems, as previously described, can also be an effective approach to establishing trust and overcoming trust barriers.[50,52] By working within already substantiated trust structures, study clinicians may efficiently reach patients who cannot access academic centers and promote a more just recruitment process in clinical research.

Improving Diversity and Equity of Clinical Trial Leaders

One of the strategies to improve enrollment and retention of patients from underrepresented minority groups is to improve the diversity of clinical trial leadership. Diversity is limited within oncology as a specialty. Indeed, in 2019, only 5.1% of radiation oncology faculty and 5.7% of medical oncology faculty registered on the Association of American Medical Colleges (AAMC) full-time Faculty Roster identified as Underrepresented in Medicine (URM).[10] Similarly, women made up 29.1% of radiation oncology faculty and 38.1% of medical oncology faculty in the same study.[53] Parallel trends are also present in surgical oncology.[54] This lack of diversity among medical faculty and leadership leads to poor recruitment of URM medical students and residents and propagates a vicious cycle of underrepresentation.[55–57]

Clinical trial leadership is also plagued by a lack of representation of women and physicians from URM backgrounds. Indeed, in a study assessing the gender of authors across 114 oncology randomized control trials, only 22.9% were women.[58] Furthermore, there was an even lower proportion of women steering committee members (20.3%), first authors (21.9%), and senior authors (10.3%). A second study assessing 598 Phase 3 therapeutic oncologic randomized clinical trials found that 17.9% of trials had a female senior author.[59] The highest rate of female senior author sites was seen in breast and head and neck cancer trials. In contrast, the lowest rates of female senior authorship were observed in gastrointestinal, genitourinary, and hematologic cancer trials. Interestingly, no female senior authors for surgical trials were identified.

In addition, structural barriers to access, fear, and mistrust of the medical establishment are thought to contribute to low clinical trial enrollment rates among URM patient. Investigator bias has also been reported, with some respondents to a qualitative interview reporting opinions that patients from ethnic and racial minorities are less promising clinical trial participants. Racial concordance has been associated with improved communication and health care utilization among patients with URM.[60–62] Involvement of URM investigators is also associated with higher rates of patient with URM enrollment and retention in clinical trials.[63–65] As a result, increasing leadership among URM oncology physicians and trial leaders would not only help to inspire the next generation of URM physicians but could also help to improve clinical trial enrollment of patients with URM.

SUMMARY

In summary, minority groups are vastly underrepresented in clinical trial participants and leadership. Because these studies provide innovative and revolutionary treatment options to patients with cancer and have the potential to extend survival, it is imperative that public and private stakeholders, as well as hospital and clinical trial leadership, prioritize equity and inclusion of diverse populations in clinical trial development and recruitment strategies. Achieving equity in clinical trials could be an important step in reducing the overall cancer burden and mortality disparities in vulnerable populations.

CLINICS CARE POINT

- Despite higher cancer mortality rates, Black/African American patients are underrepresented in clinical trials.

- Representation in clinical trials varies across different races/ethnicities, sociodemographic status, and age groups.
- Physicians can play a role in improving clinical trial enrollent and retention among underrepresented groups.

DISCLOSURE

The authors have nothing to disclose.

REFERENCES

1. Islami F, Guerra CE, Minihan A, et al. American Cancer Society's report on the status of cancer disparities in the United States, 2021. CA Cancer J Clin 2022;72(2): 112–43.
2. SEER Cancer Statistics Review, 1975-2017. National Cancer Institute SEER. Available at: https://seer.cancer.gov/csr/1975_2017/index.html. Accessed April 18, 2022.
3. Cancer Disparities in the Black Community. Am Cancer Soc. Available at: https://www.cancer.org/about-us/what-we-do/health-equity/cancer-disparities-in-the-black-community.html. Accessed April 18, 2022.
4. Duma N, Vera Aguilera J, Paludo J, et al. Representation of minorities and women in oncology clinical trials: review of the past 14 years. J Oncol Pract 2018;14(1): e1–10.
5. Bureau. National Population by Characteristics: 2010-2019. United States Census Bureau. Available at: https://www.census.gov/data/tables/time-series/demo/popest/2010s-national-detail.html. Accessed April 18, 2022.
6. 2019 Drug Trials Snapshots Summary Report. US Food & Drug Administration, Available at: https://www.fda.gov/drugs/drug-approvals-and-databases/drug-trials-snapshots Accessed April 18, 2022.
7. U.S. Census Bureau QuickFacts: United States. United States Census Bureau. Available at: https://www.census.gov/quickfacts/US. Accessed April 18, 2022.
8. Knepper TC, McLeod HL. When will clinical trials finally reflect diversity? Nature, 557(7704), 2018, 157-159.
9. Unger JM, Hershman DL, Osarogiagbon RU, et al. Representativeness of Black patients in cancer clinical trials sponsored by the National Cancer Institute compared with pharmaceutical companies. JNCI Cancer Spectr 2020;4(4). pkaa034.
10. Ramamoorthy A, Pacanowski MA, Bull J, et al. Racial/ethnic differences in drug disposition and response: review of recently approved drugs. Clin Pharmacol Ther 2015;97(3):263–73.
11. Loree JM, Anand S, Dasari A, et al. Disparity of race reporting and representation in clinical trials leading to cancer drug approvals from 2008 to 2018. JAMA Oncol 2019;5(10):e191870.
12. Nazha B, Mishra M, Pentz R, et al. Enrollment of racial minorities in clinical trials: old problem assumes new urgency in the age of immunotherapy. Am Soc Clin Oncol Educ Book 2019;39:3–10.
13. Trant AA, Walz L, Allen W, et al. Increasing accrual of minority patients in breast cancer clinical trials. Breast Cancer Res Treat 2020;184(2):499–505.

14. Amirikia KC, Mills P, Bush J, et al. Higher population-based incidence rates of triple-negative breast cancer among young African-American women: implications for breast cancer screening recommendations. Cancer 2011;117(12):2747–53.

15. Carey LA, Perou CM, Livasy CA, et al. Race, breast cancer subtypes, and survival in the Carolina Breast Cancer Study. JAMA 2006;295(21):2492–502.

16. Kohler BA, Sherman RL, Howlader N, et al. Annual Report to the Nation on the Status of Cancer, 1975-2011, Featuring Incidence of Breast Cancer Subtypes by Race/Ethnicity, Poverty, and State. JNCI J Natl Cancer Inst 2015;107(6): djv048.

17. Boyle P. Triple-negative breast cancer: epidemiological considerations and recommendations. Ann Oncol 2012;23:vi7–12.

18. Dawood S. Triple-negative breast cancer: epidemiology and management options. Drugs 2010;70(17):2247–58.

19. Hudis CA, Gianni L. Triple-negative breast cancer: an unmet medical need. Oncologist 2011;16(Suppl 1):1–11. https://doi.org/10.1634/theoncologist.2011-S1-01.

20. Schmid P, Cortes J, Dent R, et al. Event-free survival with pembrolizumab in early triple-negative breast cancer. N Engl J Med 2022;386(6):556–67.

21. Sparano JA, Gray RJ, Makower DF, et al. Adjuvant chemotherapy guided by a 21-gene expression assay in breast cancer. N Engl J Med 2018;379(2):111–21. https://doi.org/10.1056/NEJMoa1804710.

22. Collin LJ, Yan M, Jiang R, et al. Oncotype DX recurrence score implications for disparities in chemotherapy and breast cancer mortality in Georgia. NPJ Breast Cancer 2019;5:32.

23. Meyer S, Woldu HG, Sheets LR. Sociodemographic diversity in cancer clinical trials: New findings on the effect of race and ethnicity. Contemp Clin Trials Commun 2021;21:100718.

24. Abbas A, Diaz A, Obeng-Gyasi S, et al. Disparity in clinical trial participation among patients with gastrointestinal cancer. J Am Coll Surg 2022;234(4):589–98.

25. Parekh T, Desai A. Demographic and socioeconomic disparities among cancer survivors in clinical trials participation, USA, 2016–2018. J Cancer Educ 2020; 37(1):80–90.

26. Unger JM, Vaidya R, Hershman DL, et al. Systematic review and meta-analysis of the magnitude of structural, clinical, and physician and patient barriers to cancer clinical trial participation. JNCI J Natl Cancer Inst 2019;111(3):245–55.

27. Grant SR, Noticewala SS, Mainwaring W, et al. Non-English language validation of patient-reported outcome measures in cancer clinical trials. Support Care Cancer 2020;28(6):2503–5.

28. George S, Moran E, Duran N, et al., Using animation as an information tool to advance health research literacy among minority participants, AMIA Annu Symp Proc, 2013, 2013, 475-484.

29. Hunt LM, de Voogd KB. Are good intentions good enough?: Informed consent without trained interpreters. J Gen Intern Med 2007;22(5):598–605.

30. anne Hughson J, Woodward-Kron R, Parker A, et al. A review of approaches to improve participation of culturally and linguistically diverse populations in clinical trials. Trials 2016;17(1):1–10.

31. Howerton MW, Gibbons MC, Baffi CR, et al. Provider roles in the recruitment of underrepresented populations to cancer clinical trials. Cancer Interdiscip Int J Am Cancer Soc 2007;109(3):465–76.

32. Amorrortu RP, Arevalo M, Vernon SW, et al. Recruitment of racial and ethnic minorities to clinical trials conducted within specialty clinics: an intervention mapping approach. Trials 2018;19(1):115.

33. Clark LT, Watkins L, Piña IL, et al. Increasing diversity in clinical trials: overcoming critical barriers. Curr Probl Cardiol 2019;44(5):148–72.

34. Census - Social Characteristisc in the United States. United States Census Bureau. Available at: https://data.census.gov/cedsci/table?tid=ACSDP5Y2020.DP02&hidePreview=true. Accessed April 18, 2022.

35. Glickman SW, Ndubuizu A, Weinfurt KP, et al. Perspective: the case for research justice: inclusion of patients with limited English proficiency in clinical research. Acad Med 2011;86(3):389–93.

36. Michael J, Aylen T, Ogrin R. Development of a Translation Standard to support the improvement of health literacy and provide consistent high-quality information. Aust Health Rev 2013;37(4):547–51.

37. Webb DA, Coyne JC, Goldenberg RL, et al. Recruitment and retention of women in a large randomized control trial to reduce repeat preterm births: the Philadelphia Collaborative Preterm Prevention Project. BMC Med Res Methodol 2010;10(1):1–15.

38. Risk factors: age - national cancer Institute. National Cancer Institute; 2015. Available at: https://www.cancer.gov/about-cancer/causes-prevention/risk/age. Accessed April 18, 2022.

39. Hurria A, Togawa K, Mohile SG, et al. Predicting chemotherapy toxicity in older adults with cancer: a prospective multicenter study. J Clin Oncol 2011;29(25):3457–65.

40. Palaia I, Loprete E, Musella A, et al. Chemotherapy in elderly patients with gynecological cancer. Oncology 2013;85(3):168–72.

41. Javid SH, Unger JM, Gralow JR, et al. A prospective analysis of the influence of older age on physician and patient decision-making when considering enrollment in breast cancer clinical trials (SWOG S0316). Oncologist 2012;17(9):1180–90.

42. Kemeny MM, Peterson BL, Kornblith AB, et al. Barriers to clinical trial participation by older women with breast cancer. J Clin Oncol 2003;21(12):2268–75.

43. Grasso C, McDowell MJ, Goldhammer H, et al. Planning and implementing sexual orientation and gender identity data collection in electronic health records. J Am Med Inform Assoc 2019;26(1):66–70.

44. Heck NC, Mirabito LA, LeMaire K, et al. Omitted data in randomized controlled trials for anxiety and depression: A systematic review of the inclusion of sexual orientation and gender identity. J Consult Clin Psychol 2017;85(1):72.

45. Lunn MR, Capriotti MR, Flentje A, et al. Using mobile technology to engage sexual and gender minorities in clinical research. PLoS One 2019;14(5):e0216282.

46. Kim ES, Bruinooge SS, Roberts S, et al. Broadening eligibility criteria to make clinical trials more representative: American Society of Clinical Oncology and Friends of Cancer Research Joint Research Statement. J Clin Oncol 2017;35(33):3737.

47. Unger JM, Hershman DL, Till C, et al. "When offered to participate": a systematic review and meta-analysis of patient agreement to participate in cancer clinical trials. JNCI J Natl Cancer Inst 2021;113(3):244–57.

48. Sood A, Prasad K, Chhatwani L, et al. Patients' attitudes and preferences about participation and recruitment strategies in clinical trials, Mayo Clinic Proc, 2009;84(3):243–247.

49. Moreno-John G, Gachie A, Fleming CM, et al. Ethnic minority older adults participating in clinical research. J Aging Health 2004;16(5_suppl):93S–123S.

50. Curry L, Jackson J. Recruitment and retention of diverse ethnic and racial groups in health research: An evolving science. In: Curry L, Jackson J, editors. The science of inclusion: Recruiting and retaining racial and ethnic elders in health research. Washington, DC: Gerontological Society of America; 2003. pp. 1–7

51. Vesey GA. Recruitment and retention of minority elders in health-related research: A community-based approach. Sci Incl Recruit Retaining Racial Ethn Elders Health Res Wash DC Gerontol Soc Am 2003;82(9):82–9.

52. McDougall GJ Jr, Simpson G, Friend ML. Strategies for research recruitment and retention of older adults of racial and ethnic minorities. J Gerontol Nurs 2015; 41(5):14–23.

53. Kamran SC, Niemierko A, Deville C, et al. Diversity Trends by Sex and Underrepresented in Medicine Status Among US Radiation and Medical Oncology Faculty Over 5 Decades. JAMA Oncol 2022;8(2):221–9.

54. Yu AYL, Iwai Y, Thomas SM, et al. Diversity among surgical faculty, residents, and oncology fellows from 2011/2012 to 2019/2020. Ann Surg Oncol 2022;29(5): 2763–5.

55. Price EG, Gozu A, Kern DE, et al. The role of cultural diversity climate in recruitment, promotion, and retention of faculty in academic medicine. J Gen Intern Med 2005;20(7):565–71.

56. West MA, Hwang S, Maier RV, et al. Ensuring equity, diversity, and inclusion in academic surgery: an American Surgical Association white paper. Ann Surg 2018; 268(3):403–7.

57. Rodríguez JE, Campbell KM, Mouratidis RW. Where are the rest of us? Improving representation of minority faculty in academic medicine. South Med J 2014; 107(12):739–44.

58. Muquith M, Pham T, Espinoza M, et al. Representation of investigators by gender among authors of phase 3 oncology trials worldwide. JAMA Netw Open 2022; 5(2):e220031.

59. Ludmir EB, Mainwaring W, Miller AB, et al. Women's representation among lead investigators of clinical trials in oncology. JAMA Oncol 2019;5(10):1501–2.

60. Saha S, Komaromy M, Koepsell TD, et al. Patient-physician racial concordance and the perceived quality and use of health care. Arch Intern Med 1999; 159(9):997–1004.

61. Shen MJ, Peterson EB, Costas-Muñiz R, et al. The effects of race and racial concordance on patient-physician communication: a systematic review of the literature. J Racial Ethn Health Disparities 2018;5(1):117–40.

62. Laveist TA, Nuru-Jeter A. Is doctor-patient race concordance associated with greater satisfaction with care? J Health Soc Behav 2002;43(3):296–306.

63. Corbie-Smith G, Thomas SB, Williams MV, et al. Attitudes and beliefs of African Americans toward participation in medical research. J Gen Intern Med 1999; 14(9):537–46.

64. Corbie-Smith G, Thomas SB, St George DMM. Distrust, race, and research. Arch Intern Med 2002;162(21):2458–63.

65. Branson RD, Davis K, Butler KL. African Americans' participation in clinical research: importance, barriers, and solutions. Am J Surg 2007;193(1):32–9. https://doi.org/10.1016/j.amjsurg.2005.11.007 [discussion: 40].

Printed and bound by CPI Group (UK) Ltd, Croydon, CR0 4YY

03/10/2024

01040476-0006